G. Hasenfuss · H. Just (Eds.) ■ Heart rate as a determinant of cardiac function

G. Hasenfuss · H. Just

Editors

Heart rate as a determinant of cardiac function

Basic mechanisms
and clinical significance

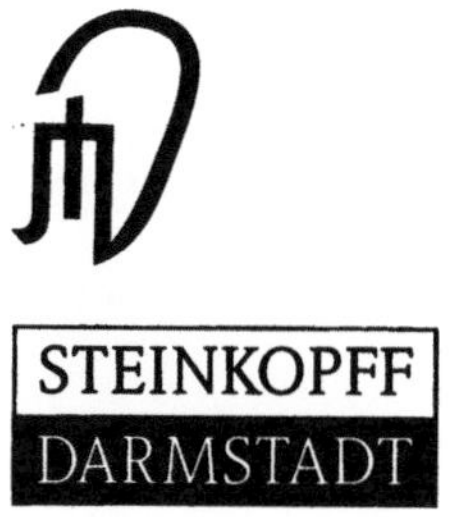

STEINKOPFF
DARMSTADT

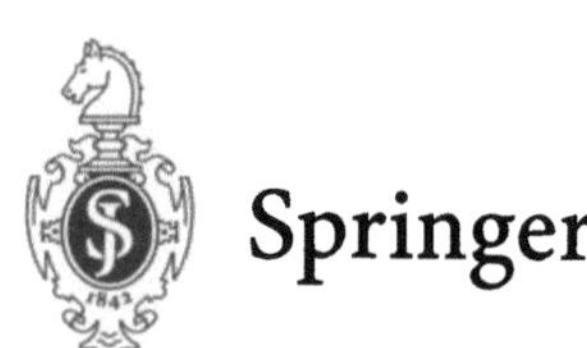

Springer

Prof. Dr. G. Hasenfuss
Abteilung Kardiologie und Pneumologie der Universität Göttingen
Robert-Koch-Straße 40, 37075 Göttingen, Germany

Prof. Dr. H. Just
Medizinische Fakultät, Ethik Kommission
Elsässer Straße 2a, Haus 1a, 79110 Freiburg, Germany

Die Deutsche Bibliothek – CIP Cataloging-in-Publication-Data
A catalogue record for this publication is available from
Die Deutsche Bibliothek

ISBN-13: 978-3-642-47072-1   e-ISBN-13: 978-3-642-47070-7
DOI: 10.1007/978-3-642-47070-7

Steinkopff Verlag is a company in the BertelsmannSpringer publishing group
© Steinkopff Verlag Darmstadt 2000
Softcover reprint of the hardcover 1st edition 2000

The use of general descriptive names, registered names, trademarks, etc. in this publication does not imply, even in the absence of a specific statement, that such names are exempt from the relevant protective laws and regulations and therefore free for general use.

Product liability: The publishers cannot guarantee the accuracy of any information about the application of operative techniques and medications contained in this book. In every individual case the user must check such information by consulting the relevant literature.

Medical Editor: Sabine Ibkendanz – English Editor: Mary K. Gossen
Production: Heinz J. Schäfer
Cover design: Erich Kirchner, Heidelberg
Typesetting: Typoservice, Griesheim

Printed on acid-free paper

Introduction

Numerous studies have indicated that in a variety of cardiac diseases the influence of heart rate on cardiac function is altered and that both heart rate and heart rate variability are of great relevance for the prognosis of cardiac patients.

Heart rate is an important determinant of cardiac function. In humans and most animal species, increased heart rate during exercise enhances cardiac output through an increased number of beats per minute as well as by its action on myocardial performance. The latter effect, termed the force-frequency relation, strength-interval relation or TREPPE (staircase) phenomenon was first observed by Bowditch in the isolated frog heart. Recent studies demonstrated that in failing human myocardium the force-frequency relation is flattened or inversed. The altered force-frequency relation results from disturbed function at the level of the myocyte due to disturbed calcium homeostasis. The latter may be the consequence of altered transsarcolemmal calcium influx, altered sarcoplasmic reticulum calcium uptake and release as well as of altered sarcolemmal sodium-calcium exchange. Knowledge of the subcellular defects underlying disturbed calcium homeostasis may allow the development of new therapeutic strategies to treat heart failure patients. In addition, the finding of an altered force-frequency relation in the failing human heart may suggest that heart rate reduction is of critical importance for patients suffering from heart failure. In this regard, the beneficial effects of β-blockers as well as of amiodarone observed in patients with congestive heart failure may be partially related to the effect of those agents on heart rate.

During the last decade many studies also demonstrated that heart rate and heart rate variability have significant impact on arrhythmogenesis and prognosis in patients with cardiac diseases. In patients with heart failure, heart rate is increased and heart rate variability and baroreceptor reflex sensitivity are decreased. All three changes reflect a relative increase of the sympathetic over the parasympathetic nervous system. The mechanisms underlying this autonomic imbalance are complex and not completely understood. Heart rate variability as a reflection of the balance of the sympathetic and parasympathetic nervous system is related to electrical stability of the myocardium. Increased vagal activity is associated with increased heart rate variability and a decrease in the high frequency band in the spectral analysis of heart rate variability. Most clinical studies observed an increase in heart rate and in low to high frequency ratio in the spectral analysis of heart rate variability prior to spontaneous episodes of ventricular tachycardia in patients after myocardial infarction. The latter indicates a decrease in vagal relative to sympathetic tone. Heart rate variability was also shown to be a good and independent predictor of mortality of patients after myocardial infarction. Furthermore, it was observed that heart rate variability is reduced in patients with heart failure within 24 hours before onset of ventricular tachycardia. Whether or not pharmacological agents which influence heart rate and heart rate variability may be associated with altered prognosis is not known yet.

In the Gargellen Conference "Heart rate as a determinant of cardiac function – Basic mechanisms and clinical significance" international experts in this field were brought together to elaborate on the interrelation between heart rate and myocardial function, arrhythmias, prognosis, and therapy of patients with cardiac diseases. Basic mechanisms as well as clinical relevance and therapeutic consequences were critically discussed.

Göttingen, May 2000   G. Hasenfuss

Contents

Physiology and pathophysiology of baroreceptor function and neuro-hormonal abnormalities in heart failure

H. R. Kirchheim, A. Just, H. Ehmke

Physiologisches Institut, Universität Heidelberg

Introduction

This review deals with the neuro-hormonal changes in congestive heart failure, a syndrome that is usually initiated by a reduction of cardiac output. In order to do this, we should like to 1) summarise previous and more recent evidence for a number of these neuro-hormonal derangement's, 2) review the experimental evidence for an abnormality in the function of the arterial- and cardiopulmonary baroreceptor reflexes and 3) discuss, whether this abnormality or an interaction with renal mechanisms might cause the neuro-hormonal derangements in congestive heart failure.

Evidence for a reduced "vagal tone" in congestive heart failure

Before presenting evidence in favor of a loss of resting "vagal tone" in heart failure, the physiology of the baroreflex and the respiratory influences on cardiac vagal activity need to be briefly reviewed.

Vagal preganglionic neurones innervating the heart (vagal cardiomotor neurones) are predominantly located in the ventrolateral part of the rostral nucleus ambiguus (NA). Baroreceptor influences are probably transmitted to these neurones through projections from the nucleus tractus solitarii (NTS) to the NA. A species dependent number of vagal preganglionic neurones located in the dorsal motor nucleus of the vagus (DMV) have also been described, but little is known whether they differ in function from those neurones in the NA (for references: see 22, 24).

Baroreceptor influence on vagal cardiomotor neurones

Baroreceptor stimulation causes excitation of vagal cardiomotor neurones and bradycardia (70, 98, 105). The central latency of this baroreflex excitation amounts to 20–110 ms only (24). Furthermore, these vagal cardiomotor neurones are more sensitive to the baroreceptor input than sympathetic neurones although they have a higher threshold than the latter (95). Recordings of efferent cardiac vagal activity have shown that in the anaesthetized

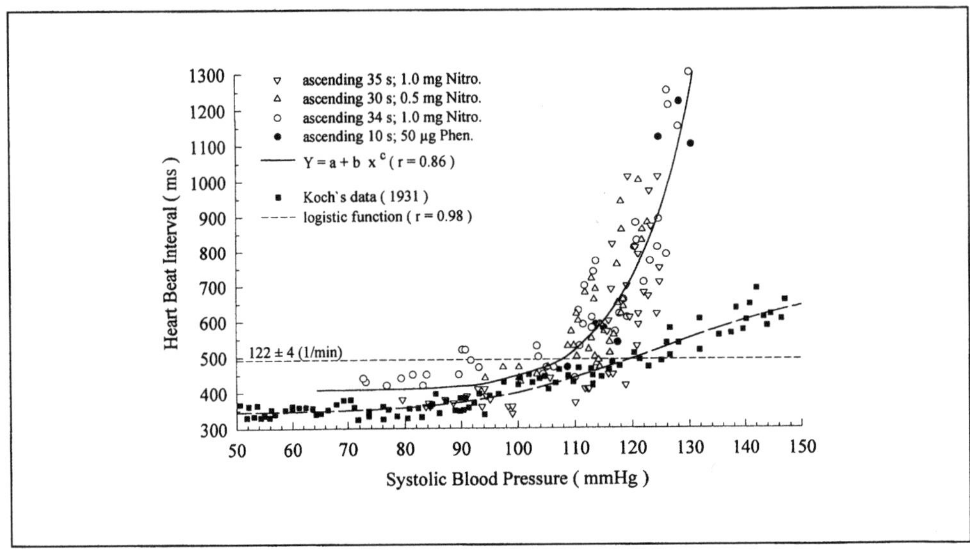

Fig. 1 Relationship between systolic blood pressure and heart beat interval in conscious (our own data) and in anaesthetized dogs (Koch's data). In conscious dogs, blood pressure was either decreased by an i.v. injection of Nitro-glycerine (Nitro; open triangels, open circles) or increased by a bolus injection of Phenylephrine (Phen.; filled circles). Nitro-glycerine-experiments: After systolic pressure had dropped to a minimum of 72–94 mmHg, systolic pressure and the first heart beat interval to follow were recorded for 30–35 seconds with increasing pressure (ascending). Phenylephrine-experiments: Systolic pressure and the first heart beat interval to follow were recorded for 10 seconds with increasing pressure (ascending). The data were approximated by the power function $Y = a + b^c$ (r = 0.86). Koch's data: Heart beat interval versus carotid sinus pressure in anaesthetized dogs (right carotid sinus preparation; left sinus nerves and both aortic nerves cut) as reported by Koch (92). The data were approximated by a 4-parameter logistic function ($Y = a+b / (x/c)^d$; r = 0.98). ----: 122 ± 4 (SEM) beats/min: Intrinsic heart rate as evaluated from 11 conscious dogs (see text).

animal these efferents show very little central activity unless blood pressure exceeds 140–150 mmHg (70, 71, 98). In Koch's data, which were also obtained during anaesthesia, heart rate is reduced below the intrinsic heart rate of a dog's sinus node (122 ± 4 beats/min) when systolic blood pressure increases above 125 mmHg (Fig. 1). Both observations may be limited by anaesthesia, which reduces "vagal tone" (see below). In our experiments in conscious dogs, heart rate is reduced below the intrinsic heart rate at a systolic blood pressure of 110 mmHg already (Fig. 1). Finally, experiments in which vagal cardiomotor neurones and cardiac sympathetic neurones were stimulated electrically have clearly shown that the response of the vagal neuroeffector junction (sinus node) is much faster (a change may be complete within 3–4 seconds) than the response to sympathetic stimulation (a maximum response may require 25–35 seconds). The "off-response" of the vagal neuro-effector junction is also much faster than their sympathetic counterpart (170, 175, 176). This has the important physiological advantage of increasing both heart rate and cardiac output within a few seconds, for instance at the onset of exercise.

Respiratory influences on cardiac vagal activity

Respiratory variations of heart rate were first described by Carl Ludwig in 1847 (for reference see 21). Early workers agreed that the arrhythmia was abolished by division of the cervical vagus nerves, thus, providing evidence as to its neural origin. Later work revealed that both central and pulmonary reflex mechanisms were involved and that the efferent pathway is largely vagal in both animals and man (21). Respiratory arrhythmia is quite striking in humans, in conscious and in morphine-chloralose-anaesthetized dogs but is weak or absent in conscious cats, rabbits, and rats. However, even in species normally presenting clear sinus arrhythmia, it is suppressed by various anaesthetic agents with vagolytic properties (21, 62, 70). In chloralose-anaesthetized dogs, central cardiac vagal activity ("vagal tone") is still present after elimination of all afferents running in the vagi, the aortic, and the sinus nerves (92). Central respiratory activity originating from medullary neurones strongly influences vagal cardiomotor discharge, which shows a pattern inverse to sympathetic efferent activity with a maximum occurring during expiration (71, 98, 105). Recording cardiac vagal efferent nerve activity Katona and co-workers (78) showed that respiratory sinus arrhythmia in the spontaneously breathing dog is due to a complete cessation of vagal efferent activity during the inspiratory phase of each respiratory cycle. The presence of this central "vagal tone", i.e., resting activity in the cardiac vagal efferent fibers, is an important prerequisite for the demonstration of respiratory arrhythmia. Iriuchijima and co-workers, also recording the activity of vagal cardiomotor neurones, observed that vagal efferent cardiomotor fibers could only be activated by the baroreceptor input during expiration (71). This is in line with the previous observation that the vagally transmitted bradycardia by electrical stimulation of the carotid sinus nerve was minimal at the early phase of inspiration and maximal at early expiration (94). In man Eckberg and collaborators found that a baroreceptor stimulus by brief neck suction increased the heart beat interval by 30 ms (minimum) during inspiration and by 220 ms (maximum) during early expiration (36).

Dependence of respiratory arrhythmia and baroreflex bradycardia on "vagal tone"

That respiratory sinus arrhythmia increases with an increasing heart beat interval was reported as early as 1935 (147). Consequently, the standard deviation of the heart beat interval, which more recently is used as an index of respiratory arrhythmia, also increases with an increasing baseline heart beat period. The relationship between the respiratory variation in the heart beat interval and baseline heart beat was found to be nearly quadratic (93, 145). This was confirmed by Katona and Jih (79), who found that a linear correlation was less appropriate. In their experiments, the respiratory variations of heart rate period reached a minimum at a heart rate period of around 550 ms (= 120/min), which is close to a dog's intrinsic heart rate (see below). These results clearly suggest that the degree of respiratory sinus arrhythmia may be used as a non-invasive indicator of the degree of prevailing central parasympathetic "vagal tone" (79).

The slope of the relationship between systolic pressure and heart beat interval after the intravenous injection of a vasoconstrictor drug (called "baroreflex sensitivity" according to the "Oxford"-method) is also a function of the baseline heart beat interval (10, 12, 16, 51, 67, 161).

Reduced "vagal tone" in heart failure

The tachycardia in patients suffering from heart failure was aleady known to E. Starling (154), but, because of the early recognition of sympathetic overactivity, traditionally was assigned to an enhanced cardiac sympathetic tone. Indirect evidence for a reduced resting vagal discharge to the heart was provided by the observation that patients with a diseased myocardium showed a depressed respiratory arrhythmia (145). Calculating an arrhythmia-index this author also reported that respiratory arrhythmia was dependent on age as well as on the resting heart rate. Using microneurography to record muscle sympathetic nerve discharge in healthy subjects and in patients with heart failure, Porter and collaborators noted a strong central respiratory modulation of sympathetic outflow, but very few signs of changes in vagal outflow, i.e., no respiratory arrhythmia (131). Short baseline R-R intervals and small standard deviations of the R-R interval indicating a decreased level of vagal cardiac nerve activity were also noted in heart failure (2, 131, 144, 151, 153). In some of the patients studied by Porter and co-workers the standard deviations of the R-R interval were almost as small as in heart transplant patients (denervated donor, denervated recipient) (3, 144). Smith and collaborators reported that the correction of heart failure by transplantation (denervated donor, innervated recipient) restored the parasympathetic control toward normal (151). More direct evidence for a reduced "vagal tone" in heart failure was provided by Eckberg and co-workers. Patients with coronary heart disease and idiopathic cardiomyopathy experienced the same degree of bradycardia (–9 to –10 beats/min) as control subjects when given propranolol intravenously, but less tachycardia after intravenous atropine sulphate (+34 beat/min versus +15 beats/min). The authors therefore suggested that in patients with heart disease the baseline vagal tone from the central nevous system was diminished (35). Similar data after intravenous application of atropine (10 µg/kg) were reported by Porter and co-workers, who observed that heart rate increased to the same level (89–92 beats/min) in both groups of subjects, but started from a lower baseline level (65 beats/min) in the healthy subjects as compared to patients suffering of heart failure (77 beats/min) (131).

Increased sympathetic nerve activity in congestive heart failure

Before presenting evidence in favor of an increased sympathetic nerve discharge to several target organs in heart failure, a few remarks should be made with regard to the origin of resting sympathetic nerve activity.

It is clear now that neurones in the rostral ventrolateral medulla (RVLM) are tonically active and generate a large component of the resting sympathetic activity in anaesthetized animals (for references see 22). A question which still remains unanswered is how this tonic activity in the RVLM neurones is generated. Three different mechanisms have been proposed (for references see 22): 1) One suggestion is that the RVLM sympathetic cells are chemosensitive and are tonically excited even at normal levels of blood pH, pO_2, and pCO_2. In support of this theory, the blood flow and capillary density within the RVLM have been shown to be significantly greater than in surrounding areas. 2) Another suggestion is that pacemaker cells in the RVLM are largely responsible for generating resting activity in sympathetic neurones. 3) A third theory suggests than an ensemble of neurones (referred to as "network oscillator") in the brain stem generates a basal level of activity which is then transmitted to the RVLM sympathoexcitatory neurones.

In many clinical studies plasma noradrenaline has been used as an index for an increased sympatho-adrenal activity in heart failure which should be commented on before discussing the increased sympathetic nerve discharge to different organs.

Plasma levels of noradrenaline are elevated and correlate with the severity of the disease in congestive heart failure (18, 158). In normal men estimations of total and organ-specific noradrenaline spillover have shown that 25 % of total spillovers have their origin in the kidneys (22 %) and the heart (3 %). The hepatomesenteric circulation (9 %), skeletal muscle (20 %), and skin (5 %) together contribute approximately 34 % of total spillover (43). Studies on the kinetics of plasma noradrenaline in heart failure have shown that cardiac (+540%) and renal (+206 %) noradrenaline spillover are increased (64). It was estimated that the elevated plasma levels were caused by an increased spillover and a reduced clearance, probably due to a reduced muscle and visceral blood flow (64). Increased spillover and reduced clearance contributed equally to the high plasma levels (23). However, a more recent study by Meredith and co-workers suggests that the increased spillover results primarily from an increased sympathetic nerve firing, not from faulty neuronal reuptake of noradrenaline (110). At least in some patients increased levels of adrenaline were also reported (64).

Cardiac sympathetic nerve activity (noradrenaline spillover)

Although there are no direct recordings of cardiac sympathetic nerve discharge in animals with heart failure, there can be little doubt from the analysis of noradrenaline spillover that sympathetic nerve discharge to the heart is enhanced. The reported increases in cardiac noradrenaline spillover of patients in comparison to healthy subjects ranges between +145 % (99) to +800 % (110), while other authors reported values between these extremes (64, 80, 81).

Sympathetic nerve acitivity to skeletal muscle

Microneurography of sympathetic action potentials in skin and muscle nerves has contributed considerably to our understanding of the function of the sympathetic nervous system (160, 169). Muscle sympathetic nerve   activity provides vasoconstrictor impulses to the resistance vessels of skeletal muscle and is strongly time-locked to the heart beat. In normotensive and hypertensive subjects and in patients with congestive heart failure, the frequency of sympathetic bursts correlated positively with forearm venous plasma noradrenaline concentration (102, 168). The strong pulse-synchronous muscle nerve activity suggests that it is dominanted by the inhibitory influences of arterial baroreceptor afferents. In this context we should like to add a few remarks on the physiology of the inhibition of sympathetic efferents by baroreceptor input, since it is an essential background for the interpretation of several clinical studies suggesting a defect in baroreflex sympathetic inhibition in heart failure.

The central latency of the baroreceptor inhibition of sympathetic neurones as determined in animals ranges from 150–200 ms (24). Electrical stimulation of the carotid sinus nerve in anaesthetized animals produces a reduction in sympathetic activity with a maximum within the first seconds (138, 149). After this early strong inhibition, sympathetic activity returns within 60 seconds to a steady-state level of less pronounced inhibition. Both, the dynamic and the static response increases with increasing stimulus frequencies up to 30–40 imp/s and remains constant at higher frequencies. The maximum in the static response is reached at frequencies of 20–30 imp/s. Interrupted impulse volleys are more effective in sympathetic inhibition (static) than the same number of impulses per time during continuous stimulation (138). The maximum static inhibition can be obtained with a high impulse frequency within a stimulus train of 220 to 500 ms duration and a repitition rate of 1 Hz. This resembles a pattern similar to the one during the pulsatile discharge of the baroreceptors under normal conditions and explains the strongly phasic discharge pattern in baroreceptor controlled sympathetic activity. Applying carotid sinus nerve stimulation this pattern of sympathetic inhibition was also reported in humans by Wallin and co-workers. Conforming observations in animals (24) these authors also found that carotid sinus nerve stimulation had no   reproducible effect on skin nerve activity (165).

Muscle nerve activity in man displays large inter-individual variations. A correlation between the blood pressure level and the "tonic level" of muscle sympathetic nerve activity has been demonstrated in essential hypertension, but it should be noted that the relationship is weak (166, 167, 169). Despite the caveats with regard to tonic activity, the microneurographic recordings provide rather good evidence that sympathetic nerve activity to skeletal muscle is higher in patients when compared with normal subjects (48, 57, 102, 131).

Sympathetic nerve discharge to skin

Sympathetic activity to the skin normally is irregular with no relation to the pressure pulse. Functionally it is composed of vasoconstrictor, vasodilator, and sudomotor activity and is very low in relaxed subjects in a thermoneutral environment. Skin nerve activity as compared with muscle sympathetic nerve activity has a more pronounced respiratory rhythmicity, is barely affected by baroreceptors, and is predominantly engaged in thermoregulatory responses (4, 73, 82, 83, 169). Recent simultaneous recordings of sympathetic skin and muscle nerve activity in 6 resting patients with severe heart failure revealed that in contrast to muscle sympathetic activity skin nerve discharge was not increased (112).

Renal sympathetic nerve activity

There is good evidence from nerve recordings or renal noradrenaline spillover in animals with congestive heart failure that renal sympathetic nerve activity is increased (28, 29, 46, 64, 96, 143).

In conscious dogs a moderate reflex activation of the renal sympathetic nerves (+ 62 %) increases the lower limit of renal blood flow- and glomerular filtration rate autoregulation as well as the threshold for pressure-dependent renin release by an α_1-adrenergic mechanism (Fig. 5); an augmented angiotensin II formation does not play a major role in mediating this resetting (128). At a constant renal perfusion pressure sympathetic activation causes a direct β_1-andrenergic stimulation of renin release. Thus, at least transiently sodium and water retention may be initiated without necessarily inducing an initial major reduction of renal blood flow and glomerular filtration rate (7, 88, 90, 91, 137, 148). If the degree of renal sympathetic activation in early congestive heart failure, indeed, is only moderate as shown in animals studies (+ 50 %) (46), it would be consistent with the hypothesis that a normal baroreceptor function could initiate these changes in early congestive heart failure (87).

Hormonal abnormalities in congestive heart failure

Activation of the renin-angiotensin-system

More than 40 years ago Merrill and co-workers reported an increased renal venous renin activity in patients with congestive heart failure (111). It is known now that the renin-angiotensin-aldosterone system plays an essential role in the sodium and water retention and the restoration of cardiac output and arterial blood pressure in congestive heart failure (34, 177). The mechanisms controlling renin release in heart failure have not been well defined in clinical studies, and in the past it seemed particularly difficult to explain the sodium retention in early heart failure when blood pressure, blood volume, and renal blood flow are apparently unchanged. Using inferior vena cava constriction to induce heart failure in dogs, Witty and collaborators (181) proposed that the renal "baroreceptor" mechanism was responsible for the early increase in plasma renin activity. Further, below we will describe the role of the pressure-dependent renin release in blood pressure control and explain how the efferent renal nerves and the renal "baroreceptor" – mechanism may interact in the early renin activation of heart failure.

Increased plasma levels of ANP

Atrial natriuretic peptide (ANP) is a circulating hormone released by distension of the left and right atrium. Thus, ANP is released by maneuvers, which change intrathoracic blood volume, such as volume loading, head-out water immersion, acute salt load, chronic salt load, change in posture, and inferior vena cava constriction. Any increase of volume in intrathoracic compartment of the low pressure system, which determines the filling of the heart (preload), can be counteracted by the following effects of ANP: 1) an increase of venous compliance, 2) an increase of sodium excretion unrelated to changes in renal blood flow or glomerular filtration rate, 3) a volume redistribution within the low pressure system away from the heart (130), and 4) an antagonistic action towards the renin-angiotensin-aldosterone system (for references see 85). However, the latter effect becomes evident only when the renin-angiotensin system is activated. Furthermore, ANP seems to modulate the actions of vasoconstrictor agents rather than having a direct and wholly independent effect on resistance vessels (40, 85). While changes in dietary sodium intake induce a 2–3 fold increase in plasma ANP, very high levels of ANP have been observed in heart failure (8–10 fold). The most prominent function of ANP in congestive heart failure is probably its antagonistic action towards the volume retaining factors (renal sympathetic nerves, angiotensin II, aldosterone, vasopressin; for references see 40, 85). This allows fluid balance to be achieved at an elevated level (compensation). More recent studies provide evidence that ANP secretion does not chronically adapt to stimulation by increased atrial pressure (150), so in congestive heart failure a reduced responsiveness of the kidney to ANP may be a more important factor inducing angoing sodium retention with a shift of the cardiovascular system from a state of compensation to one of decompensation (for references see 180).

Increased plasma levels of AVP

Arginine vasopressin (AVP) serves osmotic and hemodynamic regulation, and its release is affected by plasma osmolality, blood volume, and blood pressure (140). Small decreases in blood pressure of the order of 5–10 % usually have little effect on plasma vasopressin, whereas decreases in blood pressure of 20–30 % result in hormone levels several times those required to produce maximum antidiuresis. The AVP response to changes in blood volume appear to be quantitatively and qualitatively similar to the response to blood pressure. Little or no rise in plasma AVP can be detected until blood volume falls by 6–8 %. Beyond that point, plasma AVP begins to rise at a rapidly increasing rate in relation to the degree of hypovolemia and usually reaches levels 20–30 times normal when blood volume is reduced by 20–30 %.

In patients suffering from heart failure the plasma levels seem to be increased in proportion to the degree of their cardiac disability (185). Since AVP appears to only play a major role in blood pressure control under conditions of cardiovascular stress, including dehydration or hemorrhage (65), it seems possible that its activation during heart failure is directed towards the same goal. Seemingly normal AVP levels found in many heart failure patients are inappropriate for their plasma osmolalities and probably contribute to abnormal sodium and water retention (for references see 37). AVP also has important central actions on sympathetic nerve discharge and renin release.

Endothelial factors, defective nitric oxide-function

An increase in the circulating level of endothelin, a potent vasoconstrictor released by the endothelium, was also observed in experimental heart failure (107) as well as in patients (19, 155). An apparent decrease in the local release of endothelium-derived relaxing factor, or nitric oxide (NO) has been reported in experimental heart failure (76, 124) and in patients (97). In normal rats (142) and rabbits (63) changes in peripheral sympathetic nerve activity have been recorded after systemic inhibition of NO synthesis. A more recent study by Zanziger and co-workers in the normal anaesthetized cat suggests that endogenous NO reduces basal sympathetic tone in the RVLM and attenuates excitatory somato-sympathetic reflex responses (186). The same group of authors provided evidence that sympathetic baroreflex function is preserved during both impaired endogenous synthesis or excess exogenous supply of NO in the brainstem (187). Recording carotid sinus nerve discharge in anaesthetized cats, these authors found that neither abluminal nor intravascular administration of the NO synthase inhibitor LNNA significantly modulated baroreceptor activity (188).

Thus, aside from the influence on basal sympathetic tone, the role of nitric oxide in cardiovascular physiology seems to be largely confined to a peripheral interaction with sympathetic vasomotor tone. The role of endothelin and NO in the pathophysiology of congestive heart failure still needs to be established.

Arterial and cardiopulmonary baroreceptor abnormalities

Carotid sinus baroreceptors

Recording single unit carotid sinus baroreceptor discharge in normal dogs and in dogs with pacing-induced congestive heart failure (250 beats/min for 4 weeks), Wang and co-workers observed that threshold pressure (119 versus 91 mmHg) was increased and sensitivity was reduced (max. slope: 0.40 versus 0.63 spikes/s/mmHg). Pressure in the isolated sinus was increased in this study by slow ramp increases (2–3 mmHg/s) from zero to threshold pressure and subsequently in 25 mmHg steps lasting 10–15 s to a maximum of 250 mmHg. By measuring carotid sinus diameter, the authors further provided evidence that the decreased sensitivity was not due to a change in compliance of the carotid sinus wall (171). A similar observation had been reported before in dogs with chronic aortocaval fistulas (high-output heart failure), in which both static and dynamic characteristics of the baroreceptor afferents could be evaluated (119). The same authors more recently investigated the total number of myelinated and unmyelinated fibers in the carotid sinus nerve in dogs with pacing induced heart failure, in which the single unit baroreceptor responses to static and pulsatile pressure changes were markedly depressed. However, there was no evidence for significant changes in the number or type of fibers, indicating that desensitization is a more likely possibility to explain the depressed function than structural changes (174).

Aortic baroreceptors

Similar observations were made for the aortic baroreceptors. Aortic afferent activity was studied in open chest anaesthetized dogs, which were either sham operated or had chronic aortocaval fistulas (120). This high-output heart failure was associated with a reduced baroreceptor sensitivity and a resetting of the operating point to a higher pressure level. The authors also measured aortic diameter and strain and found that the decrease in discharge sensitivity was unrelated to wall strain. Dibner-Dunlap and Thames recorded aortic nerve multifiber activity in anaesthetized sham operated dogs and in dogs with heart failure induced by rapid ventricular pacing; blood pressure was changed by phenylephrine or nitroglycerine injections. A decrease in sensitivity by 36 % and 52 % (baseline, or after vagotomy) was observed in the heart failure group with a reduction in the range over which aortic nerve activity changed, but no alterations in threshold pressure (25). Further support was supplied recently by DiBona and Sawin, who recorded single fiber aortic nerve activity in anaesthetized normal rats and in rats with congestive heart failure due to myocardial infarction. Also changing pressure using vasoactive drugs, they found an increased threshold pressure and a decreased sensitivity (30).

Atrial receptors

Using two different approaches to induce heart failure in dogs, Greenberg and co-workers (pulmonary artery stenosis and tricuspid avulsion) and Zucker and co-workers (chronic infrarenal aortovacal fistulas) showed that atrial type-B receptor discharge sensitivity was clearly depressed (58, 189). In the study by Zucker and co-workers all receptors recorded from were located in the left atrium near the pulmonary vein – left atrial junction. Zucker and colleagues also showed that the compliance of the left atria, in which these endings were located, was reduced and that there were histological abnormalities in the unencapsulated endings, which are thought to have the anatomical features of this type of sensory receptor. In rats with congestive heart failure due to myocardial infarction DiBona and Sawin als recorded single-unit vagal nerve activity and found that the sensitivity as evaluated from the relationship between left ventricular enddiastolic pressure and vagal activity was depressed. Although the receptors were not localized, the study at least confirms a defect in vagal afferent activity in congestive heart failure (30).

Left ventricular mechanoreceptors

Although there are clinical (116) and experimental observations (8, for further references see 175, 190) suggesting an abnormality of ventricular reflexes in congestive heart failure, no work has been done up to date on the electrophysiological characteristics of ventricular mechanoreceptive and chemoreceptive afferents in any model of congestive heart failure.

Abnormalities in the baroreceptor control of sympathetic nerve activity

Consistent with the abnormalities at the receptor level, reports on experiments studying the relationship between carotid sinus- or systemic blood pressure and renal sympathetic nerve discharge or renal norepinephrine spillover in animals with congestive heart failure reported a decrease in sensitivity in dogs (172), rats (30, 31, 46), and rabbits (122). In one study in dogs no change (non-significant 5 % decrease) was observed (25). Using conscious rabbits with adriamycin-induced cardiomyopathy Sano and co-workers observed that the baro-reflex-renal norepinephrine spillover response to hypotension in an early stage of heart failure showed a significant upward shift (resetting), while in established failure there was a significant blunting of the spillover response (decreased sensitivity) (143). In many studies (25, 30, 31, 46, 122, 143) vasoactive drugs were used to change blood pressure. Since under these circumstances changes in cardiac filling pressure cannot be exluded (49, 114), the resetting or the calculated loss of sensitivity cannot be specifically attributed to arterial or cardiopulmonary receptors. In the most controlled experiments by Wang and co-workers, who studied an isolated sinus preparation of one side with all other cardio-pulmonary or baroreceptor input removed, the data show that the baroreflex sympathetic inhibition at sinus pressures above 180 mmHg was more attenuated than the reflex sym-pathetic activation observed below a sinus pressure of 80 mmHg; the slope of the relation-ship suggested a decrease in the carotid sinus-sympathetic reflex sensitivity by 24 % (172). DiBona and associates used rats with heart failure due to coronary infarction and similar to Wang and co-workers found that the failure to inhibit renal sympathetic nerve discharge was most pronounced at systemic pressures above 150 mmHg and reported decreases in gain between 41 and 49 % (30, 31). Using the same method in rats, Feng and collaborators found a decrease in sensitivity for inhibition of renal sympathetic nerve activity by 30 % between 120 and 160 mmHg (46). Thus, the receptor abnormalities, at least with regard to the efferent renal nerves, seem to cause an overall attenuation of the reflex sensitivity.

Three of the studies mentioned above also tested the "central gain" of the baroreceptor reflex in congestive heart failure. Dibner-Dunlap and colleagues used the ratio of the percent change in renal nerve activity to the percent change in aortic nerve activity and found no evidence for a central abnormality (25). This was supported by Wang and associates recording renal sympathetic nerve discharge and electrically stimulating the carotid sinus nerve (172). In the rat with cardiac failure (coronary infarction) DiBona and Sawin, measuring simultaneously afferent vagal nerve activity and efferent renal sympathetic nerve discharge, also found no evidence for a central abnormality (30).

As to the relative inhibitory influence mediated by the arterial as compared to cardiopulmonary receptors in congestive heart failure, it was suggested that in heart failure due to rapid pacing that the cardiopulmonary input is especially impaired (25, 26). In rats with heart failure induced by coronary infarction Feng and co-workers observed no significant change in renal sympathetic nerve discharge during volume expansion (48). DiBona and Sawin (32) observed that increases in renal sympathetic nerve activity after individual or combined sinuaortic denervation or vagotomy were less in cardiac failure (coronary infarction) than in normal control rats in both order sequences. In rats with heart failure vagotomy produced lesser increases in renal sympathetic nerve discharge than sinuaortic denervation in both order sequences. The authors suggested that tonic vagal restraint is always low in cardiac failure.

Finally it should be noted that almost all studies in animals were made under the influence of anaesthesia. The combination of surgical trauma (activation of viscerosomatic afferents) in acutely prepared experimental animals with a chloralose or pentobarbital anesthesia, for example, induces a strong increase of "tonic" renal sympathetic nerve activity, while Alfathesin anesthesia has only little influence (for references see 90). The operating point (resting blood pressure) on the logistic function curve relating renal nerve activity to blood pressure in these animals is located either at the midpoint (maximum sensitivity) or even further up toward a higher resting nerve activity (25, 30, 31, 172). Thus, when applied to the physiological situation, these curves would erroneously suggest equally large degrees of sympathetic activation as well as inhibition. However, in the resting conscious animal, the operating point is non-symmetrically positioned at a low resting sympathetic nerve discharge (Fig. 6), which suggests an entirely different conclusion with regard to integrative control, because it only needs a slight increase in blood pressure to induce a maximum sympathetic inhibition (90). Therefore, the function curves relating sympathetic nerve activity to blood pressure should be looked at very critically, when it comes to deciding whether an abnormality was caused by a change in tonic activity, in range or in sensitivity or whether it was due to a resetting. In a study in man, which used multiunit recordings of muscle sympathetic nerve discharge (49), patients with congestive heart failure showed a higher resting activity at a comparable mean blood pressure level (89 versus 90 mmHg) than the healthy control group (61 versus 32 bursts/min). While the sympathetic inhibition caused by a phenylephrine induced pressure rise (+10 mmHg) was identical in both groups, sympathetic activation after nitro-glycerine induced hypotension (−15 mmHg) was attenuated in the heart failure group. Thus, the impaired baroreflex control in this study might well be explained by a resetting of the function curve relating nerve activity to blood pressure toward a higher pressure level.

Effect of glycoside therapy on baroreceptor afferents or their reflexes

With regard to the mechanism responsible for the arterial and cardiopulmonary baroreceptor abnormalities, the effects of cardiac glycosides should also be shortly mentioned. It has been known for many years that cardiac glycosides posses neuroexcitatory effects (52), most likely by inhibiting Na^+-K^+-ATPase. Studies in normal animals had suggested that the administration of digitalis or digitalis-like drugs in relatively high doses can sensitize both arterial and cardiopulmonary mechanoreceptors (133, 156). Wang and co-workers demonstrated that the reduced discharge of carotid sinus baroreceptor afferents in dogs with pacing induced congestive heart failure was increased and normalized again when the sinus was perfused with 0.01 µg/ml ouabain; this effect was not observed in the normal animals (171, 192). Administration of a low dose of digitalis to the isolated carotid sinus in dogs with congestive heart failure also normalized the reduced duration of postexcitatory depression, which is described for other mechanoreceptors and is thought to be due to an increase in Na^+-K^+-ATPase (172, 192). The same group of authors have reported that aldosterone which augments Na^+-K^+-ATPase in transporting epithelium, in a low concentration (200–500 pg/ml) decreased discharge of single unit baroreceptor afferents in the isolated carotid sinus preparation of normal dogs. The effect was not associated with a change in the carotid sinus pressure-diameter relationship. The inhibitory action could not be reversed by ouabain, but was completely eliminated after removal of the endothelium or the aldosterone receptor blocker spironolactone. The authors suggested that although it remains unclear if aldosterone participates in the depression of baroreceptor discharge in heart failure, sustained hyperaldosteronemia may contribute to the depression of baroreceptor function through an endothelial cell mechanism (172, 192). The cause for the obvious increase in the Na^+-K^+-ATPase in baroreceptors in heart failure is not known.

There is also some indirect evidence in man supporting the effects of low doses of ouabain on the carotid sinus afferents; Ferguson and co-workers demonstrated that muscle sympathetic activity recorded by peroneal nerve microneurography could be reduced in patients with heart failure by the intravenous administration of a rapidly acting digitalis preparation, which was accompanied by an increased systolic (+16 %) and pulse pressure (+41 %), no change in mean pressure, an increase of cardiac output (+21 %), and a 28 % increase of forearm blood flow. No inhibition of muscle sympathetic nerve activity was reported after administration of equal inotropic doses of dobutamine, which caused no change in systolic and diastolic pressure and increased cardiac output by 34 % which suggested to the authors that the sympathetic inhibition was not due to the improvement of cardiac function. However, this conclusion is weakened by the fact that after dobutamine there were no changes of systolic blood pressure, a variable which normally is responsible for considerable phasic baroreceptor inhibition. In normal volunteers, the digitalis preparation did not change sympathetic nerve activity, while it increased systolic (+12 %), pulse- (+24 %), and mean pressure (+5 %; there was no change in forearm blood flow. The authors suggested that the effects in the patients result from afferent activation of low or high pressure baroreceptors (48). In a later study the same group of authors reported an enhanced reflex increase of sympathetic nerve activity due to low level LBNP (up to −15 mmHg) after the application of the same drug in healthy volunteers and suggested that digitalis selectively augments cardiopulmonary baroreflex control of sympathetic activity (146). The salient point in this conclusion is that at −15 mmHg LBNP the sympathetic activity (bursts/min) was similar in the control and the digitalis group, but started from a lower level after the drug, which reduced baseline resting sympathetic nerve discharge in these healthy volunteers. Altogether it remains questionable, whether the action of digitalis in man is specifically normalizing the reduced activity of baroreceptor afferents in congestive heart failure. There are several possible sites of action for digitalis.

The baroreceptor heart rate reflex

In heart failure a reduced heart rate response, especially to an increase in blood pressure, has been observed early in patients (35) and in conscious dogs with heart failure produced by tricuspid avulsion and pulmonary stenosis (67). Eckberg and associates in 1971 already had suggested that "a diminished outflow of parasympathetic nerve impulses from the central nervous system" (see above: "reduced vagal tone in heart failure") might be the mechanism for this abnormality. In a host of studies to follow, however, the interpretation of the results obtained with the rather simle "Oxford" method (see above: "Dependence of Respiratory Arrhythmia and Baroreflex Bradycardia on "Vagal Tone") mainly produced the unproven but popular notion of a decreased "baroreflex sensitivity". Therefore, in the section to follow we want to critically analyse the "Oxford" method in order to find out, whether there is unequivocal evidence for a decrease in heart rate "reflex sensitivity".

The finding that heart rate varies inversely with acute changes in arterial pressure has been appreciated since the experiments of Etienne-Jules Marey (106). "Baroreflex sensitivity" is inferred from the slope of the relationship between systolic blood pressure and the first or second heart beat interval to follow of a blood pressure elevation (first 15 seconds usually) produced by an injection of phenylephrine. In a similar fashion the systolic blood pressure – pulse interval relationship was analysed for the response to hypotension, i.e., following an injection of nitro-glycerine. Since systolic pressure is an excellent indicator of the baroreceptor stimulus (for references see 83), there is indeed some logic to use it as an independent variable.

Especially in many human studies only small pressure perturbations of systolic pressure were induced. Consequently relatively short curve-segments were analyzed which were easily fitted by a linear regression. This holds true for experiments in normal man (12, 35), in patients with heart failure (35), in normal animals, and in those with experimentally induced congestive heart failure (10, 16, 17, 67, 178). A "baroreflex sensitivity" was estimated either for only the bradycardia response due to hypertension (12, 35, 67) or for both, the tachycardia response due to hypotension, and the bradycardia response due to hypertension (10, 16, 17, 178). Probably because of the difficulty to obtain a satisfactory linear curve-fit when anazlyzing a larger pressure range (tachycardia and bradycardia response in one and the same relationship), the responses were regularly plotted in two separate graphs. The "baroreflex sensitivity" analyzed for the bradycardia response in normal dogs was always found to be larger than for the tachycardia response, so a "baroreflex sensitivity" was reported, which was 2–3 fold higher for the response to hypertension when compared with the response to hypotension (10, 16, 17). White, also working with dogs, reported an even larger difference (8-fold) (178). In this study for example one curve was plotted for the phenylephrine and a second one for the glyceryl trinitrate response in one and the same dog (dog # 256; Fig. 1). A close look at these data obviously shows that one common curve could have been plotted, which, however, would show a non-linear relationship with a high slope in the low heart rate range and a very flat slope in the high heart rate range (178).

So, in essence all these findings simply support the experiments by Koepchen and Thurau (93), who observed that over a large range of pressures the relationship between systolic blood pressure and heart beat interval in anaesthetized dogs is non-linear. A similar result had been already observed by Koch (92) who plotted heart beat interval as a function of mean carotid sinus pressure (Fig. 1). In the careful study by Koepchen and Thurau (93) this relationship at intervals between 456 and 333 ms (132–180 beats/min) was rather flat with a slope which was only 1/6 of the slope above intervals of 500 ms (120 beats/min). In its steep portion (high "baroreflex sensitivity") above 500 ms the curve was shifted along the pressure axis by the respiratory phase, i.e., during mid-end inspiration (decreased efferent vagal activity) to the right, and at end-expiration(increased efferent vagal activity) to the left (see Fig. 10 of that study). A non-linearity between heart rate and carotid sinus transmural pressure has also been reported by Thron and co-workers (159) and Wagner and co-workers (164) when they studied the heart rate reflex in normal humans subjects. The highest baroreflex slope was found with decreasing transmural pressure in a range of heart beat intervals between 632 ms (95/min) and 800 ms (72/min).

Our own data (Fig. 1) obtained in conscious dogs also show one non-linear relationship for both drug injections (phenylephrine and nitro-glycerine), demonstrating a rather flat curve above 122 beats/min and a steep rise below this value. This is the "intrinsic" or "autonomic" rate of a dog's sinus node which was determined in 11 conscious dogs between the 2nd and 3rd hour after inducing a ganglionic blockade (hexamethonium: 5 mg/kg i.v. +5 mg/kg/min infusion). The result corresponds to the data reported by others: Rigel and co-workers (139) observed 126 ± 6 beats/min in conscious dogs (after β-blockade), when the "excess tachycardia" observed after Atropin sulphate (0.1 mg/kg i.v.) was abolished by additional vagal nerve cooling. Versteeg and collaborators reported a resting heart rate of 123 ± 3 beats/min in 7 cardiac denervated conscious dogs (162).

Although there is probably a range of some overlap between sympathetic and vagal influences on the sinus node around 122 beats/min, it is obvious that the steep portion of the systolic blood pressure – pulse interval relationship below 122 beats/min is dominated by vagal efferent activity, while the rather flat portion above 122 beats/min is mainly due to an elevated sympathetic efferent activity. Studying the effects of drugs acting on the peripheral vascular bed in anaesthetized or conscious dogs and in humans Glick and Braunwald (53) observed already that when arterial pressure rises above control, the decrease in heart rate was mediated by vagal efferents, withdrawal of sympathetic activity playing no detectable role. In healthy subjects the bradycardia due to the i.v. injection of phenylephrine remained unchanged after cardiac sympathetic blockade by thoracic epidural anaesthesia, while the tachycardia due to nitro-glycerine i.v. was significantly attenuated (55). This is also consistent with the fact that Koch's data only differ from our results (unanaesthetized dogs) in the range above 122 beats/min (Fig. 1), which may be explained by the well known vagolytic properties of anaesthesia.

Altogether the studies in dogs with experimental congestive heart failure present unequivocal evidence for a defect in the vagal component of the baroreceptor heart rate reflex, i.e., the linearized slope of the systolic blood pressure – pulse interval relationship below 122 beats/min or above a systolic pressure of 110–120 mmHg (phenylephrine) is reduced by 30 % to 95 % (10, 16, 17, 67, 178). This is consistent with the observation of a reduced "vagal tone" in patients with congestive heart failure and is supported by Sopher and collaborators (153), who used a baroreceptor stimulus by brief (5 s) neck suction in heart failure patients and in healthy subjects in order to induce a reflex change in the R-R interval. The peak response in the R-R interval was smaller in patients suffering from heart failure than in the healthy subjects (+ 95 versus + 178 ms). The baseline R-R interval during normal breathing was 1006 ms in healthy subjects and 866 ms in patients with heart failure; the standard deviation of the R-R interval was significantly smaller in patients with heart failure. The authors suggested that the baroreflex malfunction in heart failure is predicted by low baseline levels of vagal cardiac outflow.

In heart failure the linearized heart beat interval-systolic pressure relationship was also evaluated separately for the tachycardia response to nitroglycerine only (see:"The baroreceptor-heart rate reflex") and this slope was also reported to be reduced. However, the reported absolute reduction in slope was usually very slight (10, 16, 17, 178) and much less convincing than the slope reduction reported for the bradycardia due to a phenylephrine injection. This is easily explained by the fact that the slope after nitroglycerine in the normal dogs was determined for intervals between 536 and 730 ms (resting heart rate: 112–82 beats/min), while the slope in dogs with heart failure was determined in the range below 454 ms (resting heart rate: above 132 beats/min) (Fig. 1). In a study by Dibner-Dunlap and Thames (25), who used cardiac pacing to induce heart failure in morphin- α-chloralose-anaesthetized dogs (which preserves cardiac "vagal tone"), it was observed that the baro-reflex change of R-R interval was only attenuated when assessed by blood pressure elevation, but not by reduction. Consequently these authors concluded that there was an abnormal parasympathetic but a preserved cardiac sympathetic control of heart rate. Altogether the studies which evaluated both the tachycardia due to hypotension (nitro-glycerine) and the bradycardia due to hypertension (phenylephrine) provide no unequivo-cal evidence for a defect in the sympathetic component of the baroreceptor heart rate reflex.

In Fig. 2 we have used the data of a number of publications and plotted the slope of the systolic blood pressure – pulse interval relationship ("baroreflex sensitivity") as a function of baseline heart rate. The graph shows that in the healthy animal as well as in congestive heart failure "baroreflex sensitivity" is reduced whenever heart rate increases, particularly at a heart rate between 50 and 120 beats/min, which is dominated by the vagal efferents to the sinus node. Of note, the data by Bristow and collaborators, who reported a decrease in the "baroreflex slope" in man with increasing loads of exercise (heart rate reached 150 beats/min) would also fit into this graph (12).

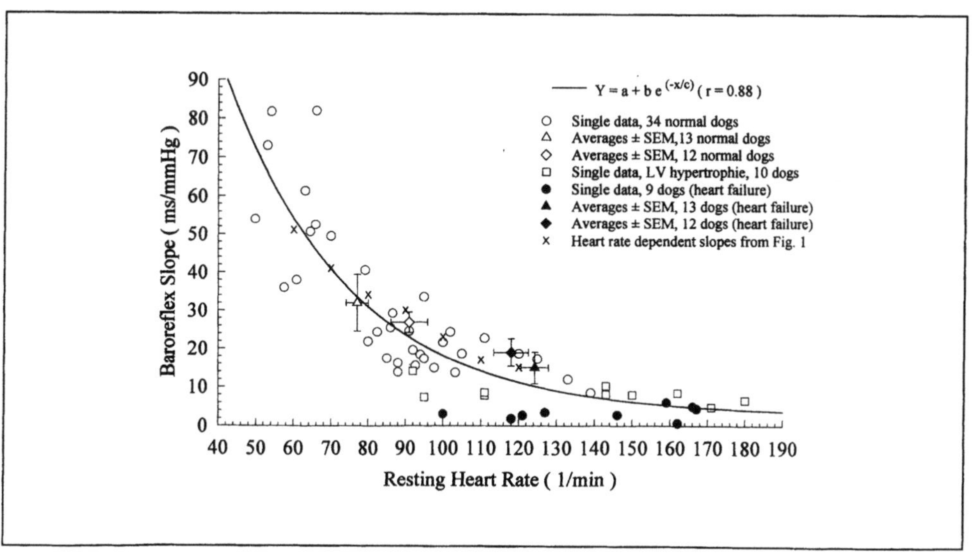

Fig. 2 Baroreflex slope ("baroreflex sensitivity" as calculated from the relationship between heart beat interval and systolic blood pressure) in conscious dogs plotted as a function of baseline heart rate. Open circles: 34 normal dogs (51, 67, 161). Open triangles: Averaged data ± SEM from 13 normal dogs (16). Open diamonds: Averaged data ± SEM from 12 normal dogs (10). Open squares: 10 dogs with left ventricular hypertrophy (tricuspid avulsion and progressive pulmonary stenosis) (67). Filled circles: 9 dogs with heart failure (tricuspid avulsion and progressive pulmonary stenosis) (67). Filled triangles: Averaged data from 13 dogs with heart failure (due to pacing) (16). Filled diamonds: Averaged data ± SEM from 12 dogs with heart failure (due to pacing) (10). Slope at 70, 80, 90, 100, 110 and 120 beats/min from experiments shown in Fig. 1. Data were approximated by the exponential function $Y = a + b\,e^{(-x/c)}$; r = 0.88.

With regard to the mechanism of the reduced baroreflex bradycardia two further studies need to be shortly mentioned here: Higgins and co-workers showed in dogs that the impaired baroreflex bradycardia in heart failure was not associated with an efferent or an end-organ defect, since the sinuatrial node in these dogs reacted normally to direct electrical vagal stimulation (68). Ellenbogen and co-workers (42) demonstrated normal slowing of the native sinus node during pharmacologically induced increases of arterial pressure in heart transplant recipients (donor denervated, recipient innervated) who had advanced heart failure before transplantation.

In summary there is unequivocal experimental evidence that congestive heart failure is associated with an impairment of the vagally mediated baroreflex bradycardia, while the evidence for a similar defect in the baroreflex sympathetic tachycardia is not convincing at all. The low resting discharge rate of vagal cardiomotor neurones at a normal systolic blood pressure level or above seems to be the dominating factor causing this abnormality. In contrast to the often repeated and unfortunately still very popular notion of a reduced "baroreflex sensitivity", these studies by no means prove that the activating afferent baroreceptor input to vagal and sympathetic cardiomotor neurones is impaired in a sense which would grant this generalized conclusion. To our knowledge the relationship between afferent baroreceptor activity and vagal or sympathetic cardiomotor efferent discharge has not been compared yet between normals and animals with congestive heart failure. It is interesting to note in this context that chemically activated cardiac reflexes (bradycardia due to intracoronary injections of 0.01, 0.1 and 0.4 µg/kg Veratridine) in conscious dogs with pacing induced heart failure are enhanced rather than attenuated (17); in sinuaortic denervated dogs with the same form of heart failure this was also observed after intracoronary injections of prostacyclin (PGI_2) (8). This is consistent again with a low resting vagal activity in heart failure.

Abnormalities in the baroreceptor control of vasomotor responses

Only a few authors have studied the baroreflex control of peripheral resistance in animals with congestive heart failure. In an often cited early study by Higgins and collaborators (67) in conscious dogs with heart failure (tricuspid avulsion and progressive pulmonary stenosis), it was observed that the increase in blood pressure in response to bilateral carotid occlusion as well as the increase in mesenteric and renal vascular resistance was smaller than in normal dogs. It was concluded that the regional circulatory adjustments to baroreceptor unloading were attenuated by congestive heart failure. For the following reasons this conclusion is not tenable: the smaller pressure response in the dogs with heart failure (+ 26 versus + 52 mmHg) was paralleled by a smaller increase in heart rate also (88 to 119 versus 125 to 138 beats/min), while mesenteric and renal blood flow were not changed. Thus it cannot be excluded that the reduced vagal restraint in the heart failure dogs probably also reduced the increase in heart rate, cardiac output, and blood pressure. Consequently the calculated increase in renal and mesenteric vascular resistance was larger in the normal dogs, which showed a larger pressure rise, and this probably was mediated by autoregulation of blood flow. This is consistent with a more recent investigation in conscious dogs with pacing induced heart failure, in which the authors analyzed the open-loop relationships between carotid sinus pressure and blood pressure, heart rate, cardiac output, and total peripheral resistance (123). It was shown that heart failure depressed baroreflex control of blood pressure through a concurrent reduction in the reflex control of heart rate and cardiac output, whereas the reflex control of vascular resistance was not consistently affected. A normal reaction in hindlimb vascular resistance to a phenylephrine-induced increase or a nitroglycerine-induced fall in blood pressure in anaesthetized dogs with pacing-induced congestive heart failure was also shown by Wilson and co-workers (179). Thus, there is no good evidence for an attenuated vasomotor response due to baroreceptor unloading in heart failure.

Studies in man have been concerned with the effects of orthostasis, lower body negative pressure (LBNP) or blood loss on forearm, splanchnic, and renal blood flow in congestive heart failure.

Before discussing these interventions in patients with congestive heart failure, a peculiarity in normal man as compared to dog should be mentioned: for the cardiopulmonary reflexes, which in man may be rather selectively inactivated by graded LBNP (up to −20 mmHg: no or little effect on aortic pulse pressure, mean pressure, dP/dt, and heart rate), not only the splanchnic vascular bed and renal sympathetic nerves but, contrary to animals, also the muscle (forearm) vascular bed seems to be a major target organ (1, 74; for further references see 141). For the kidney the effects of an enhanced sympathetic nerve discharge (unloading of cardiopulmonary receptors) on renin release and sodium reabsorption have to be quantitatively dissociated from vasomotor effects. In animals and probably also in man it needs a comparatively stronger activation of the renal nerves, i.e., by the simultaneous unloading of the arterial baroreceptors, in order to induce renal vasomotor effects. Larger changes in LBNP (−20 to −45 mmHg), which also affect carotid sinus and aortic baroreceptors in man, induce reflex vasomotor changes of a similar magnitude as orthostasis induced by 90° head up tilt. Thus, in normal man a low level of LBNP (−20 mmHg) induces decreases in splanchnic blood flow by 10 to 15 %, a slight increase in plasma renin activity (PRA), an increase of muscle sympathetic nerve discharge (for references see 141) and a reduction in forearm blood flow in the range of −20 to −30 % (47, 69). A similar reduction in forearm blood flow (−21 %) with only a −7 % fall in renal blood flow (positron emission tomography) was reported in normal subjects after a blood loss of 450 ml, which did not change heart rate and mean arterial blood pressure (113). Reductions in renal and splanchnic blood flow (around −10 %) in normal man are usually not observed until more negative values of LBNP are attained, which also affect sinoaortic baroreceptor afferents (−20 to −40 mmHg) (69). In normal man the largest changes in renal (−11 % to −30 %) and hepatic plasma flow (−14 % to − 39 %) were reported during orthostasis (103, 141).

In patients with congestive heart failure there is evidence for a reduced baseline blood flow to several regions: blood flow to the forearm is reduced by 25 % − 56 % (47, 56, 113, 115), to the calf by 44 % (184), to the liver by 36 % (103), and to the kidney by 41 to 44 % (103, 113) in spite of little changes (a few mmHg) in mean arterial blood pressure. In patients with congestive heart failure the renal blood flow response due to low level LBNP and due to blood loss (−450 ml) is either normal (18) or slightly enhanced (−12.5 % versus −7 %) (113). The response in splanchnic blood flow to low level LBNP is also normal in patients with congestive heart failure (20). Orthostasis or high level LBNP also induced similar renal and mesenteric or hepatic blood flow responses in patients as compared with the healthy control group (20, 103). Although due to the methods in human studies the evidence is rather indirect with regard to the differentiation between the cardiopulmonary or the arterial baroreflex, it can be concluded that in man also there is no evidence for a defect in the baro- or cardiopulmonary reflex renal or splanchnic vasomotor response in congestive heart failure.

With regard to the reaction of forearm blood flow to head-up tilt, it is known that patients with congestive heart failure respond with a paradox vasodilatation instead of showing a vasoconstriction (11). This has been confirmed by a number of studies using blood loss, orthostasis or low and high level of LBNP. No change or a slight increase (+5 %) of forearm blood flow was reported (20, 47, 56, 113, 115). A paradox vasodilatation during orthostasis was also observed in man in calf subcutaneous blood flow representing blood flow to muscle (182 183, 184). This group of authors recently reported that the abnormal reflex dilatation in calf subcutaneous flow is normalized to a vasoconstriction after cardiac transplantation (parts of the posterior atrial wall of the recipient remains intact) (184).

The reason behind this abnormal response of muscle blood flow in the extremities in congestive heart failure in man is unclear, but one of the more recent hypothesis shall be mentioned: a part of the vasoconstriction observed in subcutaneous tissue and skeletal muscle during orthostasis depends on a local "veno-arteriolar reflex" (66) which may be blocked by local anaesthesia, an α-antagonist, or by external counterpressure to reduce venous transmural pressure (for references see 141). In patients with congestive heart failure this "local reflex" seems to be still intact (182, 184). However, when the baroreceptor and this "local reflex" are activated simultaneously in patients, the local mechanism was unable to prevent the paradoxical vasodilatation, which was suggested to be a central nervous system mediated β-adrenergic vasodilator reflex, since it was abolished by proximal nerve block and local β-receptor blockade (77).

Interaction between the arterial- and cardiopulmonary baroreceptor reflexes and hormonal control in congestive heart failure

Altogether congestive heart failure is associated with an abnormality in the receptor transduction process of the carotid sinus- and aortic baroreceptors probably unrelated to possible changes in the mechanical properties of the vessel wall. The afferent activity from the low pressure system of the circulation is even more depressed, probably, because in addition the mechanical compliance of the receptor-carrying structures are affected (see "Arterial and cardiopulmonary baroreceptor abnormalities") which may be responsible for the associated histological defects at the receptor endings (atria). This obviously is due to the chronic volume overload. In part these changes may explain the decreased sensitivity between receptor stimulation and reflex sympathetic inhibition. The repeatedly observed failure to further increase sympathetic nerve activity with unloading of the receptors suggests that other factors than receptor defects in addition disturb the tonic regulation of sympathetic nerve discharge. This is also supported by the fact that there is an early defect in the tonic vagal discharge to the heart (see "Evidence for a reduced vagal tone in congestive heart failure"). Up to now there has been little evidence for a decrease in the central gain of the arterial- or cardiopulmonary baroreceptor reflex. In contrast to the result-

Fig. 3 Effects of congestive heart failure (CHF; due to pacing) on mean arterial pressure (MAP) heart rate (HR), left atrial pressure (LAP), and plasma norepinephrine concentration (Plasma NE) in 9 intact and 9 sinu-aortic denervated (SAD) conscious dogs. *: P < 0.05 CHF versus control. ....: P < 0.05 SAD versus control [Redrawn from data in (9)]

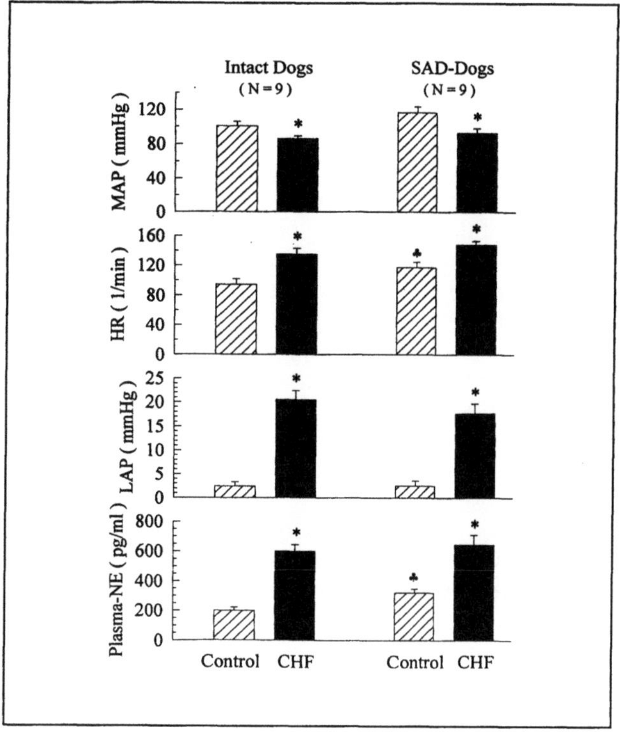

ing abnormality in the rapidly acting neural control of cardiac output with reduced receptor activation, the baroreflex control of vasomotor tone in the kidney, and the mesenteric circulation seems largely unaffected. An exception seems to be the unexplained peculiar behavior of skeletal muscle vascular tone in man (see "Abnormalities in the baroreceptor control of vasomotor responses"). The largely intact reflex increase in renal and mesenteric vascular resistance points to a possible involvement of tonically acting hormonal vasomotor influences in congestive heart failure. So altogether it remains questionable, whether there is any causal relationship between these abnormalities in the cardiovascular reflexes and the neuro-hormonal changes observed in congestive heart failure. An interesting experiment with regard to a possible causal relationship between abnormalities in the cardiovascular reflexes and the neur-hormonal changes should be mentioned (9). The authors looked for the changes in plasma norepinephrine in chronically sinuaortic denervated dogs in which heart failure was induced by rapid pacing. They found that without sinuaortic receptors there was still a significant increase in plasma norepinephrine (Fig. 3). Unfortunately this does not exclude that a possible defect in the remaining cardiopulmonary receptors was responsible for the increase in plasma noradrenaline in heart failure.

Next we will summarize some previous and more recent evidence from animal experiments with some supporting observations in man, which suggest that the kidney via angiotensin II and its action in the central nervous system may determine the tonic level of sympathetic and parasympathetic nerve discharge and cause a resetting of the baroreceptor reflexes.

Central effects of angiotensin II

It is generally accepted that Ang II-induced chronic hypertension is not mediated via a direct action of Ang II on vascular smooth muscle, rather than it appears that this type of hypertension requires time (hours to days) to develop and involves a central mechanism (134, 136). There is also an abundance of evidence suggesting that Ang II acts in the central nervous system to decrease vagal motor activity to the heart and to increase the level of activation of the sympathetic nervous system (6, 14, 15, 72, 75, 100, 104, 121, 132, 135).

Several authors have reported that an intravenous infusion of Ang II in anaesthetized animals reduces the slope of the relationship between mean arterial blood pressure and heart rate (15, 60, 101). Other studies using conscious dogs or rabbits have failed to observe an alteration in slope, but have suggested a resetting toward a higher blood pressure (13, 109, 135). In part this difference may be related to the dose of Ang II and different species (6). In spite of the latter inconsistencies there is general agreement that Ang II resets the heart rate reflex towards higher pressures, which was prevented in rabbits by lesioning the area postrema. This suggests that the resetting of cardiac baroreflex by Ang II involved an action at the are postrema (108).

In contrast to the acute resetting of the baroreceptor heart rate reflex, the resetting of the baroreflex control of sympathetic nerve activity by Ang II has been shown to be a chronic effect. In reviewing the recent literature Bishop and co-workers (6) stated: "Acute administration of Ang II has a direct vasoconstrictor action to increase arterial pressure, which initiates a baroreflex response to inhibit sympathetic nerve activity. At that point in time, ganglionic blockade has little effect on the pressor response. Subsequently, as the arterial baroreflex resets toward higher pressures, sympathetic nerve activity increases back towards the control level. Now ganglionic blockade causes a greater fall in arterial pressure, suggesting a neurogenic mechanism." In support of the central origin of this mechanism it has been found that Ang II-induced hypertension in the rat and in the rabbit was prevented by ablation of the area postrema (for references see 6). Whether the tonic sympathetic nerve discharge of a conscious normotensive animal at rest may be influenced by the intravenous application of a converting enzyme inhibitor is not yet clear. While Noshiro and co-workers reported no change in the renal norepinephrine spillover in the conscious rabbit after enalapril (121), Zucker and calloborators after captopril observed a 26% decrease in resting renal sympathetic nerve discharge in the conscious dog although mean arterial pressure decreased by 7 mmHg (191). In conclusion there is evidence that by a central action Ang II reduces tonic vagal discharge to the heart, acutely resets the baroreceptor-heart rate reflex towards a higher pressure level, and with some latency (~1–1.5 hours) causes the same resetting of the baroreceptor-sympathetic nerve activity reflex (6).

Pressure-dependent renin release as a blood pressure stabilizing system

Regarding the pathophysiology of congestive heart failure in principle only three mechanisms of renin release need to be considered:

Pressure-dependent renin release ("renal baroreceptor") is a mechanism located in the renal vasculature itself and, therefore, is also tightly coupled to renal autoregulation.

The renal sympathetic nerves may influence renin release via two different mechanism. Their activity can either directly influence the innervated juxtaglomerular cells via a β_1-adrenergic pathway or they can modulate pressure-dependent renin release by an α_1-adrenergic vasomotor mechanism. The β_1-adrenergic pathway can, of course, also be activated by circulating epinephrine. The neural α_1-adrenergic resetting occurs in both, pressure-dependent renin release and in autoregulation of renal blood flow and glomerular filtration rate. The resetting in autoregulation documents itself in a shift of the lower limits towards a higher blood pressure level (for references see 88, 89). This hemodynamic sympathetic resetting is obviously little affected by a possible secondary formation of angiotensin II (128). Altogether these observations support the coupling between autoregulation and pressure-dependent renin release. It seems likely that the α_1-adrenergic vasoconstriction of the larger preglomerular resistance vessels is resetting pressure-dependent renin release and autoregulation by affecting the myogenic response of the preglomerular vessels located more downstream towards the glomerulum (39, 61, 87, 88, 90, 91, 128).

A low *sodium diet* or the administration of a converting enzyme inhibitor has been shown to increase only the steep slope of the curve describing pressure-dependent renin release (44, 45).

Autoregulation of renal blood flow and pressure-dependent renin release as observed in a resting conscious dog is depicted in Fig. 4. This stimulus-response curve reveals a characteristic pattern: a flat section or plateau in the high pressure range and a very steep section in the low pressure range. When this stimulus-response curve is approximated by two straight lines, a threshold pressure (P_{th}) may be easily defined. The average threshold pressure in these 8 conscious dogs was 91 mmHg and the increase in renin release occurs without major alterations of renal blood flow (Fig. 4). Previous experiments conducted by other authors in anaesthetized dogs and our own data obtained in conscious dogs provide unequivocal evidence that the maximum of pressure-dependent renin release coincides very accurately with the lower limit of renal blood flow autoregulation (60–70 mmHg). Below

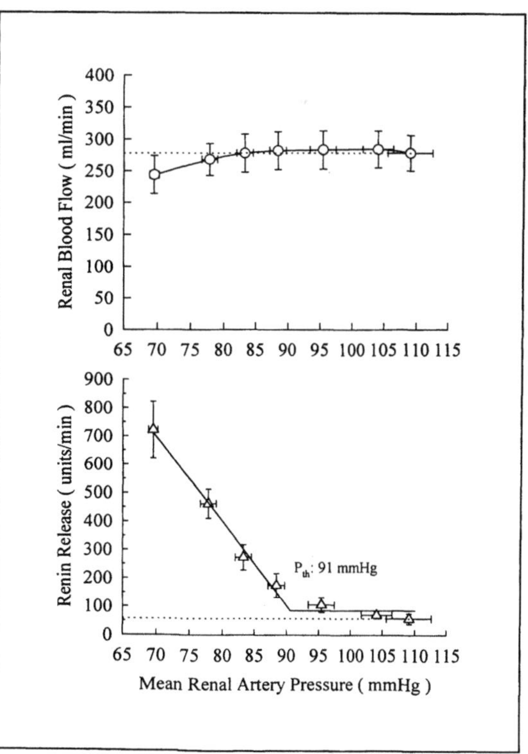

Fig. 4 Renal blood flow and renin release (renal-venous minus arterial plasma renin activity multiplied by renal plasma flow) of the left kidney as a function of mean renal artery pressure in 8 conscious dogs (renal perfusion pressure was reduced without changing aortic blood pressure in steps of 10 min duration). Threshold pressure (P_{th}) of pressure dependent renin release was approximated by two linear regression lines. Note that below P_{th} renin release was doubled for a fall of blood pressure by 2.6 mmHg [Data redrawn from (38)]

this pressure range a further increase of renin release is not observed (41, 50). The very high sensitivity of this mechanism is indicated by the fact that below threshold it needs a pressure drop of 2–3 mmHg only to double renin release (Fig. 4). The direct β_1-adrenergic modular effect on renin release is much less effective. It may slightly increase the slope of the curve below threshold (89) and elevates the suprathreshold plateau level only moderately when renal perfusion pressure is kept constant (59). Up to now we have determined the threshold pressure in 135 experiments conducted in 35 individual foxhounds and have observed that it was rather stable over time in the individual dog but varied between the dogs from 82 to 106 mmHg (average: 92.2 ± 1 mmHg). For averaging purposes we have selected 7 conscious dogs with individual threshold pressures between 96 and 99 mmHg and fitted the plot by a four parameter logistic dose-response curve (Fig. 5). The normal operating point on this curve, i.e., the resting blood pressure was 110 mmHg and, thus, only 12 mmHg above threshold. In a previous study in 14 conscious dogs the difference between long-term mean arterial blood pressure and threshold pressure on average was 12.5 mmHg (38). Since the lower limit of autoregulation of glomerular filtration rate (84 mmHg) is significantly higher when compared to renal blood flow autoregulation (67 mmHg) (86), threshold pressure for pressure-dependent renin release is very close to the pressure level below which glomerular filtration rate begins to fall. The α_1-adrenergic resetting of threshold pressure by a moderate activation of the renal sympathetic nerves, which did not change renal blood flow significantly, is also depicted in Fig. 5 (39, 61, 84, 87, 88, 90, 128).

Comparing the stimulus-response curve for pressure-dependent renin release (Fig. 5) with the arterial- and cardiopulmonary baroreceptor characteristic relating sympathetic nerve discharge to mean arterial blood pressure (Fig. 6), it becomes evident that in a normal

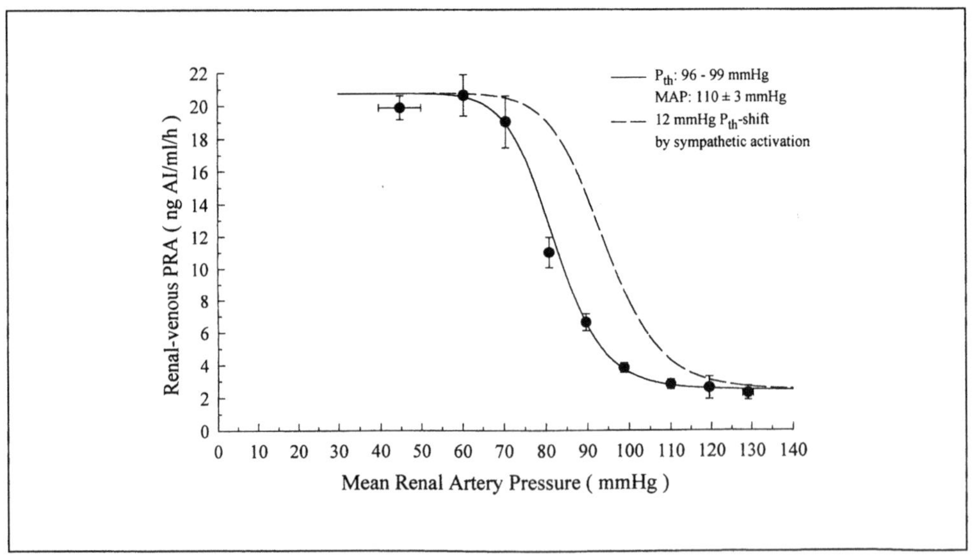

Fig. 5 Relationship between renal-venous plasma renin activity and mean renal artery pressure of left kidney as evaluated from 33 experiments in 7 conscious dogs (renal perfusion pressure was reduced without changing aortic blood pressure in steps of 5 min duration). Since in a total number of 35 dogs we observed that threshold pressures (P_{th}) varied from dog to dog between 82 and 106 mmHg, for averaging purposes 7 dogs were selected for this graph, which had a P_{th} between 96 and 99 mmHg. The data were approximated by a four parameter logistic function $Y = a + b / (x/c)^d$, $r = 0.99$ MAP: average resting mean arterial blood pressure ± SEM.

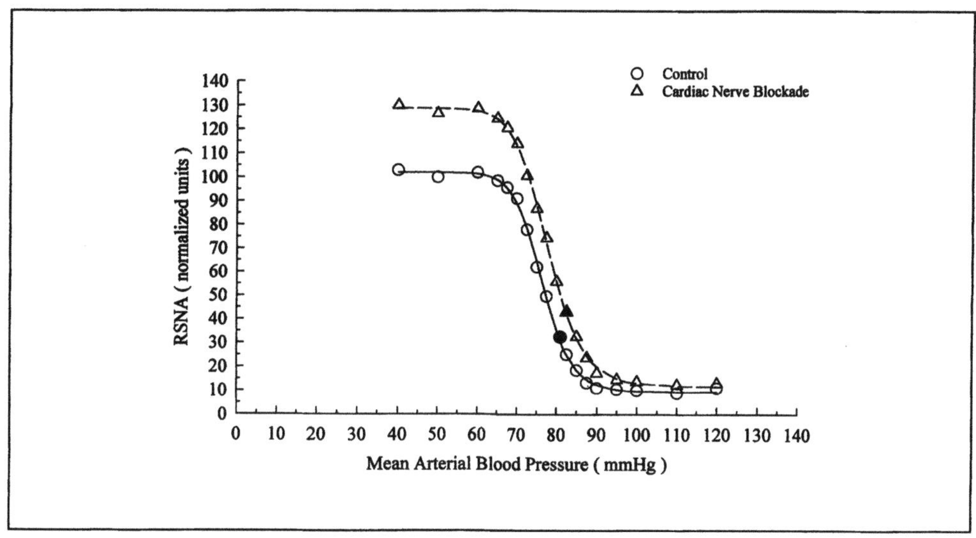

Fig. 6 Relationship between integrated multiunit renal sympathetic nerve activity (R.S.N.A.) and mean arterial blood pressure obtained 6 days after electrode implantation in 7 conscious rabbits (see 90). Cardiac nerve blockade (open triangle) was achieved by intrapericardial instillation of procaine. In both the control and the cardiac nerve blockade experiment the sinu-aortic receptor areas remained intact. Filled symbols: Resting blood pressure [Redrawn from (90)]

conscious animal at rest the location of both operating points suggests that a normal resting blood pressure is associated with a low tonic sympathetic nerve discharge (Fig. 6) and a minimum renin release (Fig. 5), constituting two systems, which obviously protect the body only against a fall in blood pressure. At the same time the highest capillary pressure (45–50 mmHg) in the cardiovascular system, i.e., glomerular capillary pressure, is protected from decreasing below a level, which would compromise renal function. Furthermore it is easily conceived that due to the α_1-adrenergic threshold shift the effect of even a slight fall of arterial blood pressure on renin release will be potentiated by the concomitant baroreflex increase in sympathetic nerve discharge (Fig. 5).

An important role of pressure-dependent renin release in the medium-term (1–4 hours) blood pressure control has been proposed in a previous study from our laboratory (38). A close correlation between mean arterial blood pressure and threshold pressure was found. Hence, the prevailing blood pressure may depend on the variables which describe pressure-dependent renin release, i.e., slope and threshold pressure. A causal relationship between mean arterial blood pressure and this renin release has been proposed, involving the following mechanism: the prevailing mean arterial blood pressure is usually above threshold pressure. However, for about 15 % of the time mean arterial pressure falls below this threshold due to the endogenous variability of blood pressure. These episodes of low mean arterial blood pressure induce renin release, which in turn increase blood pressure (38).

In a later study we have provided direct evidence for the function of this feedback mechanism under physiological closed-loop conditions. A feedback device was developed (117) which allowed us to maintain a constant pressure difference between systemic and renal artery pressure. Both kidneys were, thus, subjected to a pressure reduction without decreasing systemic mean arterial blood pressure. In this way our method constituted a closed-loop preparation in which any subsequent increase in systemic blood pressure also induced the same increase in renal perfusion pressure. Hence, it was possible to quantify directly the exact amount of compensation by the kidney, i.e., the closed-loop gain of this control system in conscious dogs. Using converting-enzyme inhibition, we could quantify the contribution of the renin-angiotensin system to this compensation (129).

The major results of this study are depicted in Fig. 7. In A it is demonstrated that in a time control of 6 dogs there was no clear trend in blood pressure. In B and C the effects of

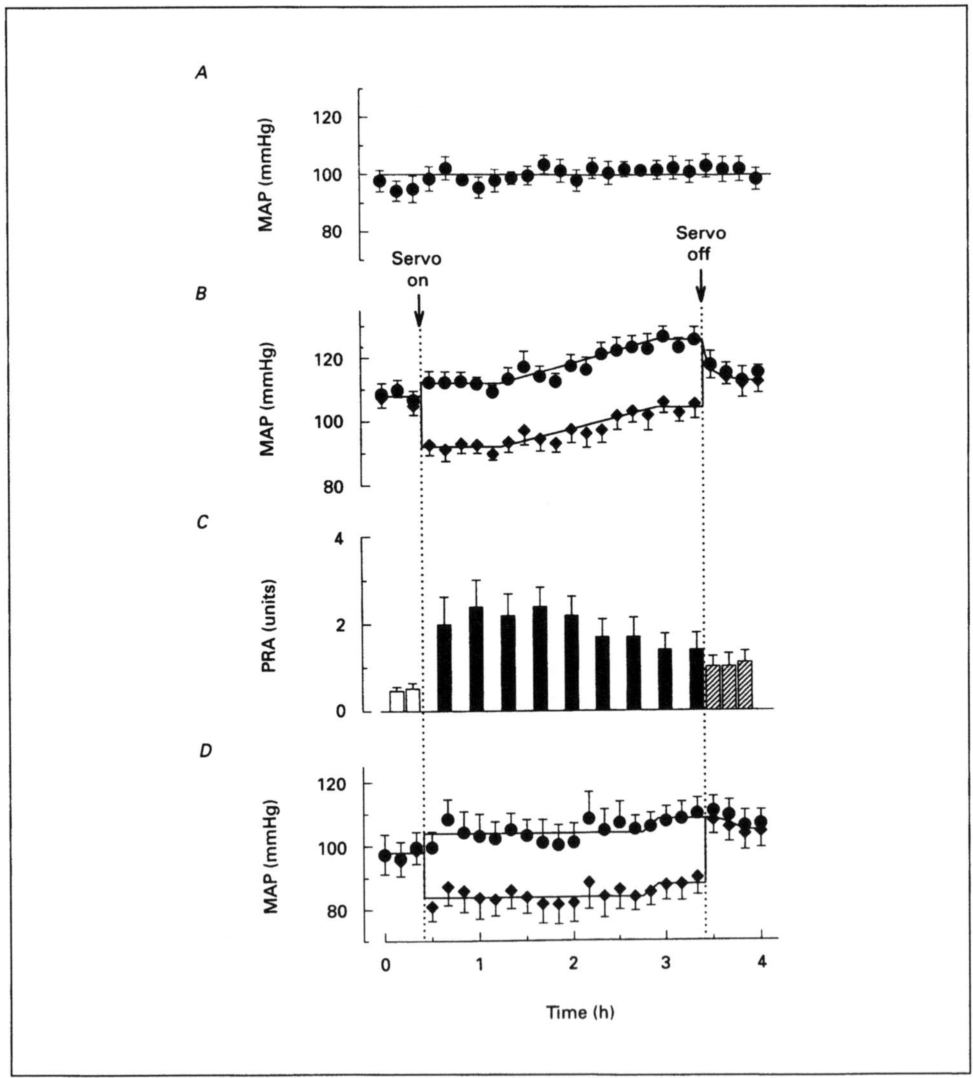

Fig. 7 A) Time control of mean arterial blood pressure (MAP) in 6 conscious dogs. **B)** Effect of servo-control of 20 mmHg pressure difference between systemic blood pressure and renal perfusion pressure. Filled circles: mean aortic pressure above the aortic cuff. Filled diamonds: mean aortic pressure below the cuff. **C)** Plasma renin activity during experiment as shown in B. **D)** Effect of servo-control as shown in B after converting enzyme inhibition [Fig. 2 from (129)]

servo-control of a 20 mmHg pressure difference between systemic blood pressure and renal perfusion pressure in 6 dogs are depicted. During the last 30 minutes of servo-controlling the pressure-difference, a new steady state was obtained in all six dogs. Plasma renin activity increased immediately and decreased again during the rising phase of blood pressure. The closed-loop gain was 0.63 i.e., 63 % of the 20 mmHg error signal was compensated for. In D the same experiment was conducted in six dogs during converting enzyme inhibition; from this protocol a closed-loop gain of 0.15 was calculated. It can be concluded from these experiments that the kidneys play an important role in the medium-term blood pressure control, most probably via the renin-angiotensin system. In these experiments two until now unexplained observations are interesting to note: 1) although plasma renin activity increased immediately as renal perfusion pressure was reduced below threshold, it took roughly 1 hour after blood pressure started to rise. 2) Although renal perfusion pressure was compensated for by 63 %, plasma renin activity did not return to its initial value during the steady state.

We should like to put forward the following hypothesis to explain these observations: 1) the pressor effect of the angiotensin II formed immediately after the reduction of renal perfusion pressure is initially compensated for by a reflex sympathetic inhibition due to the normal function of the arterial and cardiopulmonary reflexes. Subsequently the slow central action of angiotensin II at the area postrema after approximately 1 hour (see above: "central effects of Ang II") starts to reset the arterial and cardiopulmonary reflexes towards a higher pressure level, readjusting a normal sympathetic nerve discharge to a higher blood pressure level (see Fig. 6). 2) Depending on the exact location of the operating point (Fig. 6), the amount of this readjustment of sympathetic nerve discharge may not be complete, so there might be a remaining nervous resetting of pressure-dependent renin release with a slightly elevated plasma renin level during the new steady state. This hypothesis is consistent with the known central actions of angiotensin II but of course still needs experimental verification.

There can be no doubt that plasma renin activity rises early in congestive heart failure (for references see 118). According to the experimental data described in the last section, this early increase in plasma renin activity has to be considered a normal physiological response. Even a slight decrease in stroke volume will be noted by the high dynamic sensitivity of the arterial baroreceptors via the changes in aortic dP/dt, systolic pressure, and pulse pressure (83) resulting in a moderate increase in renal sympathetic nerve discharge. Thus, even without any change in aortic mean blood pressure renin release will be activated due to the increase of threshold pressure (Fig. 5). Consequently early renal denervation in the thoracic caval constriction model of congestive heart failure can decrease plasma renin activity by 50 % (181). This stimulatory influence of the renal nerves will be potentiated when accompanied by a fall in mean arterial blood pressure (Fig. 5). The selective chronic reduction of renal perfusion per se to 75–80 % of control, which in conscious dogs has no effect on glomerular filtration rate, is sufficient to initiate sodium and water retention and increase total body sodium within 24 hours. This sodium and volume retention by the way will go on unlimited for days, when the normally occurring downregulation of Ang II and Aldosterone, which brings back the animals into sodium balance, is prevented by infusing these hormones (7, 137, 148). The increase in extracellular fluid volume, of course, via the Frank-Starling mechanism may improve cardiac function (compensation). As long as the low pressure system receptors are functioning their potent inhibitory action on the renal sympathetic nerves will bring back threshold pressure and, thus, renin release to normal. The downregulation of Ang II and Aldosterone, which was described above, may also contribute to compensation. Thus, even severe cardiac dysfunction with an extensive elevation of total body sodium and water may be associated with a completely normal plasma renin activity. The importance of blood pressure as a major stimulus for the activation of the renin-angiotensin system in congestive heart failure was demonstrated by Dzau and co-worker; in three groups of patients with similar reductions in cardiac output and comparable elevations in pulmonary capillary wedge pressure plasma renin activity was inversely correlated with mean arterial blood pressure. A normal plasma renin activity was only found in one of the groups, in which mean arterial blood pressure had reached a normal level, even though evidence for severe cardiac dysfunction still persisted (33).

Actions of angiotensin II in congestive heart failure

As already mentioned there is a reduced "vagal tone" in congestive heart failure, and there is convicing evidence that in normal animals angiotentin II via an action at the area postrema causes withdrawal of "vagal tone". Thus, the reduced "vagel tone" observed in congestive heart failure may very well at least in part be caused by a central action of angiotensin II. There is circumstantial evidence from clinical studies to support this suggestion; studying the reflex bradycardia in patients with the neck-suction technique Vogt and co-workers reported an enhanced response 24 hours after the application of converting enzyme inhibitor (163). Osterziel and co-workers, recognizing that the amount of reflex bradycardia ("Baroreflex sensitivity") due to neck-suction was an indicator of "vagal tone", observed that the reflex bradycardia in patients with congestive heart failure was inversely correlated with plasma renin activity (126). Furthermore they noted that converting enzyme inhibition increased "vagal tone" significantly in congestive heart failure (125, 127). A decrease in the high frequency component of heart rate variability, which was taken to indicate an augmentation of "vagal tone", was also found after therapy with a converting enzyme inhibitor in patients of congestive heart failure (5).

There is some indirect and some direct evidence in the most recent literature to support the hypothesis that in congestive heart failure there is an abnormality of arterial- and cardiopulmonary reflexes, which is caused by a central action of angiotensin II.

In conscious rabbits with cardiomyopathy induced by doxorubicin Noshiro and associates observed that the blunted mean arterial pressure-renal norepinephrine spillover relationship as well as the blunted relationship between mean arterial pressure and total norepinephrine spillover was returned close to normal after intravenous converting enzyme inhibition. The authors suggested that the renin-angiotensin system contributes significantly to the attenuated baroreflex response in heart failure (122). Using vasomotor drugs to decrease or increase blood pressure while recording renal sympathetic nerve discharge in conscious normal rats as well as in rats with congestive heart failure (ligation of the left coronary artery), DiBona and associates studied the relationship between blood pressure and renal nerve activity (31). The authors further examined the effects of intravenously or intracerebroventricular angiotensin II AT_1-receptor blockade (losartan) on these function curves. Rats suffering from congestive heart failure as compared to the normal animals showed a reduced range of sympathetic control and a decrease in maximum gain but no resetting of the function curve. While the intravenous or intracerebroventricular application of losartan did not affect the function curve in the normal rats, it restored the reduced gain in congestive heart failure to reach 80 % of that observed in the control rats. Although it should be considered that renal sympathetic nerve discharge for methodological reasons had to be plotted in % of control, a comparison of the function curves in congestive heart failure before and after losartan in Fig. 3 of the study even suggests some resetting. However, the most important finding in the study was that losartan administration to conscious rats with heart failure decreased renal sympathetic nerve discharge at an unchanged arterial blood pressure (31).

There is also support from a most recent observation in man; converting enzyme inhibition decreased systolic pressure in patients with heart failure and in control subjects. However, sympathetic nerve activity to skeletal muscle (microneurography) decreased in patients and increased in control subjects. The baroreflex responses (phenylephrine, sodium nitroprusside, lower body negative pressure, and head down tilt) were enhanced by converting enzyme inhibition in patients but not in normal control subjects (27).

Conclusions

Altogether there is growing evidence that at least with regard to the loss of vagal control of heart rate and the enhanced sympathetic nerve discharge, the renin-angiotensin-system seems to play an essential role in congestive heart failure by setting the tonic level of sympathetic nerve discharge. Due to their high dynamic sensitivity the arterial baroreceptors can detect even slight changes in arterial pulse contour. The resulting disinhibition of the renal sympathetic nerves will in concert with the pressure-dependent mechanism activate the renin-angiotensin system. This activation may be switched off as soon as the resulting sodium and water retention has found a new steady-state in total body sodium and water. By signalling the state of filling of the low pressure system and by their inhibitory action on the renal nerves, the cardiopulmonary afferents are probably participating in the setting of this steady state, but other factors downregulating Ang II and Aldesterone are probably also involved. In this way even the failing heart is able to stabilize blood pressure at a level which inhibits renin release and prevents severe decreases in glomerular filtration. However, when in spite of the volume expansion the failing heart is unable to provide a minimal perfusion pressure for the brain and the kidneys, renin activation and volume retention seems to go on unlimited finally leading to decompensation. The angiotensin-dependent increase in tonic sympathetic discharge may be especially important in the latter situation, constituting a last line of defence. It needs more integrative studies in experimental animals and man to provide evidence for this hypothesis and several other speculations in this review.

Acknowledgments   The studies from our laboratory which were mentioned in this review were generously supported by the German Research Foundation within the SFB 320 (project A/1), the Graduiertenkolleg "Experimentelle Nieren- und Kreislaufforschung", Heidelberg, and the projects Ki 151/5–2 and Ki 152/5–3. We would also like to thank Professor J. O. Arndt, Düsseldorf, for critically reading the manuscript.

References

1. Abboud FM, Eckberg DL, Johannsen UL, Mark AL (1979) Carotid and cardiopulmonary baroreceptor control of splanchnic and forearm vascular resistance during venous pooling in man. J Physiol 286: 173–184
2. Arai Y, Saul JP, Albrecht P, Hartley LH, Lilly LS, Cohen RJ, Colucci WS (1989) Modulation of cardiac autonomic activity during and immediately after exercise. Am J Physiol 256: H132–H141
3. Beck W, Barnard CN, Schrire V (1969) Heart rate after cardiac transplantation. Circulation 40: 437–445
4. Berne C, Fagius J (1993) Metabolic regulation of sympathetic system activity: lessons from intraneural nerve recordings. Int J Obes Relat Metab Disord 17: Suppl 3: S2–S6

5. Binkley PF, Haas GJ, Starling RC, Nunziata E, Hatton PA, Leier CV, Cody RJ (1993) Sustained augmentation of parasympathetic tone with angiotensin-converting enzyme inhibition in patients with congestive heart failure. J Am Col Cardiol 21: 655–661

6. Bishop VS, Shade RE, Haywood JR (1991) Hormonal modulation of baroreceptor reflexes. In: PB Persson & HR Kirchheim (ed) Baroreceptor Reflexes. Integrative Functions and Clinical Aspects. Springer, Berlin Heidelberg New York, pp 226–236

7. Boemke W, Seeliger E, Rothermund L, Corea M, Pettker R, Mollenhauer G, Reinhardt HW (1995) ACE inhibition prevents Na and water retention and MABP increase during reduction of renal perfusion pressure. Am J Physiol 269: R481–R489

8. Brändle M, Wang W, Zucker IH (1994) Ventricular mechanoreflex alterations in chronic heart failure. Circ Res 74: 262–270

9. Brändle M, Patel KP, Wang W, Zucker IH (1996b) Hemodynamic and norepinephrine response to pacing-induced heart failure in conscious sino-aortic denervated dogs. J Appl Physiol 81: 1855–1862

10. Brändle M, Wang W, Zucker IH (1996a) Hemodynamic correlates of baroreflex impairment of heart rate in experimental canine heart failure. Bas Res Cardiol 91: 147–154

11. Bridgen W, Sharpey-Schafer EP (1950) Postural change in peripheral blood flow in cases with left heart failure. Clin Sci 9: 93–100

12. Bristow JD, Brown Jr EB, Cunningham DJC, Howson MG, Strange Petersen E, Pickering TG, Sleight P (1971) Effect of bicycling on the baroreflex regulation of pulse interval. Circ Res 28: 582–592

13. Brooks VL, Reid IA (1986) Interaction between angiotensin II and the baroreceptor reflex in the control of adrenocorticotropic hormone secretion and heart rate in conscious dogs. Circ Res 58: 816–828

14. Bunag RD, Erisson L, Tanabe S (1990) Baroreceptor reflex enhancement by chronic intracerebroventricular infusion of enalapril in normotensive rats. Hypertension 15: 284–290

15. Campagnole-Santos MJ, Heringer SB, Batisda EN, Khosa MC, Santos RA (1992) Differential baroreceptor reflex modulation by centrally infused angiotensin peptides. Am J Physiol 263: R89–R94

16. Chen JS, Wang W, Bartholet Th, Zucker IH (1991) Analysis of baroreflex control of heart rate in conscious dogs with pacing-induced heart failure. Circulation 83: 260–267

17. Chen JS, Wang W, Cornish KG, Zucker IH (1992) Baro- and ventricular reflexes in conscious dogs subjected to chronic tachycardia. Am J Physiol 263: H1084–H1089

18. Chidsey CA, Harrison DC, Braunwald E (1962) Augmentation of the plasma norepinephrine response to exercise in patients with congestive heart failure. N Engl J Med 267: 650–654

19. Cody RJ, Haas GJ, Binkley PF, Caspers Q, Kelley R (1992) Plasma endothelin correlates with the extent of pulmonary hypertension in patients with chronic congestive heart failure. Circulation 85: 504–509

20. Creager MA, Hirsch AT, Dzau VJ, Nabel EG, Cutler SS, Colucci WS (1990) Baroreflex regulation of regional blood flow in congestive heart failure. Am J Physiol 258: H1409–H1414

21. Daly M de B (1986) Interactions between respiration and circulation. In: Handbook of Physiology, Section III, volume 2, part II, Cherniak NS, Widdicombe JG (eds.) Am Physiol Soc, Bethesda, pp 529–594

22. Dampney RAL (1994) Functional organisation of central pathways regulating the cardiovascular system. Physiol Rev 74: 232–264

23. Davis DD, Baily R, Zelis R (1988) Abnormalities in systemic norepinephrine kinetics in human congestive heart failure. Am J Physiol 254: E760–E766

24. Dembowsky K, Seller H (1995) Arterial baroreceptor reflexes. In: Vaitl D and Schandry R (eds) From the Heart to the Brain – The Psychophysiology of Circulation – Brain Interaction. Peter Lang GmbH, Frankfurt, Berlin, Bern, New York, Paris, Wien, pp 35– 60

25. Dibner-Dunlap ME, Thames MD (1989) Baroreflex control of renal sympathetic nerve activity is preserved in heart failure despite reduced arterial baroreceptor sensitivity. Circ Res 65: 1526–1535

26. Dibner-Dunlap ME, Thames MD (1992) Control of sympathetic nerve activity by vagal mechanoreflexes is blunted in heart failure. Circulation 86: 129–1934

27. Dibner-Dunlap ME, Smith ML, Kinugawa T, Thames M (1996) Enalapril augments arterial and cardiopulmonary baroreflex control of sympathetic nerve activity in patients with heart failure. J Am Coll Cardiol 27: 358–364

28. DiBona GF, Herman PF, Sawin LL (1988) Neural control of renal function in oedema-forming states. Am J Physiol 254: R1017–R1024

29. DiBona GF, Sawin LL (1991) Role of renal nerves in sodium retention of cirrhosis and congestive heart failure. Am J Physiol 260: R298–R305

30. DiBona GF, Sawin LL (1994) Reflex regulation of renal nerve activity in cardiac failure. Am J Physiol 266: R27–R39

31. DiBona GF, Jones SY, Brooks VL (1995) Ang II receptor blockade and arterial baroreflex regulation of renal nerve activity in cardiac failure. Am J Physiol 38: R1189–R1196

32. DiBona GF, Sawin LL (1995) Increased renal nerve activity in cardiac failure: arterial vs. cardiac baroreflex impairment. Am J Physiol 268: R112–R116

33. Dzau VJ, Colucci WS, Hollenberg NK, Williams GW (1981) Relation of the renin-angiotensin-aldosterone system to clinical state in congestive heart failure. Circulation 63: 645–651

34. Dzau VJ, Pratt RE (1986) Renin-angiotensin system: Biology, Physiology, and Pharmacology. In: Fozzard HA, Haber E, Jennings BB, Katz AM, Morgan HE (eds) The Heart and Cardiovascular System, New York, Raven Press, pp 1631–1662

35. Eckberg DL, Drabinsky M, Braunwald E (1971) Defective cardiac parasympathetic control in patients with heart disease. N Engl J Med 285: 877–883

36. Eckberg DL, Kifle YT, Roberts VL (1980) Phasic relationship between normal human respiration and baroreflex responsiveness. J Physiol 304: 489–502

37. Eckberg DL, Sleight P (eds.) Human Baroreceptor Reflexes in Health and Disease, Oxford University Press (1992) pp 413–418

38. Ehmke H, Persson PB, Kirchheim H (1987) A physiological role for pressure-dependent renin release in long-term blood pressure control. Pflügers Arch 410: 450–456

39. Ehmke H, Persson P, Fischer S, Hackenthal E, Kirchheim H (1989) Resetting of pressure-dependent renin release by intrarenal alpha1-adrenoceptors in conscious dogs. Pflügers Arch 413: 261–266

40. Ehmke H, Persson PB, Just A, Nafz B, Seyfarth M, Hackenthal E, Kirchheim H (1992) Physiological concentrations of ANP exert a dual regulatory influence on renin release in conscious dogs. Am J Physiol 263: R529–R536

41. Eide I, Løyning E, Kiil F (1977) Evidence for hemodynamic autoregulation of renin release. Circ Res 32: 237–243

42. Ellenbogen KA, Mohanty PK, Szentpetery S, Thames MD (1989) Arterial baroreflex abnormalities in heart failure: Reversal after orthotopic cardiac transplantation. Circulation 79: 51–58

43. Esler M, Jennings G, Leonard P, Sacharias N, Burk F, Johns J, Blombery P (1984) Contribution of individual organs to total noradrenaline in humans. Acta Physiol Scand: Suppl 527: 11–16

44. Farhi ER, Cant JR, Barger AC (1983) Alterations of renal baroreceptor by salt intake in control of plasma renin activity in conscious dogs. Am J Physiol 245: F119–F122

45. Farhi ER, Cant JR, Paganelli WC, Dzau VJ, Barger AC (1987) Stimulus-response curve of the renal baroreceptor: effect of converting enzyme inhibition and changes in salt intake. Circ Res 61: 670–677

46. Feng QP, Carlsson S, Thoren P, Hedner T (1994) Characteristics of renal sympathetic nerve activity in experimental congestive heart failure in the rat. Acta Physiol Scand 150: 259–266

47. Ferguson DW, Abboud FM, Mark AL (1984) Selective impairment of baroreflex-mediated vasoconstrictor responses in patients with ventricular dysfunction. Circulation 69: 451–460

48. Ferguson DW, Berg WJ, Sanders JS, Roach PJ, Kempf JS, Kienzle MG (1989) Sympathoinhibitory response to digitalis glycosides in heart failure patients. Direct evidence from sympathetic neural recordings. Circulation 80: 65–77

49. Ferguson DW, Berg WJ, Roach PJ, Oren RM, Mark AL (1992) Effects of heart failure on baroreflex control of sympathetic neural activity. Am J Cardiol 69: 523–531

50. Finke R, Gross R, Hackenthal E, Huber J, Kirchheim HR (1983) Threshold pressure for the pressure-dependent renin release in the autoregulating kidney of conscious dogs. Pflügers Arch 399: 102–110

51. Frankel RA, Metting PJ, Britton SL (1993) Evaluation of spontaneous baroreflex sensitivity in conscious dogs. J Physiol 462: 31–45

52. Gillis RA, Quest JA (1978) Neural actions of digitalis. Ann Rev Med 29: 73–79

53. Glick G, Braunwald E (1965) Relative role of sympathetic and parasympathetic nervous system in the reflex control of heart rate. Circ Res 16: 363–375

54. Göbel U, Schröck H, Seller H, Kuschinsky W (1990) Glucose utilization, blood flow and capillary density in the ventrolateral medulla of the rat. Pflügers Arch 416: 477–480

55. Goertz A, Heinrich H, Seeling W (1992) Baroreflex control of heart rate during high thoracic epidural anaesthesia. A randomised clinical trial on anaesthetised humans. Anaesthesia 47: 984–987

56. Goldsmith SR, Francis GS, Levine TB, Cohn JN (1983) Regional blood flow response to orthostasis in patient with congestive heart failure. J Am Coll Cardiol 1: 1391–1395

57. Grassi G, Seravalle G, Cattaneo BM, Lanfranchi A, Vailati S, Giannattasio C, Delbo A, Sala C, Bolla GB, Pozzi M, Mancia G (1995) Sympathetic activation and loss of reflex sympathetic control in mild congestive heart failure. Circulation 92: 3206–3211

58. Greenberg TT, Richmond WH, Stocking RA, Gupta PD, Meehan JP, Henry JP (1973) Impaired atrial receptor responses in dogs with heart failure due to tricuspid insufficiency and pulmonary artery stenosis. Circ Res 32: 424–433

59. Gross R, Hackenberg HM, Hackenthal E, Kirchheim H (1981) Interaction between perfusion pressure and sympathetic nerves in renin release by carotid baroreflex in conscious dogs. J Physiol (Lond) 313: 237–250

60. Guo GB, Abboud FM (1984) Angiotensin II attenuates the baroreflex control of heart rate and sympathetic activity. Am J Physiol 246: H80–H89

61. Hackenthal E, Paul M, Ganten D, Taugner R (1990) Morphology, physiology, and molecular biology of renin secretion. Physiol Rev 70: 1067–1116

62. Halliwill JR, Billman GE (1992) Effect of general anaesthesia on cardiac vagal tone. Am J Physiol 262: H1719–H1724

63. Harada S, Tokunaga S, Momohara M, Masaki H, Tagawa T, Imaizumi T, Takeshita A (1993) Inhibition of nitric oxide formation in the nucleus tractus solitarius increases renal sympathetic nerve activity in rabbits. Circ Res 72: 511–516

64. Hasking G, Esler MD, Jennings GL, Burton D, Johns JA, Korner PI (1986) Norepinephrine spillover to plasma in patients with congestive heart failure: evidence of increased overall and cardiorenal sympathetic nervous activity. Circulation 4: 615–621

65. Hasser EM, Bishop VS (1988) Neurogenic and humoral factors maintaining arterial pressure in conscious dogs. Am J Physiol 255: R693–R698

66. Henriksen O (1977) Local sympathetic reflex mechanism in regulation of blood flow in human subcutaneous adipose tissue. Acta Physiol Scand 101 (Suppl 450): 7–48

67. Higgins CB, Vatner SF, Eckberg DL, Braunwald E (1972a) Alterations in the baroreceptor reflex in conscious dogs with heart failure. J Clin Invest 51: 715–724, 1972

68. Higgins CB, Vatner SF, Franklin D, Braunwald E (1972 b) Effects of experimentally produced heart failure on the peripheral vascular response to severe exercise in conscious dogs. Circ Res 31: 186–194

69. Hirsch AT, Levenson DJ, Dzau VJ, Cutler SS, Doherty AR, Creager MA (1989) Regional vascular response to prolonged lower body negative pressure in normal subjects. Am J Physiol 257: H219–H225

70. Iriuchijima J, Kumada M (1963) Efferent cardiac vagal discharge of the dog in response to electrical stimulation of sensory nerves. Jap J Physiol 13: 599–605

71. Iriuchijima J, Kumada M (1964) Activity of single vagal fibres efferent to the heart. Jap J Physiol 14: 479–487

72. Ismay MJ, Lumbers ER, Stevens AD (1979) The action of angiotensin II on the baroreflex response of the conscious ewe and the conscious fetus. J Physiol (Lond) 288: 467–479

73. Jänig W (1985) Organisation of the lumbar sympathetic outflow to skeletal muscle and skin of the cat hindlimb and tail. Rev Physiol Biochem Pharmacol 102: 119–213

74. Johnson JM, Rowell LB, Niederberger M, Elsman MM (1974) Human splanchnic and forearm vasoconstrictor responses to reduction of right atrial and aortic pressure. Circ Res 34: 515–524

75. Joy MD, Lowe RD (1970) Evidence that the area postrema mediates the central cardiovascular response to angiotensin II. Nature 228: 1003–1304

76. Kaiser L, Spickard RC, Olivier NB (1989) Heart failure depresses endothelium-dependent response in canine femoral artery. Am J Physiol 256: H962–H967

77. Kassis E (1989) Baroreflex control of the circulation in patients with congestive heart failure. Dan Med Bull 36: 195–211

78. Katona PG, Poitras JW, Barnett GO, Terry BS (1970) Cardiac vagal efferent activity and heart rate period in carotid sinus reflex. Am J Physiol 218: 1030–1037

79. Katona PG, Jih F (1975) Respiratory sinus arrhythmia: non-invasive measure of parasympathetic cardiac control. J Appl Physiol 39: 801–805

80. Kaye DM, Lambert GW, Lefkovits J, Morris M, Jennings G, Esler MD (1994) Neurochemical evidence of cardiac sympathetic activation and increased central nervous system norepinephrine turnover in severe congestive heart failure. J Am Coll Cardiol 23: 570–578

81. Kaye DM, Lefkovits J, Jennings GL, Bergin P, Broughton A, Esler MD (1995) Adverse consequences of high sympathetic nervous activity in the failing human heart. J Am Coll Cardiol 26: 1257–1263

82. Kendrick E, Öberg B, Wennergren G (1972) Extent of engagement of various cardiovascular effectors to alterations of carotid sinus pressure. Acta Physiol Scand 86: 410–418

83. Kirchheim HR (1976) Systemic arterial baroreceptor reflexes. Physiol Rev 56: 100–176

84. Kirchheim HR, Finke R, Hackenthal E, Löwe W, Persson P (1985) Baroreflex sympathetic activation increases threshold pressure for the pressure dependent renin release in conscious dogs. Pflügers Arch 405: 127–135

85. Kirchheim, HR (1987) Physiological significance of atrial natriuretic factor in cardiovascular control. In: Christiansen C, Riss BJ (eds.) Highlights on Endocrinology, Nørhaven Bogtrykker A/S, pp 165–172

86. Kirchheim HR, Ehmke H, Hackenthal E, Löwe W, Persson P (1987) Autoregulation of renal blood flow, glomerular filtration rate and renin release in conscious dogs. Pflügers Arch 410: 441–449 (1987)

87. Kirchheim HR, Ehmke H, Persson P (1988) Physiology of the renal baroreceptor-mechanism of renin release and its role in congestive heart failure. Am J Cardiol 62: 68E–71E

88. Kirchheim HR, Ehmke H, Persson P (1989) Sympathetic modulation of renal hemodynamics, renin release and sodium excretion. Klin Wochenschr 67: 858–864

89. Kirchheim H, Ehmke H, Persson PB (1990) Role of blood pressure in the control of renin release. Acta Physiol Scand 139 (Suppl. 591): 40–47

90. Kirchheim HR (1991) Baroreceptor regulation of renal function. In: PB Persson & HR Kirchheim (eds) Baroreceptor Reflexes. Integrative Functions and Clinical Aspects. Springer, Berlin Heidelberg New York, pp 181–208

91. Kirchheim HR, Ehmke H (1994) Vasoactive Hormones: modulators of renal function. Clin Investig 72: 685–687

92. Koch E (1931) Die reflektorische Selbststeuerung des Kreislaufs, Theordor Steinkopff, Dresden und Leipzig, pp 211–217

93. Koepchen HP, Thurau K (1959) Über die Entstehungsbedingungen der atemsynchronen Schwankungen des Vagustonus (Respiratorische Arrhythmie) Pflügers Arch 269: 10–30

94. Koepchen HP, Wagner PH, Lux HD (1961) Über die Zusammenhänge zwischen zentraler Erregbarkeit, reflektorischem Tonus und Atemrhythmus bei der Steuerung der Herzfrequenz. Pflügers Arch 273: 443–465

95. Kollai M, Koizumi K (1989) Cardiac vagal and sympathetic nerve responses to baroreceptor stimulation in the dog. Pflügers Arch 413: 365–371

96. Kon VA, Yared A, Ichikawa I (1985) Role of renal sympathetic nerves in mediating hypoperfusion of renal cortical microcirculation in experimental congestive heart failure and acute extracellular volume depletion. J Clin Invest 76: 1913–1920

97. Kubo SH, Rector TS, Bank AJ, Williams RE, Heifetz SM (1991) Endothelium-dependent vasodilatation is attenuated in patients with heart failure. Circulation 84: 1589–1596

98. Kunze DL (1972) Reflex discharge patterns of cardiac vagal efferent fibres. J Physiol 222: 1–15

99. Lambert GW, Kaye DM, Lefkovits J, Jennings GL, Turner AG, Cox HS, Esler MD (1995) Increased central nervous system monoamine neurotransmitter turnover and its association with sympathetic nervous activity in treated failure patients. Circulation 92: 1813–1818

100. Lee WB, Ismay MJ, Lumbers ER (1980) Mechanism by which angiotensin II affects the heart rate of conscious sheep. Circ Res 47: 286–292

101. Lee WB, Lumbers ER (1981) Angiotensin and the cardiac baroreflex response to phenylephrine. Clin Exp Pharmacol Physiol 8: 109–117

102. Leimbach WN, Wallin BG, Victor RG, Aylward PE, Sundlöf G, Mark AL (1986) Direct evidence from intra-neural recordings for increased central sympathetic outflow in patients with heart failure. Circulation 73: 913–919

103. Lilly LS, Dzau VJ, Williams GH, Rydstedt L, Hollenberg NK (1984) Hyponatremia in congestive heart failure: implications for neurohumoral activation and responses to orthostasis. J Clin Endocrinol Metab 59: 924–930

104. Lumbers ER, Potter EK (1982) The effects of vasoactive peptides on the carotid cardiac baroreflex. Clin Exp Pharmacol Physiol (Suppl.) 7: 45–49

105. MacAllen RM, Spyer KM (1978) The baroreceptor input to cardiac vagal motoneurones. J Physiol 282: 365–374

106. Marey EJ (1859) Recherches sur le poulse au moyen d'un nouvel appareil enregistreur: le sphygmographe. Mémoires lus a la Société de Biologie, 281–309

107. Margulies KB, Hildebrand Jr FL, Lerman A, Perrella MA, Bornett Jr JC (1990) Increased endothelin in experimental heart failure. Circulation 82: 2226–2230

108. Matsukawa S, Reid IA (1990) Role of area postrema in the modulation of the baroreflex control of heart rate by angiotensin II. Circ Res 67: 1462–1473

109. Matsumura Y, Hasser EM, Bishop VS (1989) Central effect of angiotensin II on baroreflex regulation in conscious rabbits. Am J Physiol 256: R694–R700

110. Meredith IT, Eisenhofer G, Lambert GW, Dewar EM, Jennings GL, Esler MD (1993) Cardiac sympathetic nervous activity in congestive heart failure. Evidence for increased neuronal norepinephrine release and preserved neuronal uptake. Circulation 88: 136–145

111. Merrill AJ, Morrison JL, Brannon ES (1946) Concentration of renin in renal venous blood in patients with chronic heart failure. Am J Med 1: 468–472

112. Middlekauff HR, Hamilton MA, Stevenson LW, Mark AL (1994) Independent control of skin and muscle sympathetic nerve activity in patients with heart failure. Circulation 90: 1794–1798

113. Middlekauff HR, Nitzsche EU, Hamilton MA, Schelbert HR, Fonarow GC, Moriguchi JD, Hage A, Saleh S, Gibbs GG (1995) Evidence for preserved cardiopulmonary baroreflex control of renal cortical blood flow in humans with advanced heart failure. Circulation 92: 395–401

114. Minisi AJ, Dibner-Dunlap ME, Thames MD (1989) Vagal cardiopulmonary baroreflex activation during phenylephrine infusion. Am J Physiol 257: R1147–R1153

115. Mohanty PK, Arrowood JA, Ellenbogen KA, Thames MD (1989) Neurohormonal and hemodynamic effects of lower body negative pressure in patients with congestive heart failure. Am Heart J 118: 78–85

116. Mukharji J, Thames MD, Newton M, Hirsh PD, Lewis SA, Rehr RB, Cowley MJ, Hess ML, Hastillo A, Lower RR, Vetrove GW (1987) Contrast injection bradycardia during coronary angiography: effects in the denervated heart. J Heart Transplant 6: 44–48

117. Nafz B, Persson P, Ehmke H, Kirchheim HR (1992) A servo-control system for open and closed loop blood pressure regulation. Am J Physiol 262: F320–F325

118. Nicholls MG, Riegger AJG (1993) Renin in cardiac failure. In: Robertson JA & Nicholls MG (eds.) The Renin-Angiotensin-System. Gower Medical Publishing, London, New York, pp 76.1–76.21

119. Niebauer M, Zucker IH (1985) Static and dynamic responses of carotid sinus baroreceptors in dogs with chronic volume overload. J Physiol 369: 295–310

120. Niebauer M, Holmberg MJ, Zucker IH (1986) Aortic baroreceptor characteristics in dogs with chronic high output failure. Basic Res Cardiol 81: 111–122

121. Noshiro T, Way D, McGrath BP (1991) Effect of angiotensin-converting enzyme inhibition on renal norepinephrine spillover rate and baroreflex responses in conscious rabbits. Clin Exp Pharmacol Physiol 18: 375–378

122. Noshiro T, Way D, Miura Y, McGrath BP (1993) Enalapril restores sensitivity of baroreflex control of renal and total noradrenaline spillover in heart failure rabbit. Clin Exp Pharmacol Physiol 20: 373–376

123. Olivier NB, Stephenson RB (1993) Characterization of baroreflex impairment in conscious dogs with pacing-induced heart failure. Am J Physiol 265: R1132–R1140

124. Ontkean MT, Gay R, Greenberg B (1991) Diminished endothelium-derived relaxing factor activity in an experimental model of chronic heart failure. Circ Res 69: 1088–1096

125. Osterziel KJ, Dietz R, Schmid W, Mikulaschek K, Manthey J, Kübler W (1990) ACE-inhibition improves vagal reactivity in patients with heart failure. Am Heart J 120: 1120–1129

126. Osterziel KJ, Hänlein D, Willenbrock R, Dietz R (1993) Beziehung zwischen Reninsystem und parasympathischem Nervensystem bei Herzinsuffizienz. Z Kardiol 82: 406–410

127. Osterziel KJ, Dietz R (1996) Improvement of vagal tone by ACE inhibition: a mechamism of cardioprotection in patients with mild-to-moderate heart failure. J Cardiovasc Pharmacol 27 (Suppl. 2): S25–S30

128. Persson PB, Ehmke H, Nafz B, Kirchheim HR (1990) Resetting of renal autoregulation in conscious dogs: angiotensin II and alpha1-adrenoceptors. Pflügers Arch 417: 42–47

129. Persson BP, Ehmke H, Kirchheim H, Lempinen M, Nafz B (1993) The role of the kidney in canine blood pressure control: direct assessment of the closed-loop gain. J Physiol (Lond) 464: 121–130

130. Peters J, Neuser D, Schaden W, Arndt JO (1992) Atrial natriuretic peptide decreases hepatic and cardiac blood content, but increases intestinal blood content in supine humans. Bas Res Cardiol 87: 250–262

131. Porter Th R, Eckberg DL, Fritsch JM, Rea RF, Beightol LA, Schmedtje Jr JF, Mohanty PK (1990) Autonomic pathophysiology in heart failure patients. Sympathetic-cholinergic interrelations. J Clin Invest 85: 1362–1371

132. Potter EK, Reid IA (1985) Intravertebral angiotensin II inhibits cardiac vagal efferent activity in dogs. Neuroendocrinology 40: 493–496

133. Quest JA, Gillis RA (1974) Effect of digitalis on carotid sinus baroreceptor activity. Circ Res 35: 247–255

134. Reid IA (1984) Actions of angiotensin II on the brain: mechanisms and physiologic role. Am J Physiol 246: F533–F543

135. Reid IA, Chou L (1990) Analysis of the action of angiotensin II on the baroreflex control of heart rate in conscious rabbits. Endocrinology 126: 2749–2756

136. Reid IA (1992) Interactions between ANGII, sympathetic nervous system, and baroreceptor reflexes in regulation of blood pressure. Am J Physiol 262: E763–E778

137. Reinhardt HW, Corea M, Boemke W, Pettker R, Rothermund HL, Scholz A, Schwietzer G, Persson PB (1994) Resetting of 24-h sodium and water balance during 4 day of servo-controlled reduction of renal perfusion pressure. Am J Physiol 266: H650–H657

138. Richter DW, Keck W, Seller H (1970) The course of inhibition of sympathetic activity during various patterns of carotid sinus nerve stimulation. Pflügers Arch 317: 110-123

139. Rigel DF, Lipson D, Katona PG (1984) Excess tachycardia: heart rate after antimuscarinic agents in conscious dogs. Am J Physiol 246: H168–H173

140. Robertson GL (1992) Regulation of Vasopressin Secretion. In: Seldin DW, Giebisch G (eds.) The Kidney: Physiology and Pathophysiology, Raven Press Ltd., New York, pp 1595–1613

141. Rowell LB (1993) Human cardiovascular control. Oxford University Press, New York Oxford

142. Sakuma I, Togashi H, Yoshioka M, Saito H, Yanagida M, Tamura M, Kobayashi T, Yasuda H, Gross SS, Levi R (1992) Ng-Methyl-L-Arginine, an inhibitor of L-arginine-derived nitric oxide in vivo: A role for nitric oxide in the central regulation of sympathetic tone? Circ Res 70: 607–611

143. Sano N, Way D, McGrath BP (1990) Renal norepinephrine spillover and baroreflex responses in evolving heart failure. Am J Physiol 258: F1516–F1522

144. Saul JP, Arai Y, Berger RD, Lilly LS, Colucci WS, Cohen RJ (1988) Assessment of autonomic regulation in chronic congestive heart failure by heart rate spectral analysis. Am J Cardiol 61: 1292–1299

145. Schlomka G (1937) Untersuchungen über die physiologische Unregelmäßigkeit des Herzschlages. III Mitteilung. Über die Abhängigkeit der respiratorischen (Ruhe)-Arrhythmie von der Schlagfrequenz und vom Lebensalter. Zeitschrift für Kreislaufforschung 29: 510–524

146. Schobel HP, Oren RM, Roach PJ, Mark AL, Ferguson DW (1991) Contrasting effects of digitalis and dobutamine on baroreflex sympathetic control in normal humans. Circulation 84: 1118–1129

147. Schweitzer A (1935) Zur Frage der respiratorischen Arrhythmie. Verhandl Deutsch Gesellsch Kreislaufforsch 8: 148–154

148. Seeliger E, Boemke W, Corea M, Encke T, Reinhardt HW (1997) Mechanisms compensating Na and water retention induced by long-term reduction of renal perfusion pressure. Am J Physiol 273 (2 Pt 2): R646–54

149. Seller H, Richter DW (1971) Some quantitative aspects of the central transmission of the baroreceptor activity. In: Kao FF, Koizumi K, Vasalle F (eds.) Research in Physiology, Aulo Gaggi Publishers, Bologna pp 541–549

150. Shin Y, Lohmeier ThE, Hester RL, Kivlighin SD, Smith Jr MJ (1991) Hormonal and circulatory responses to chronically controlled increments in right atrial pressure. Am J Physiol 261: R1176–R1187

151. Smith ML, Ellenbogen KA, Eckberg DL, Szentpetery S, Thames MD (1989) Subnormal heart period variability in heart failure: effect of cardiac transplantation. J Am Coll Cardiol 14: 106–111

152. Smyth HS, Sleight P, Pickering GW (1969) Reflex regulation of arterial pressure during sleep in man: quantitative method of assessing baroreflex sensitivity. Circ Res 24: 109–121

153. Sopher AM, Smith ML, Eckberg DL, Fritsch JM, Dibner-Dunlap ME (1990) Autonomic pathophysiology in heart failure: carotid baroreceptor-cardiac reflexes. Am J Physiol 259: H689–H696

154. Starling EH (1897) Some points in the pathology of heart disease. Lancet 1: 569–572

155. Stewart DJ, Cernacek P, Costello KB, Rouleau JL (1992) Elevated endothelin-1 in heart failure and loss of normal response to postural change. Circulation 85: 510–517

156. Thames MD, Waickman LA, Abboud FM (1980) Sensitization of cardiac receptors (vagal afferents) by intracoronary acetylstrophanthidin. Am J Physiol 239: H628–H635

157. Thames MD, Dibner-Dunlap ME (1991) Baroreflexes in congestive heart failure. In: PB Persson & HR Kirchheim (eds.) Baroreceptor Reflexes. Integrative Functions and Clinical Aspects. Springer, Berlin, Heidelberg, New York, pp 181-208

158. Thomas JA, Marks BH (1978) Plasma norepinephrine in congestive heart failure. Am J 41: 233–243

159. Thron HL, Brechmann W, Wagner J, Keller K (1967) Quantitative Untersuchungen über die Bedeutung der Gefäßdehnungsreceptoren im Rahmen der Kreislaufhomoiostase beim wachen Menschen. I. Das Verhalten von arteriellem Druck und Herzfrequenz bei abgestufter Veränderung des transmuralen Blutdrucks im Bereich des Carotsisinus. Pflügers Arch 293: 68–99

160. Vallbo AB, Hackbarth KE, Torebök HE, Wallin BG (1979) Somatosensory, proprioceptive and sympathetic activity in human peripheral nerves. Physiol Rev 59: 919–957

161. Van Vliet B, Hall JE, Mizelle HL, Montani JP, Smith Jr MJ (1995) Reduced parasympathetic control of heart rate in obese dogs. Am J Physiol 269: H629–H637

162. Versteeg PGA, Noble MIM, Stubbs J, Elzinga G (1983) The effect of cardiac denervation and beta-blockade on control of cardiac output in exercising dogs. Pflügers Arch 52: 62–68

163. Vogt A, Unterberg C, Kreuzer H (1987) Acute effects of the new converting enzyme inhibitor ramipril on hemodynamics and carotid sinus baroreflex activity in congestive heart failure. Am J Cardiol 59: 149D–154D

164. Wagner J, Wackerbauer J, Hilger HH (1968) Arterieller Blutdruck und Herzfrequenzverhalten bei Hypertonikern unter Änderung des transmuralen Druckes im Karotissinusbereich. Zeitschr. Kreislaufforschg. 8: 701–712

165. Wallin BG, Sundlof G, Delius W (1975) The effects of carotid sinus nerve stimulation on muscle and skin nerve sympathetic activity in man. Pflügers Arch 358: 101–110

166. Wallin BG, Fagius J (1986) The sympathetic nervous system in man – aspects derived from microelectrode recordings. Trends Neurosci 9: 63–67

167. Wallin BG, Mörlin C, Hjelmdahl P (1987) Muscle sympathetic activity and venous plasma noradrenaline concentrations during static exercise in normotensive and hypertensive subjects. Acta Physiol Scand 129: 489–497

168. Wallin BG (1988) Intraneural recordings of normal and abnormal sympathetic activity in man. In: Bannister R (ed) Autonomic failure: a textbook of clinical disorders of the autonomic nervous system, Oxford University Press, Oxford, New York, Tokyo, pp 177–195

169. Wallin BG, Elam M (1994) Insights from intraneural recordings of sympathetic nerve traffic in humans. NIPS 9: 203–201

170. Wang SC, Borison HL (1947) An analysis of the carotid sinus cardiovascular reflex mechanism. Am J Physiol 150: 712–728

171. Wang W, Chen JS, Zucker IH (1990) Carotid sinus baroreceptor sensitivity in experimental heart failure. Circulation 81: 1959–1966

172. Wang W, Chen JS, Zucker IH (1991) Postexcitatory depression of baroreceptors in dogs with experimental heart failure. Am J Physiol 260: H1160–H1165

173. Wang W, McClain JM, Zucker IH (1992) Aldosterone reduces baroreceptor discharge in the dog. Hypertension 19: 270–277

174. Wang W, Han HY, Zucker IH (1996) Depressed baroreflex in heart failure is not due to structural changes in carotid sinus nerve fibres. J Auton Nerv System 57: 101–108

175. Warner HR, Cox A (1962) A mathematical model of heart rate control by sympathetic and vagal efferent information. J Appl Physiol 17: 349–355

176. Warner HR, Russell RO (1969) Effect of combined sympathetic and vagal stimulation on heart rate in the dog. Circ Res 24: 567–573

177. Watkins L, Burton JA, Haber E, Cant JR, Smith FW, Barger AC (1976) The renin-angiotensin-aldosterone system in congestive heart failure in conscious dogs. J Clin Invest 57: 1606–1617

178. White CR (1981) reversibility of abnormal arterial baroreflex control of heart rate in heart failure. Am J Physiol 241: H778–H782

179. Wilson JR, Lanoce V, Frey MJ, Ferraro N (1990) Arterial baroreceptor control of peripheral vascular resistance in experimental heart failure. Am Heart J 119: 1122–1130

180. Winaver J, Hoffman A, Abassi Z, Haramati A (1995) Does the heart's hormone ANP, help in congestive heart failure? NIPS 10: 247–253

181. Witty RT, Davis JO, Shade RE, Johnson J A, Prewitt RL (1972) Mechanisms regulating renin release in dogs with thoracic caval constriction. Circ Res 31: 339–347

182. Wroblewski H, Kastrup J, Mortensen SA, Haunsø S (1993) Abnormal baroreceptor mediated vasodilatation of the peripheral circulation in congestive heart failure secondary to idiopathic dilated cardiomyopathy. Circulation 87: 849–856

183. Wroblewski H (1994) Sustained paradoxical vasodilation during orthostasis in heart failure: a factor in the edema pathogenesis? Am J Physiol 267: 443–448

184. Wroblewski H, Mortensen SA, Haunsø S, Kastrup J (1994) Orthotopic cardiac transplantation reverses abnormal reflex regulation of the microvasculature in the lower leg. Cardiovasc Res 28: 1707–1712

185. Yamane Y (1968) Plasma ADH level in patients with chronic congestive heart failure. Japan Circ J 32: 745–759

186. Zanzinger J, Czachurski J, Seller H (1995a) Inhibition of basal and reflex-mediated sympathetic activity in the RVLM by nitric oxide. Am J Physiol 268: R958–R962

187. Zanzinger J, Czachurski J, Seller H (1995b) Effects of nitric oxide on sympathetic baroreflex transmission in the nucleus tractus solitarii and caudal ventrolateral medulla in cats. Neuroscience Letters 197: 199–202

188. Zanzinger J, Czachurski J, Seller H (1996) Lack of nitric oxide sensitivity of carotid sinus baroreceptors activated by normal blood pressure stimuli in cats. Neuroscience Letters 208: 121–124

189. Zucker IH, Earle AM, Gilmore JP (1977) The mechanisms of adaptation of left atrial stretch receptors in dogs with chronic congestive heart failure. J Clin Invest 60: 323–331

190. Zucker IH (1991) Baro- and cardiac reflex abnormalities in chronic heart failure. In: Zucker IH, Gilmore JP (eds.) Reflex control of the circulation. CRC Press, Boca Raton, Ann Arbor, Boston, pp. 849–873

191. Zucker IH, Chen JS, Wang W (1991) Renal sympathetic nerve and hemodynamic responses to captopril in conscious dogs: role of prostaglandins. Am J Physiol 260: H260–H266

192. Zucker IH, Wang W, Brändle M (1993) Baroreflex abnormalities in congestive heart failure. NIPS 8: 87–90

Author's address:
H. R. Kirchheim
Physiologisches Institut
der Ruprecht-Karls-Universität Heidelberg
Im Neuenheimer Feld 326
69120 Heidelberg
Germany

A mechanistic analysis of the force-frequency relation in non-failing and progressively failing human myocardium

N. R. Alpert[1], B. J. Leavitt[2], F. P. Ittleman[2], G. Hasenfuss[3], B. Pieske[3], L. A. Mulieri[1]

[1] Dept. Molecular Physiology and Biophysics, University of Vermont, Burlington, USA
[2] Dept. Surgery, University of Vermont, Burlington, USA
[3] Medizinische Klinik III, Universität Freiburg

Abstract

This review focuses on the role of the myocardial force-frequency relation (FFR) in human ventricular performance and how changes in the FFR can reduce cardiac output and, ultimately, can contribute to altering the stability of the in-vivo cardiovascular system in a way that contributes to the progression of heart failure. Changes in the amplitude, shape, and position of the myocardial FFR occurring in various forms of heart failure are characterized in terms of maximal isometric twitch tension, slope of the ascending limb (myocardial reserve), and position of the peak of the FFR on the frequency axis (optimum stimulation frequency). All three of these parameters decline according to severity of myocardial disease in the following order: non-failing atrial septal defect, non-failing coronary artery disease, non-failing coronary artery disease with diabetes mellitus, failing mitral regurgitation, failing viral myocarditis, failing idiopathic dilated cardiomyopathy. Evidence is presented supporting a sarcoplasmic reticulum Ca-pump based mechanism for this progressive depression of the FFR. Intracellular calcium cycling and concentration and Ca-pump content all diminish in proportion to degree of depression of the FFR. Additional evidence from myocyte culture studies suggests a cause of diminished Ca-pump content is sustained, elevated levels of plasma norepinephrine. A hypothesis is presented to explain the mechanism of myocardial failure and its progression in terms of changes in the cardiovascular feedback control system that are triggered by reduced moycardial reserve. Sustained elevation of plasma norepinephrine levels depresses expression of sarcoplasmic reticulum Ca-pump protein causing depression of the FFR and this causes a compensatory further increase in norepinephrine levels and a further depression of Ca-pump protein.

Key words Force-frequency relation – myocardial reserve – Ca-pump – norepinephrine – progression of heart failure

Introduction

This review focuses on the role of the myocardial force-frequency relation in human ventricular performance and how changes in it can reduce cardiac output and, ultimately, can contribute to altering the stability of the in-vivo cardiovas-cular system in a way that contributes to progression of heart failure.

The contribution of frequency treppe to cardiac output

The inherent ability of ventriular myocardium to increase its strength of contraction (independent of neurohormonal intervention) in response to an increase in contraction frequency is known as frequency treppe. This myocardial property causes contractile force to rise as contraction frequency is increased from 60 to about 180 beats per minute (bpm) and to then decline with further increase in frequency (the force-frequency relation "FFR", see Fig. 1). The importance of this myocardial property in vivo is demonstrated by the following cardiovascular response to exercise. In normal subjects producing maximal work output on an upright exercise bicycle, cardiac output is increased 3-fold above its resting level. About 70 % of this increase results directly from increased number of ejections per minute at the higher exercise heart rate. The remaining 30 % results from an increase in stroke volume that is brought about by a 50 % decrease in left ventricular endsystolic volume (10, 23). Although the Frank-Starling relation of the myocardium causes this decrease in ventricular volume to reduce contractile strength, the presence of a normal frequency treppe (i.e., a positively sloped myocardial FFR) causes an increase in contractile strength and this

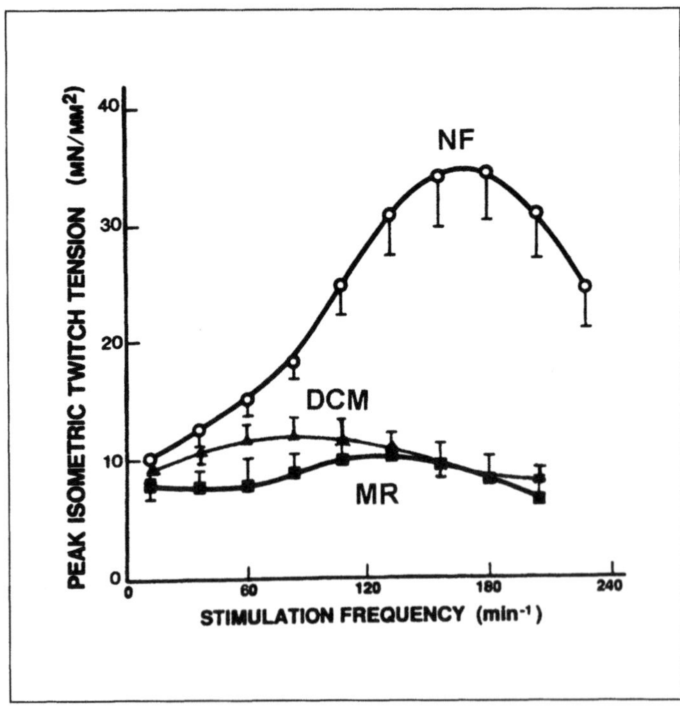

Fig. 1 Average steady-state isometric twitch tension vs. stimulation frequency in non-failing and failing myocardium. Each point represents the mean ± SEM for non-failing (NF, n = 8), mitral regurgitation failing (MR, n = 8) (17), and idiopathic dilated cardiomyopathy failing (DCM, n = 6) (15) myocardial strips at 37 °C.

compensates for the Frank-Starling effect. This suggests, as much as 40 % of the increase in cardiac output that occurs with exercise may depend on an intact FFR in normal myocardium (10). In this light the frequency treppe of the myocardium can be considered to be an important, built-in "stroke volume reserve" capable of increasing ventricular ejection independent of the Frank-Starling relation and independent of the systemic neurohumoral control system or its receptors in the myocyte membranes (24).

Myocardial biopsy and dissection
of strip preparations

Subepicardial tissue was obtained from the anterior segment of the left ventricular wall of patients undergoing coronary artery bypass surgery, mitral valve surgery, or cardiac transplant. Control myocardium was obtained from coronary artery bypass patients who had normal left ventricular wall motion and normal left ventricular function (i.e., ejection fraction greater than 0.60). A subset of these patients had insulin-dependent diabetes mellitus. Failing myocardium was obtained from patients undergoing mitral valve surgery (NYHA Class II-III failure, mean LV ejection fraction = 0.64 ± 0.05) and from hearts explanted from idiopathic dilated cardiomyopathy patients (NYHA Class IV failure, mean LV ejection fraction = 0.13 ± 0.01).

Surgical biopsies were obtained shortly after cardioplegic arrest (16). Patients gave informed, written consent before participating in the study which was approved by the Committee on Human Research of the University of Vermont. There were no complications resulting from the biopsy procedure in any patient. The excised tissue was immediately submerged in room temperature, pre-oxygenated BDM-protective solution. The BDM-protective solution for dissection consisted of Krebs-Ringer solution plus 30 mmol/l 2,3-butanedione monoxime (14). After a 60 min recovery from surgical trauma the biopsy was dissected into thin strips approximately 0.2 to 0.4 mm in diameter (16). All measurements were made in Krebs-Ringer solution after washing out the protective solution. Forskolin was dissolved in 95 % ethanol and introduced into the 90 ml muscle baths in 2 uL aliquot to give 0.5 uM Forskolin and not higher than 20 uM ethanol.

Apparatus and measurements

Isometric twitch tension was measured at the peak of the tension-length relation (L_{max}) in each muscle strip preparation using the same apparatus, methods, and protocols as described previously (15). The steady-state force-frequency relation of each strip was obtained at 37 °C with 5 min of stimulation at each frequency starting at 0.2 Hz (12 min^{-1}) and increasing in 0.2 Hz increments. Peak twitch tension of the steady-state myograms was measured by digital readout and averaged at each frequency across all strips in each group. The length at Lmax (3.5 to 4 mm) and the blotted weight (0.2 to 0.6 mg) of the active portion of each muscle strip was measured and the quotient was used to calculate its cross-sectional area.

The FFR in non-failing human myocardium

Although the heart rate dependence of myocardial contractility has been well documented for most animal species (11), it has only been since the advent of open heart surgery and cardiac transplantation that such information has become available for human myocardium. Our dissection method produces viable myocardial strips that are thin enough to be adequately oxygenated in an aqueous muscle bath at physiological temperature and contraction frequencies (14, 16). The validity of assessing myocardial function from surgically isolated strips of left ventricular human myocardium is supported by our finding of good agreement between the in vitro frequency treppe obtained from strips prepared from non-failing hearts and ventricular function curves obtained by others from non-failing hearts in vivo (13). The average force-frequency relation obtained in vitro from non-failing myocardium at 37 °C is shown in Fig 1.

The FFR in failing human myocardium

Fig. 1 shows the average FFR curves for failing left ventricular myocardium obtained in vitro at 37 °C. Expression of the peak isometric twitch amplitude in tension units (force per unit cross-section of strip preparation) allows averaging of curves from all patients with the same diagnosis. There are clear depressions of both the maximal tension and the frequency at the peak of the FFR (optimum stimulation frequency) in the failing preparations. This depression in itself is expected to severely limit the maximal systolic performance of these ventricles. In addition to the depression at any given heart rate, it is also important to note the additional loss resulting from the accompanying blunting of the rising phase of the FFR in heart failure. This decrease in slope of the ascending limb of the FFR ("blunting of the treppe response") at frequencies between resting and optimum heart rates may play an important role in progression of heart failure as described below.

As an index of relative strength of the treppe response we define myocardial reserve as the percent increase in in vitro contractile strength occurring when contraction frequency is increased from 60 to 120 bpm (see Fig. 2). A decrease in slope of the myocardial FFR represents a loss of stroke volume reserve in the ventricle. We consider this myopathic because decreased myocardial reserve would not adequately support the increased ventricular function needed during exercise. Fig. 3 shows average values of myocardial reserve measured in both non-failing myocardium and various types and degrees of heart failure.

Note that even though all three right hand histograms in Fig. 3 are from groups of patients with normal LV wall motion and normal ejection fraction, there is a clear decline in myocardial reserve between patients with atrial septal defect (ASD), coronary artery disease (CAD), and coronary artery disease with diabetes mellitus (CAD + DM). Of particular note is the finding of considerable depression in myocardial reserve (about 50 %) in the diabetic CAD's compared with the non-diabetic coronary artery disease group (CAD). This suggests that in the diabetic CADs, systemic compensatory effects in vivo may mask a depressed myocardial contractility, restoring normal resting LV function but leaving the diabetic heart less capable of surviving future coronary obstructions or other increased demands for myocardial reserve.

Fig. 2 Method of calculating myocardial reserve and optimal stimulation frequency from myocardial force-frequency curves. Myocardial reserve is defined as the percent increase in steady-state peak twitch tension when stimulation frequency is raised from 60 bpm to 120 bpm.

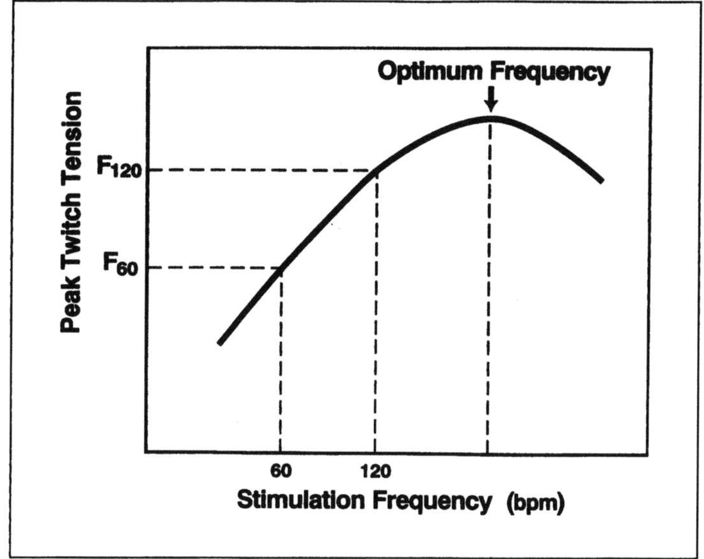

More severe depression of moycardial reserve is present in the three groups of patients in heart failure (Fig. 3). The patients in the mitral regurgitation group (MR) were in NYHA Class II-III failure and had about 60 % depression of myocardial reserve at the time of mitral valve surgery in spite of their near normal values of ejection fraction. Those in the viral

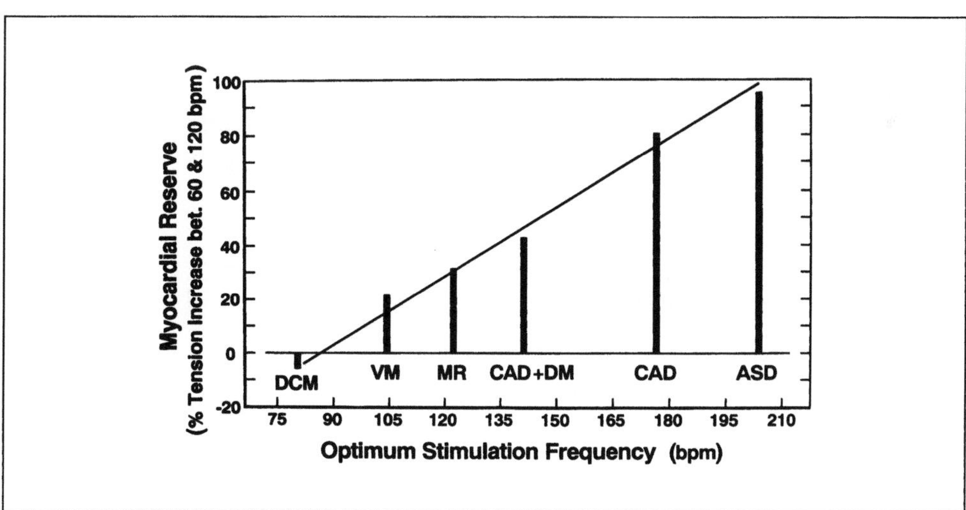

Fig. 3 Variation in myocardial reserve and optimal stimulation frequency in proportion to presence and severity of heart failure. Patients without heart failure and with normal, in-vivo left ventricular function and wall motion: Atrial-septal defect (ASD), 4 strips from 1 heart; Coronary artery disease (CAD), 8 strips from 4 hearts; Coronary artery disease with insulin dependent diabetes mellitus (CAD+DM), 6 strips from 6 hearts. Patients with heart failure: Mitral regurgitation (MR), NYHA II-III, 8 strips from 4 hearts; Viral Myocarditis (VM), NYHA IV, 8 strips from 3 hearts; Idiopathic dilated cardiomyopathy (IDCM), NYHA IV, 6 strips from 6 hearts. Values of maximal peak twitch tension (mN/mm^2) and optimal contraction frequency (bpm) are, respectively, ASD (18), 23.1, 204; CAD (17), 34.1, 173; CAD+DM (18), 21.3, 142; MR (18), 10.1, 128; VM (21), 17.5, 105; IDCM (15), 14.2, 81.

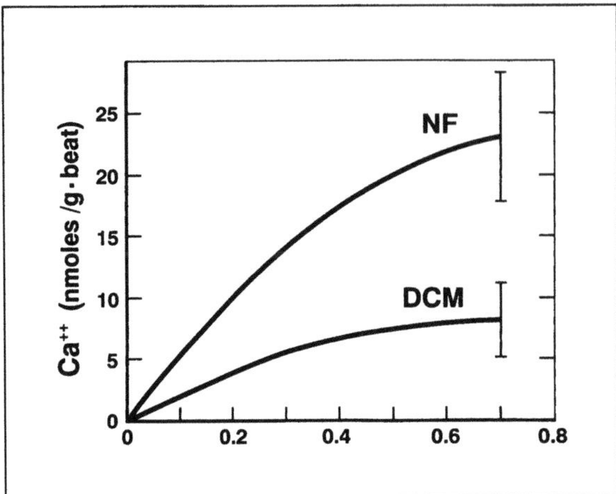

Fig. 4 Time course of intracellular calcium uptake during a steady-state twitch in non-failing and DCM-failing myocardium. To construct these curves tension independet heat was measured by thermopile myothermometry (8) and was converted to an equivalent quantity of sarcoplasmic reticulum calcium uptake using 17 kJ/mole Ca^{2+} pumped as the enthalpy of the SR Ca-ATPase and subtracting 13 % to allow for Na^+ extrusion.

cardiomyopathy (VM) and dilated cardiomyopathy (DCM) groups were in NYHA Class IV, end-stage failure at the time of cardiac transplantation. Note the extreme depression in the DCM group in which the average myocardial reserve has actually reversed to about -7 %, a negative treppe, indicating weakening of the myocardium with tachycardia.

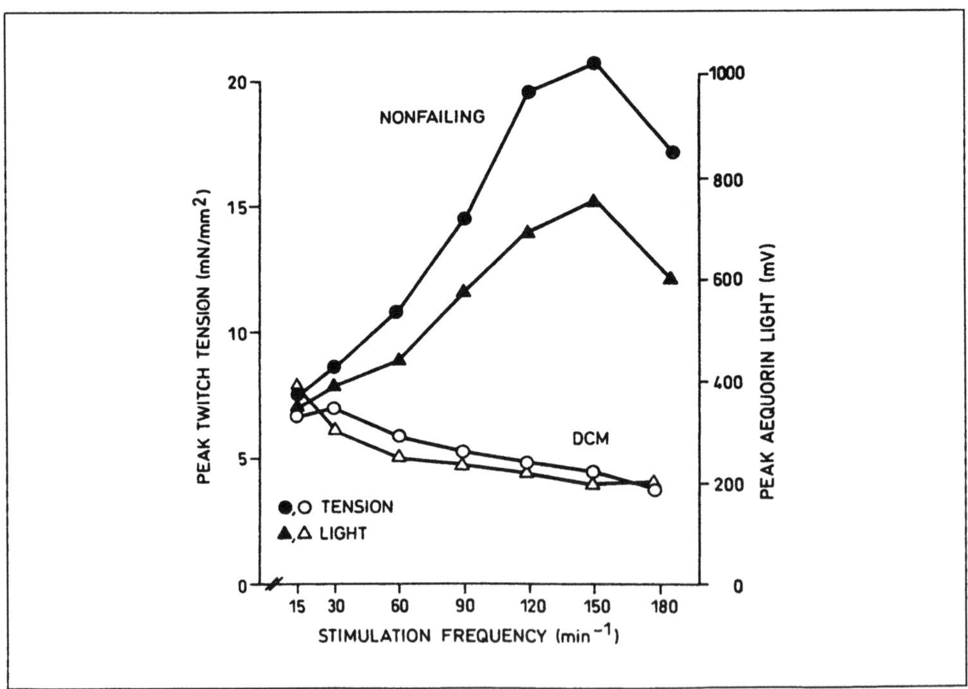

Fig. 5 Influence of stimulation frequency on intracellular Ca^{2+} transients and isometric twitch tension in a muscle strip from a non-failing heart and from a heart with end-stage failing dilated cardiomyopathy (DCM). Changes in the Ca^{2+} transients, as reflected by the aequorin light emission (triangles), are given in mV (right ordinate); changes in the isometric twitch tension (circles) are given in mN/mm^2 (left ordinate). From Fig. 2 of Pieske et al. (22) with permission.

The histograms in Fig. 3 have been positioned along the horizontal axis according to the contraction frequency at which each group's FFR peaks (see Optimum Frequency axis in Fig. 3). The presence of a direct correlation between the optimum frequency and the myocardial reserve suggests both are governed by the same (or a number of tightly coupled) intracellular mechanisms within the myocytes. Our myothermal measurements of tension independent heat, an index calcium cycled per twitch in DCM and non-failing CAD myocardium, suggest the cellular mechanism underlying depression of the FFR in failing myocardium involves alterations in the calcium handling system. Fig. 4 shows both quantity of calcium cycled per beat and the rate of its removal from the cytoplasm to be diminished by about 70 % in DCM failure (8).

More recent, direct measurements of intracellular calcium transients (Fig. 5) using the aequorin method indicate the depression in quantity of calcium cycled per twitch is accompanied by similar depressions in intracellular calcium concentration in DCM myocardium compared with normal myocardium (22). In addition to depressed calcium delivery during a twitch, the data in Fig. 5 show the negative twitch tension treppe DCM is underlaid by a corresponding negative treppe in the calcium transients as seen when stimulation frequency is increased. In non-failing myocardium (Fig. 5) the peak calcium signal increased by 58 % between 60 and 120 bpm while peak twitch tension rose by 80 %. In the DCM-failing myocardium the peak calcium signal fell by 11 % while peak twitch tension fell by 15 % over the same frequency range. In both groups the change in twitch tension per change in calcium signal was 1.37 giving evidence that altered calcium cycling is the main mechanism of force-frequency treppe and for its depression in DCM failure.

The majority of calcium ions required to activate a systolic contraction are supplied by the sarcoplasmic reticulum in adult myocardium. The amount released depends on the beat-to-beat storage of calcium and this depends, in turn, on the calcium uptake velocity of calcium pump. The frequency treppe is likely caused by a speeding up of the sarcoplasmic reticulum calcium pump due to increased phosphorylation of its control proteins by calcium dependent calmodulin kinase (18, 25). Changes in the action potential and in phosphorylation of surface membrane calcium channels may also contribute to the treppe mechanism.

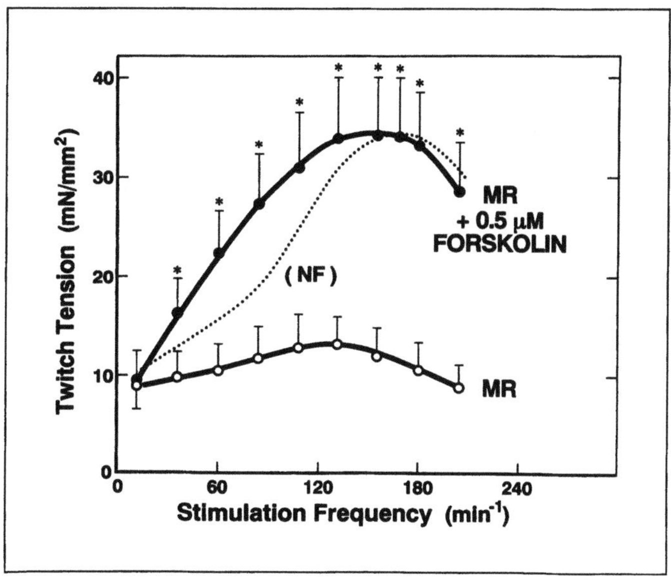

Fig. 6 Effects of forskolin on the average steady-state isometric twitch tension versus stimulation frequency relation in MR-failing myocardium. Each point represents the mean ± SEM of eight non-failing (NF) and eight MR-failing preparations (MR) (17).

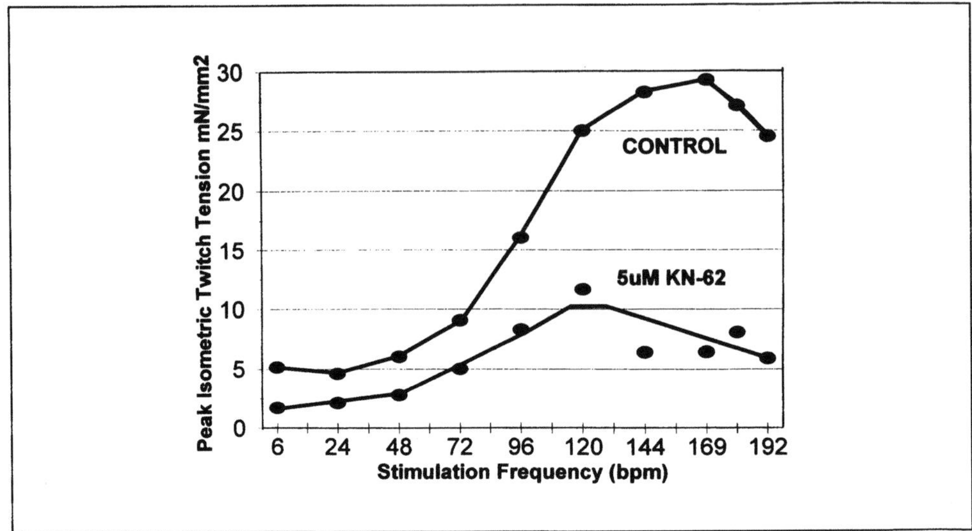

Fig. 7 Pharmacological depression of myocardial reserve and optimal stimulation frequency in NF myocardium. Average steady-state force-frequency curves from NF myocardium before (Control) and after depression of Ca^{2+}/Calmodulin kinase II with 5 µM KN-62 (Seikagaku America, Inc.). Average of three strips from one NF heart at 37 °C.

The findings of depressed calcium cycling in failing myocardium suggest interventions that increase calcium cycling should restore the depressed myocardial reserve to non-failing values. Conversely, depression of calcium cycling in non-failing myocardium should

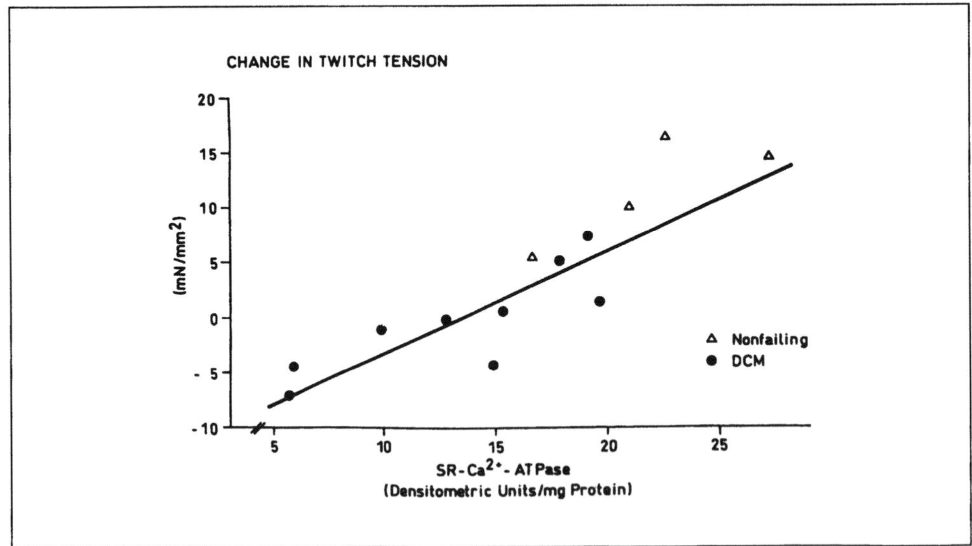

Fig. 8 Correlation between myocardial reserve and calcium pump content in NF and end-stage, DCM-failing myocardium. Myocardial reserve is calculated as the change in peak twitch tension between 120 bpm and 30 bpm ("Change in Twitch Tension"). Calcium pump content is measured as sarcoplasmic reticulum Ca^{2+}-ATPase normalized per total protein. Adapted from Fig. 5 of Hasenfuss et al. (9).

depress its myocardial reserve similar to that of the failing myocardium. These expectations are borne out as shown in Fig. 6 and 7. In MR-failing myocardium addition of forskolin, believed to increase calcium pump function by increasing cycling-AMP activated phosphorylation of phospholamban, there is a significant reversal of the depressed FFR including increase in the myocardial reserve and optimum stimulation frequency to near normal values (Fig. 6 and (21)). Conversely, depression of calcium pump function by addition of the drug KN-62, a specific inhibitor of the Ca^{2+} activated, calmodulin-kinase mediated activation of the Thr^{17} site in phospholamban, depresses the myocardial reserve and optimal stimulation frequency of non-failing myocardium to mimic that of MR-failing myocardium (Fig. 7).

These experimental demonstrations of calcium pump dependence of the FFR are supported by the finding (Fig. 8) of a direct correlation between the activity of the sarcoplasmic reticulum calcium pump and the myocardial reserve (or optimal frequency) of the FFR in samples from both DCM-failing and non-failing donor hearts (9).

Evidence supporting the role of the decreased calcium pump protein (SERCA2) as a strong contributor to decreased calcium pump ATPase and to depression of the FFR in human myocardium is seen in Fig. 9 (12). Calcium pump protein levels are depressed by 40 % on a total protein basis and by 25 % with respect to phospholamban content. This suggests in DCM-failing myocardium, in-vivo calcium pump function would be depressed both by reduction of pump content and also by having relatively more inhibition (at any given level of phosphorylation) due to an increased amount of phospholamban protein compared with calcium pump protein.

As seen in Fig. 10 there is an increase in relative content of the Na^+/Ca^{2+} exchanger protein in DCM-failing myocardium. This increase may compensate to some extent for

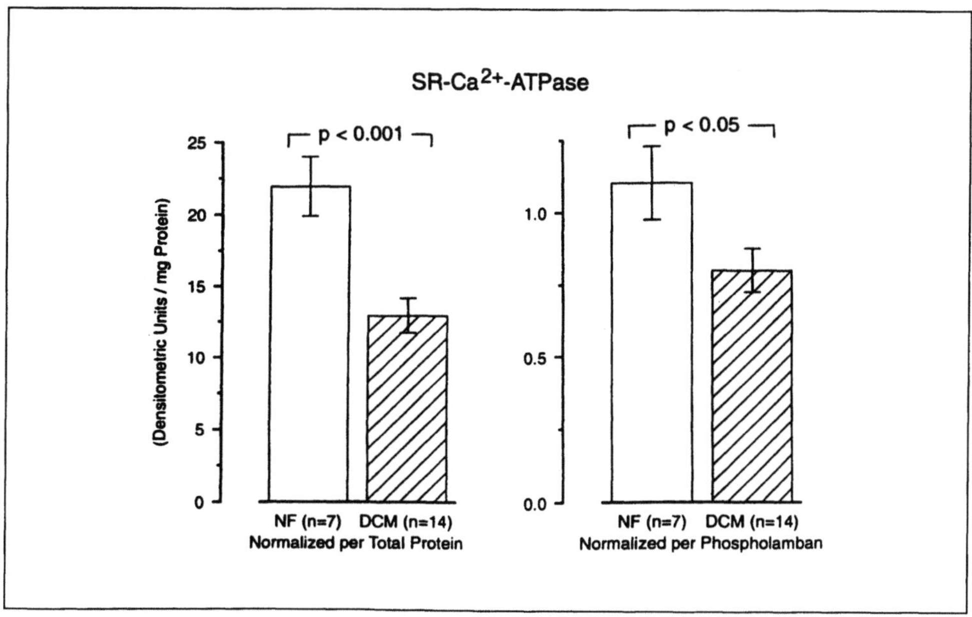

Fig. 9   Protein levels of sarcoplasmic reticulum Ca^{2+}-ATPase in non-failing and end-stage DCM-failing myocardium. Left histograms normalized per total protein recovered per gram wet weight. Right histograms were normalized per protein levels of phospholamban (pentameric form). Adapted from Fig. 4 and 6 of Meyer et al. (12).

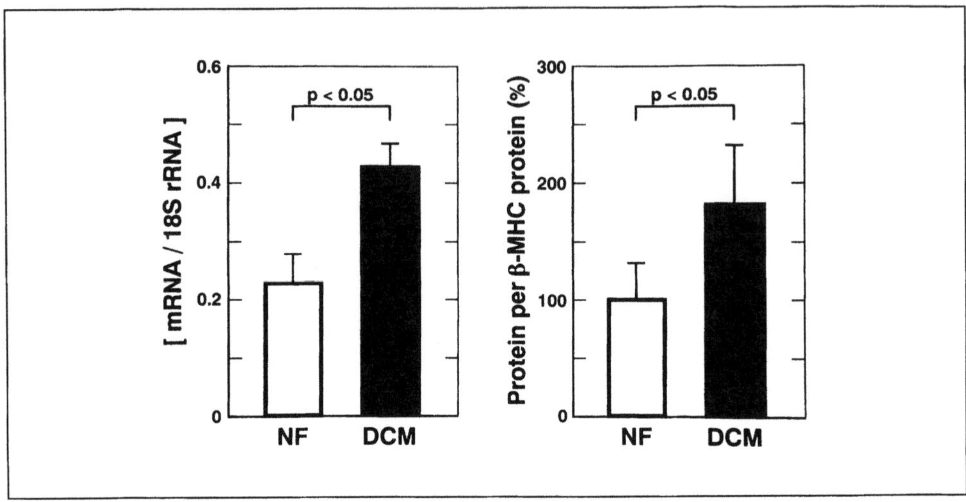

Fig. 10 Protein and mRNA levels of Na/Ca-exchanger in non-failing and end-stage DCM-failing myocardium. Adapted from Fig. 2 and 6 of Studer et al. (26).

possible increases in diastolic calcium levels resulting from the loss of calcium pumping capacity when calcium pump content is reduced.

Since these data strongly suggest that the reduction in sarcoplasmic reticulum calcium pump protein content in failing myocardium is an important contributor to reduction of myocardial reserve it is important to investigate possible mechanisms that may contribute to reduction of calcium pump content. A likely candidate is suggested by the consistent finding of elevated plasma norepinephrine (NE) levels in heart failure. In mitral or aortic valve disease or in idiopathic cardiomyopathy, plasma NE levels at rest are about twice normal. Also, with exercise, NE levels increase three to four times higher than in patients without

Fig. 11 Effects of norepinephrine on sarcoplasmic reticulum expression in cultured neonatal rat cardiomyocytes. Down-regulation of mRNA levels for calcium pump Ca^{2+}-ATPase (SRC) and phospholamban (PLN) but not calsequestrin (CSQ) occurs in response to 2 μM norepinephrine in presence of 0.1 nM T3 (1).

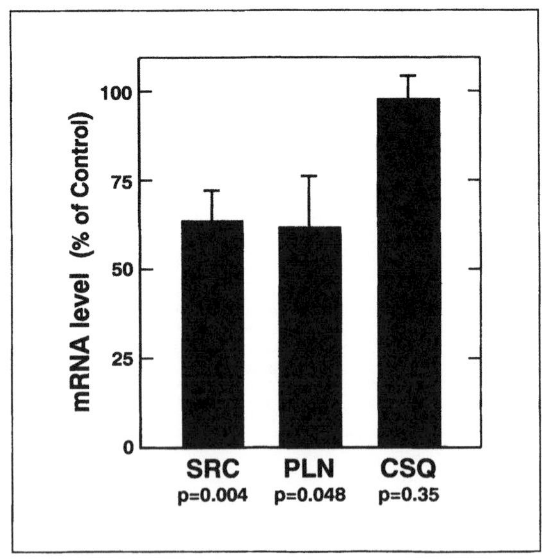

heart failure (3). Plasma NE concentration correlates strongly with left ventricular dysfunction (27) and with mortality (4) in congestive heart failure patients. Since neuroendocrine activation was observed to occur before clinical heart failure ensues (6), a causal relation between elevated plasma NE levels and progression of heart failure is suggested.

This suggestion is supported experimentally by recent findings (see Fig. 11) in tissue culture preparations showing that presence of NE in the culture medium for 2–3 days causes a 40 % depression in levels of mRNA for calcium pump protein, SERCA2, and for phospholamban in rat myocytes (1, 2, 5). This coupling between sustained elevation of NE levels and reduced SERCA2 synthesis may be an important contributor to reduced sarcoplasmic reticulum calcium pump content in the early stages of heart failure in vivo and it may also be a mechanism of progression of heart failure as described next.

Positive feedback hypothesis of progression of heart failure

Since the heart is anatomically and functionally a "component" in a number of feedback control systems in the body (e.g., hemodynamic, hormonal, neuronal), it seems worthwhile to explore the possible role of marked alterations in the dynamic function of diseased myocardium in altering the function of these feedback loops. The transition from a compensated cardiovascular system to a progressively decompensated one may result from conversion of a feedback control system that is stable because of negative feedback (i.e., the system responds to a perturbation by minimizing the effect of the perturbation) to a feedback control system that is unstable because the feedback has become positive (i.e., the system responds to a perturbation by enhancing the effect of the perturbation).

We propose that depression and eventual inversion (i.e., negative treppe) of the myocardial FFR is a mechanism of converting from negative to positive feedback control in the diseased cardiovascular system. The details of the basis for this hypothesis are shown in Fig. 12.

The inner circle in Fig. 12 represents the cardiovascular system functioning under normal conditions. With a transient increase in demand (left top: DEMAND, Transient) for cardiac output (CO), plasma norepinephrine rises (vertical arrow beside norepinephrine). This increases heart rate (see arrow between 70 and 120 bpm on HR axis of the force-frequency plot in Fig. 12). The normal frequency treppe of the myocardium (top FFR curve) causes contractility to rise from 17 to 28 units, therefore stroke volume (SV) increases. The product of increased SV and increased HR increases CO just sufficient to meet the transient demand requiring no further increase in plasma NE. Note that if the lowest FFR were present in this heart (e.g., as in the MR hearts in Fig. 6), the same increase in plasma norepinephrine would cause only about 20 % as much increase in myocardial contractility. In this case the product of increased HR times increased SV would not equal the increased demand for CO, and a further increase in plasma norepinephrine would occur in order to meet the increased demand. The question of the mechanism of progression of heart failure may be the same as the question: how did the lower force-frequency relations get blunted?

On a short term basis elevation of plasma norepinephrine is not detrimental in itself. However, if the demand for increased CO is sustained, a degenerative condition can be established as follows. Refer now to the outer circle in the Fig. 12 representing the case of

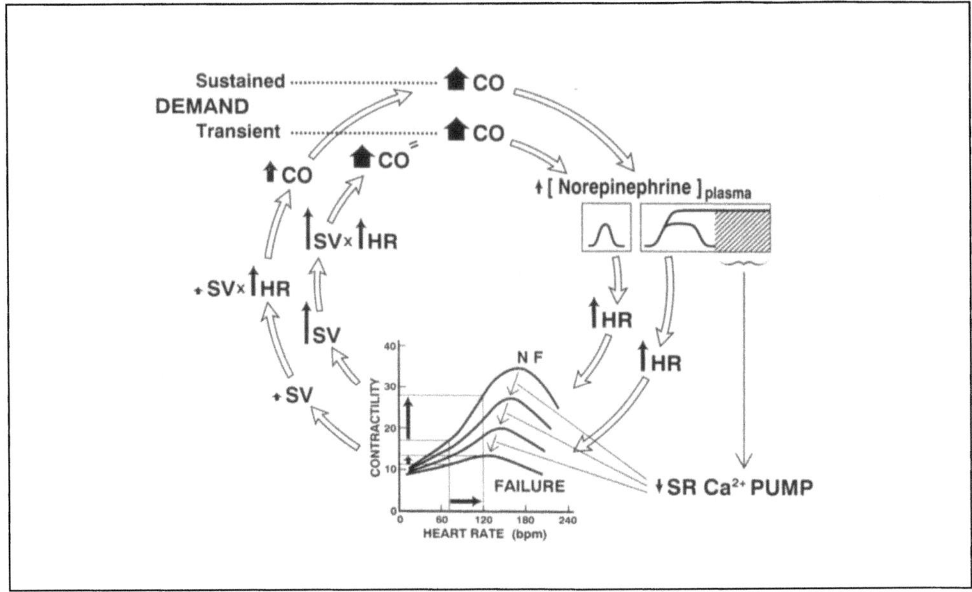

Fig. 12 Proposed role of FFR depression in the progression of heart failure. Circular pathways depict the response of the in vivo cardiovascular system to a transient (inner circle) or a sustained plus transient increase in demand for cardiac output (outer circle). Alterations in the myocardial reserve and optimal stimulation frequency of the myocardium are proposed to result from a sustained elevation of plasma norepinephrine (hatched region at upper right) which leads to further elevation of plasma norepinephrine levels (see text for details). The following abbreviations are used: CO, cardiac output; [Norepinephrine]$_{plasma}$, plasma norepinephrine concentration; HR, heart rate; SV, stroke volume; vertical arrows indicate amount of increase in associated parameters.

a sustained demand for increased CO. The new factor that comes into play is a norepinephrine-induced decrease in Ca-pump protein of the sarcoplasmic reticulum as shown at the lower right in Fig. 12. Hypothesis: sustained (e.g., 2 to 14 days) elevation of in-vivo plasma norepinephrine above a critical level (about 1–2 μM) causes the force-frequency relation to be blunted and left-shifted. This hypothesis suggests the following scenario for development of a depressed force-frequency relation and for progression of myocardial failure: Initially some acute systemic event (e.g., myocarditis or chordal rupture) or a sustained external challenge requires plasma norepinephrine levels to remain elevated in order to maintain adequate cardiac output. If the elevated levels persist above the critical concentration (hatched region in Fig. 12, right), this compensatory response eventually depresses the myocyte Ca-pump mRNA and consequently the Ca-pump content. This blunts the frequency treppe of the myocardium. With the latter alteration the cardiovascular feedback control system, which is still a stable, negative feedback control system (i.e., system reponse compensates for perturbations), now brings about a larger than normal increases in plasma norepinephrine in response to normal activity-related, moment-to-moment changes in demand for increased cardiac output. Hence with each transient increase in activity, the average plasma norepinephrine concentration is elevated even more than is required to compensate for the original systemic event. This additional increase causes further depression of Ca-pump protein concentration and further blunting and shifting of the force-frequency relation. Note that this process constitutes a positive feedback process working at the level of the molecular composition of components in the cardiovascular control system (i.e., the response of the altered system to perturbations causes increased alteration in the molecular composition of the system). Transient periods of increased physical activity now become even more effective in degrading myocyte contractility. This eventually results in a rapid, vicious-cycle phase (decompensation) that starts when the continued blunting and left-shifting of the force-frequency curve results in a negative-sloped region at or near the patient's resting heart rate. At this point we have positive feedback around the signal pathway of the control system (i.e., $\uparrow$ norepinephrine $\rightarrow$ $\uparrow$ HR $\rightarrow$ $\downarrow$ SV $\rightarrow$ $\downarrow$ CO $\rightarrow$ $\uparrow$ norepinephrine) as well as positive feedback around the molecular composition pathway (i.e., $\uparrow$ norepinephrine $\rightarrow$ $\downarrow$ Ca-pump mRNA $\rightarrow$ $\downarrow$ Ca-pump protein $\rightarrow$ $\downarrow$ CO $\rightarrow$ $\uparrow$ norepinephrine). With positive feedback in both pathways the control system is now wildly unstable and can quickly self-destruct.

Discussion and summary

The positive treppe response of the myocyte following an increase in contraction frequency constitutes an important component (the chronotropic component) of myocardial reserve. This and the Frank-Starling relation (the inotropic component) are the major mechanisms that provide sufficient cardiac reserve to increase cardiac output three- to four-fold above resting levels in response to systemic demands of exercise or other challenges. Depression or blunting of the myocardial treppe response due to myocyte remodeling limits this chronotropic component of myocardial reserve and increases use of the Frank-Starling relation and elevated sympathetic drive in order to meet increased systemic demands. The latter two compensatory actions, although effective and adequate in the acute situation, carry potentially damaging side effects when they persist for protracted periods. Increasing contractile strength by ventricular dilatation carries the risk of excessive myocardial oxygen demand because of the increased ventricular wall stress at the larger diameters. In addition, there is risk of possible remodeling of the wall architecture to accommodate a persistently larger ventricular diameter. Sustained sympathetic over-drive carries the risk of toxic effects of excess catecholamine levels.

Previously it has been postulated that heart failure develops when the compensatory hemodynamic and neurohumoral mechanisms are overwhelmed or exhausted (19) and that the inability of our current therapeutic measures to arrest progression of heart failure results from failure to treat the abnormalities in the neurohormonal system when they begin exerting adverse effects (20). Our positive feedback hypothesis suggests a detailed subcellular mechanism by which the normally compensatory effects of increased plasma and myocardial norepinephrine levels become adverse effects that cause loss of myocardial reserve. This mechanism suggests progression of heart failure involves conversion of the cardiovascular feedback control system from a stable one to an unstable one in which the instabilities contribute to an accelerated destabilization of the control system.

We have described the way in which changes in the slope of the myocardial force-frequency relation and the frequency at which the curve peaks interact with the systemic neurohormonal control system to govern the increments in plasma norepinephrine that occur in response to a given demand for increased cardiac output. The lower the slope of the force-frequency relation or myocardial reserve, the higher the increment in plasma norepinephrine needs to be to satisfy a given demand for increased cardiac output. We propose that the transition to the state where norepinephrine has adverse rather than compensatory effects occurs because a sufficiently large and sustained increase in myocardial norepinephrine levels results in altered phenotypic expression of excitation-contraction coupling proteins. This alteration in expression includes reduction in calcium pump protein levels which, in turn, results in a blunting of the slope of the myocardial force-frequency relation. This blunting in itself results in still larger increments in plasma norepinephrine levels for a given increment in cardiac output and further blunting of the force-frequency relation. With severe blunting the frequency treppe becomes negative causing positive feedback which then changes the characteristics of both the systemic control system that acutely regulates cardiac output and the one regulating longer-term remodeling of the intracellular components that modulate myocardial contractility. We propose that the resulting instability in both of these systems may be a major contributor to progression of heart failure in its early stages as well as in the later stages when other factors such as desensitization of atrial and aterial baroreceptors, excessive renin release, sodium retention, vasoconstriction, and increased intravascular volume also contribute to cardiovascular deterioration.

There is growing evidence that β-blocker therapy is effective in reversing cardiomegaly and in improving myocardial function and quality of life in patients with dilated cardiomyopathy (7, 28). These beneficial effects have been attributed to a bradycardia-related increased filling time, reduced myocardial oxygen demand, and recovery of β-receptor function. However not all patients respond to this therapy. In view of the detrimental effects of a negative treppe as described above, it is possible that an important part of the beneficial effects of β-blocker therapy may also result from interaction of its bradycardiac effect per se with the FFR. If the bradycardia is sufficient to move the operating range of heart rates to low enough values with respect to peak of the existing force-frequency relation, the negative-sloped region and its detrimental effects may be avoided or less frequently traversed throughout daily activity.

There is considerable between-patient variation in the optimum frequency of the FFR in NYHA Class IV, DCM (10–132 bpm, average 72 ± 17 bpm (16)). In a patient whose resting HR is 80 bpm and whose myocardial force-frequency relation begins its descending limb at this frequency, exertion moves the operating range to the negative-sloped region. The bradycardiac action of β-blockade will reduce the number of these negative-slope bouts per day. However, if in another patient the negative-sloped region begins at 120–130 bpm, there will be fewer excursions into the negative-sloped region per day and consequently a smaller chance for the bradycardiac effect to avoid these excursions. Thus, between-patient variation in the position of the descending limb of the FFR may be a factor contributing to the between-patient variation in efficacy of β-blocker therapy. If avoidance of negative-slope operation is the basis for a significant part of the beneficial effect of β-blocker therapy, the efficacy of this intervention should be predictable by examining the patient's in-vivo (or in-vitro) force-frequency relation. According to this hypothesis the beneficial effect of β-blocker therapy should be greater, the closer the resting HR is to the negative-sloped region of the patient's FFR.

Acknowledgment Grant support: USPHS: 1 R01 HL55641 & 28001-10/P1.

References

1. Aquilla TT, Absher M, Alpert NR, Rovner AS (1997) Norepinephrine reduces the expression of SERCA2 and PLN in vitro in both the presence and absence of T3. Biochem J (in press)
2. Aquilla TT, Rovner AS, Absher M, Fisher SA, Periasamy M, Alpert NR (1995) Catecholamines decrease the expression of Ca2+ cycling protein mRNAs in cultured cardiomyocytes. (Abstract) J Mol Cell Cardiol 27: ((5) May) A35

3. Chidsey CA, Harrison DC, Braunwald E (1962) Augmentation of the plasma nor-epinephrine response to exercise in patients with congestive heart failure. New England J Medicine 267: 650–4

4. Cohn JN, Levine TB, Olivari MT, Garberg V, Lura D, Francis GS, Simon AB, Rector T (1984) Plasma norepinephrine as a guide to prognosis in patients with chronic congestive heart failure. N Engl J Med 311: 819–23

5. Fisher SA, Buttrick PM, Sukovich D, Periasamy M (1993) Characterization of promoter elements of the rabbit cardiac sarcoplasmic reticulum Ca(2+)-ATPase gene required for expression in cardiac muscle cells. Circ Res 73: 622–8

6. Francis GS, Benedict C, Johnstone DE, Kirlin PC, Nicklas J, Liang CS, Kubo SH, Rudin-Toretsky E, Yusuf S (1990) Comparison of neuroendocrine activation in patients with left ventricular dysfunction with and without congestive heart failure. A substudy of the Studies of Left Ventricular Dysfunction (SOLVD). Circulation 82: 1724–9

7. Gilbert EM, Abraham WT, Olsen S, Hattler B, White M, Mealy P, Larrabee P, Bristow MR (1996) Comparative hemodynamic, left ventricular functional, and antiadrenergic effects of chronic treatment with metoprolol versus carvedilol in the failing heart. Circulation 94: 2817–25

8. Hasenfuss G, Mulieri LA, Leavitt BJ, Allen PD, Haeberle JR, Alpert NR (1992) Alteration of contractile function and excitation-contraction coupling in dilated cardiomyopathy. Circ Res 70: 1225–32

9. Hasenfuss G, Reinecke H, Studer R, Meyer M, Pieske B, Holtz J, Holubarsch C, Posival H, Just H, Drexler H (1994) Relation between myocardial function and expression of sarcoplasmic reticulum Ca(2+)-ATPase in failing and nonfailing human myocardium. Circ Res 75: 434–42

10. Higginbotham MB, Morris KG, Williams RS, McHale PA, Coleman RE, Cobb FR (1986) Regulation of stroke volume during submaximal and maximal upright exercise in normal man. Circ Res 58: 281–91

11. Koch-Weser J, Blinks JR (1963) The influence if the interval between beats on myocardial contractility. Pharmacol Rev 15: 601–52

12. Meyer M, Schillinger W, Pieske B, Holubarsch C, Heilmann C, Posival H, Kuwajima G, Mikoshiba K, Just H, Hasenfuss G (1995) Alterations of sarcoplasmic reticulum proteins in failing human dilated cardiomyopathy. Circulation 92: 778–84

13. Mulieri LA, Alpert NR (1997) The role of myocardial force-frequency relation in left ventricular function and progression of human heart failure. In: Altschuld R, Haworth R (eds.) Heart metabolism in failure. Greenwich, Connecticut: JAI Press, 2

14. Mulieri LA, Hasenfuss G, Ittleman F, Blanchard EM, Alpert NR (1989) Protection of human left ventricular myocardium from cutting injury with 2,3-butanedione monoxime. Circ Res 65: 1441–9

15. Mulieri LA, Hasenfuss G, Leavitt B, Allen PD, Alpert NR (1992) Altered myocardial force-frequency relation in human heart failure. Circulation 85: 1743–50

16. Mulieri LA, Leavitt BJ, Hasenfuss G, Allen PD, Alpert NR (1992) Contraction frequency dependence of twitch and diastolic tension in human dilated cardiomyopathy (tension-frequency relation in cardiomyopathy). Basic Res Cardiol 87 Suppl 1: 199–212

17. Mulieri LA, Leavitt BJ, Martin BJ, Haeberle JR, Alpert NR (1993) Myocardial force-frequency defect in mitral regurgitation heart failure is reversed by forskolin. Circulation 88: 2700–4

18. Mulieri LA, Leavitt BJ, Wright RK, Alpert NR (1997) Role of cAMP in modulating relaxation kinetics and the force-frequency relation in mitral regurgitation heart failure. Basic Res Cardiol 92 (Suppl 1): 95–103

19. Packer M (1992) The neurohormonal hypothesis: a theory to explain the mechanism of disease progression in heart failure (editorial). J Am Coll Cardiol 20: 248–54

20. Packer M (1992) Pathophysiology of chronic heart failure. Lancet 340: 88–92

21. Pieske B, Hasenfuss G, Holubarsch C, Schwinger R, Bohm M, Just H (1992) Alterations of the force-frequency relationship in the failing human heart depend on the underlying cardiac disease. Basic Res Cardiol 87 Suppl 1: 213–21

22. Pieske B, Kretschmann B, Meyer M, Holubarsch C, Weirich J, Posival H, Minami K, Just H, Hasenfuss G (1995) Alterations in intracellular calcium handling associated with the inverse force-frequency relation in human dilated cardiomyopathy. Circulation 92: 1169–78

23. Plotnick GD, Becker LC, Fisher ML, Gerstenblith G, Renlund DG, Fleg JL, Weisfeldt ML, Lakatta EG (1986) Use of the Frank-Starling mechanism during submaximal versus maximal upright exercise. Am J Physiol 251: H1101–5

24. Ricci DR, Orlick AE, Alderman EL, Ingels NB Jr, Daughters GT 2d, Kusnick CA, Reitz BA, Stinson EB (1979) Role of tachycardia as an inotropic stimulus in man. J Clin Invest 63: 695–703

25. Schouten VJ (1990) Interval dependence of force and twitch duration in rat heart explained by Ca2+ pump inactivation in sarcoplasmic reticulum. J Physiol (Lond) 431: 427–44

26. Studer R, Reinecke H, Bilger J, Eschenhagen T, Bohm M, Hasenfuss G, Just H, Holtz J, Drexler H (1994) Gene expression of the cardiac Na(+)-Ca2+ exchanger in end-stage human heart failure. Circ Res 75: 443–53

27. Thomas JA, Marks BH (1978) Plasma norepinephrine in congestive heart failure. Am J Cardiol 41: 233–43
28. Waagstein F, Bristow MR, Swedberg K, Camerini F, Fowler MB, Silver MA, Gilbert EM, Johnson MR, Goss FG, Hjalmarson A (1993) Beneficial effects of metoprolol in idiopathic dilated cardiomyopathy. Metoprolol in Dilated Cardiomyopathy (MDC) Trial Study Group (see comments). Lancet 342: 1441–6

Author's address:
N. R. Alpert
Dept. Molecular Physiology and Biophysics
Given Building
University of Vermont
Burlington, VT 05405
USA

Post-rest contraction amplitude in myocytes from failing human ventricle

K. Davia, S. E. Harding

Imperial College of Science, Technology and Medicine, Royal Brompton Campus, London, UK

Abstract

It has been reported that the balance between the two main Ca^{2+} removal systems in the cardiac cells, the sarcoplasmic reticulum (SR) and Na^+/Ca^{2+} exchanger, is altered in failing human heart. We have studied post-rest contraction behaviour as a non-invasive probe of the amount of Ca^{2+} stored in the SR in myocytes from failing and non-failing human ventricle. The first beat following a rest interval, as a percentage of the preceding steady state (B1/SS), was larger and more variable in cells from failing heart, indicating some accumulation of Ca^{2+} in the SR during rest. This could be mimicked by treatment of myocytes with digoxigenin, a compound which increases intracellular Na^+, suggesting that alterations in the Na^+ balance of the cell might contribute to the effect. Isoprenaline, which stimulates Ca^{2+} uptake by the SR while the myocyte is beating, prevented SR Ca^{2+} accumulation during rest in susceptible myocytes. We hypothesize that loss of SR function in the failing heart is partially compensated for by increased Ca^{2+} extrusion via the Na^+/Ca^{2+} exchange in the contracting myocyte, leading to increased intracellular Na^+ during activity. This Na^+ is lost at rest, predisposing the cells to accumulate Ca^{2+} in the SR. Experiments to test this hypothesis are proposed.

Key words Human – myocyte – sodium frequency

Introduction

The frequency response of single myocytes isolated from human ventricle parallels that of intact myocardium, with a strong positive staircase in non-failing tissue but not in failing (8). We have shown that inhibition of sarcoplasmic reticulum (SR) Ca^{2+} uptake, using thapsigargin, prevents the positive staircase in non-failing cells and abolishes the difference between myocytes from failing and non-failing hearts at physiological rates of beating (6). In this study we move towards the extremes of low frequency stimulation and examine the rested state beats of human ventricular myocytes. The first beat following a rest interval is thought to be mainly dependent on the Ca^{2+} remaining in the SR, and the decay or potentiation of this contraction relative to steady state has been used as a measure of the remaining SR Ca^{2+} load. Parallel experiments using interventions such as caffeine pulses or rapid cooling, which are known to release SR Ca^{2+} completely, have confirmed that post-rest contraction is directly related to the amount of Ca^{2+} stored (20). Biochemical evidence suggests that the SR Ca^{2+}-ATPase may be compromised in the failing heart, although agreement has not been reached on this point (1, 11, 13–15, 17). Post-rest experiments therefore represent a potential non-invasive method for investigating SR function in human myocytes.

We have previously shown that there are marked differences in post-rest behaviour between myocytes from failing and non-failing hearts (6). In the present study we have performed experiments using two interventions which have been at least partially successful in normalising the responses of muscle strips from failing human heart to high frequency stimulation. Forskolin (16), or isoprenaline in low (but not high) doses (3, 18) restored a positive component to the frequency staircase in muscle strips, despite the fact that β-adrenoceptor responses are desensitised in heart failure (9). The effects of isoprenaline and forskolin may be due to a normalisation of the intracellular cyclic AMP levels, which are decreased in failing compared to non-failing human ventricle in the absence of catecholamines (4, 5, 21). Treatment with agents that raise intracellular Na$^+$ has also been successful in reestablishing a positive staircase in muscle from failing human heart (3, 18). We have examined the effects of submaximal isoprenaline concentrations, and of digoxigenin, on the post-rest characteristics of myocytes from failing and non-failing human ventricle. Digoxigenin was chosen over digoxin because of the discovery that several of the cardiac glycosides have direct actions on the cardiac SR Ca^{2+} release channel (12): digoxigenin does not have these effects. We show that both isoprenaline and digoxigenin modify rest-dependent behaviour, but in opposing directions.

Methods

The patient group used in the present study are as previously described (6), with the addition of one patient with heart failure and two subjects with non-failing hearts. Myocytes were isolated from failing and non-failing left ventricular myocardium according to our standard protocol for large and biopsy-sized samples (8). Contraction amplitude was measured using a video motion detector, as before (8, 10). Myocytes contracting at the basal frequency of 0.2 Hz (32 °C) were allowed to equilibrate for 10 min or more. When the contraction amplitude was stable, rest intervals of 10 s, 30 s or 3 min were interposed; contraction was allowed to recover for 1–5 min between rests. Cells were then exposed to increasing concentrations of isoprenaline (from 0.01 nM) or digoxigenin (from 1 μM) until amplitude at least doubled from control values, and the rest protocol repeated. In selected cases, the inotropic agent was washed out, and a third rest protocol performed in a concentration of Ca^{2+} which matched the inotropic effect of the agent. When used, thapsigargin (1 μM) was applied to contracting cells for 20 min before rest protocols were performed.

Statistics

When data were obtained from more than one myocyte from each preparation the results were pooled, so that values are mean ± sem where n = patients (except for Fig. 3 where results from individual myocytes are shown). Results were compared by paired or unpaired t-test, with correction for unequal variances where appropriate. Data were tested for normality, and where this was not confirmed the non-parametric Mann-Whitney test was used instead of the two-sample t-test. Analysis of variance and linear regression were performed on pooled data using the MINITAB program (Pennsylvania).

Results

Post-rest contraction in myocytes from failing and non-failing ventricle

The size of the first post-rest contraction, relative to the previous steady-state is shown in Fig. 1 for myocytes from 27 failing and 20 non-failing ventricles; these data are updated from Davia et al. (6). There was no significant change in the steady state contraction over the course of the rest protocols, and amplitude returned to this level within 1 min of resumption of stimulation. There was pronounced post-rest decay in myocytes from non-failing ventricle, of a similar order to that we have observed in guinea-pig or rabbit myocardium (7). Post-rest decay was less pronounced in cells from failing heart, with post-rest contraction amplitude significantly higher than non-failing at 10 s (P < 0.01), 30 s

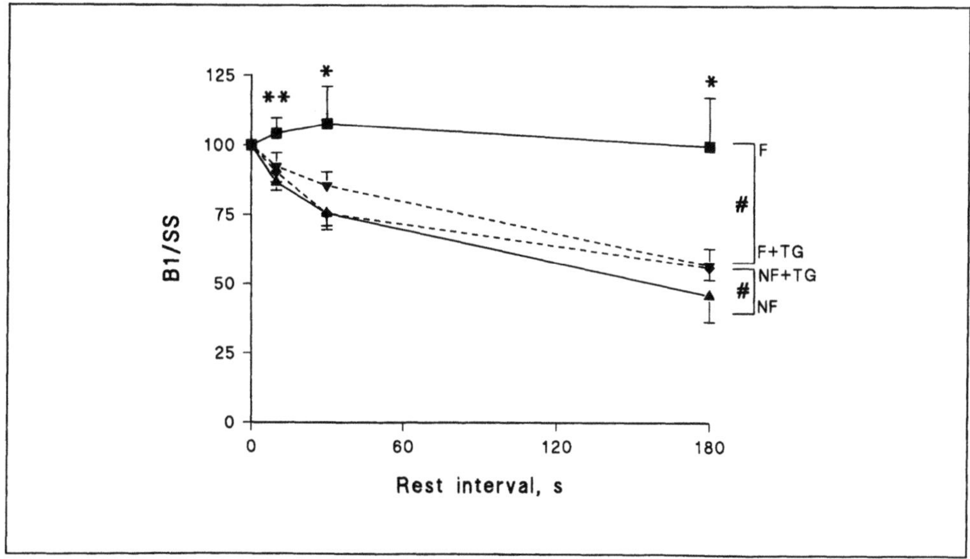

Fig. 1 First post-rest beat, as a percentage of steady state contraction (B1/SS) for increasing rest intervals in the absence of thapsigargin (solid lines) in myocytes from non-failing (NF, n = 20 subjects) and failing (F, n = 27) hearts and in the presence of thapsigargin (dashed lines) in myocytes from non-failing (NF + TG, n = 10) and failing (F + TG, n = 7) hearts. Significantly different from non-failing (without thapsigargin) **P < 0.01, *P < 0.05, significantly different between ± thapsigargin #P<0.01.

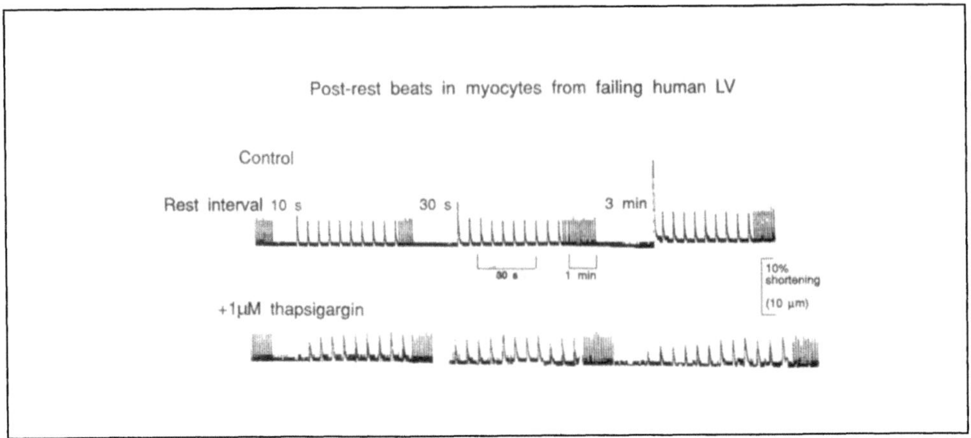

Fig. 2   Sample trace of the effect of thapsigargin on post-rest potentiation in a myocytes from failing human ventricle, at rest intervals of 10s, 30s and 3 min. Stimulation frequency was 0.2 Hz before and after rest; the first post-rest beats are shown on an expanded time scale. Steady state contraction amplitude in this myocyte (cell length 102 µm) was 5.7 µm before and 6.2 µm after thapsigargin.

($P < 0.05$) or 3 min ($P < 0.02$) (Fig. 1). The differences between failing and non-failing groups were SR-related, since they were abolished following treatment with 1 µM thapsigargin (Fig. 1, and sample trace in Fig. 2). It should be noted that there was a residual post-rest decay in the presence of thapsigargin, indicating that there is a non-SR dependent rest-sensitive mechanism in human ventricle which does not change with heart failure.

There was a marked increase in variability in post-rest beat size in cells from failing heart. This did not relate to the disease aetiology or drug treatment of the patient (although a weak

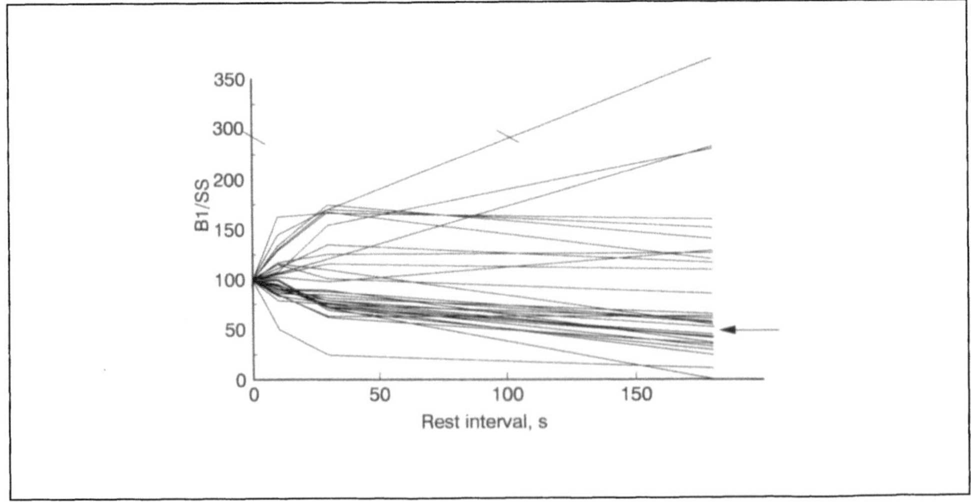

Fig. 3   First post-rest beat, as a percentage of steady state contraction (B1/SS) for increasing rest intervals in 34 individual myocytes from 27 failing hearts. The arrow indicates the average B1/SS value at 3 min in the presence of thapsigargin. Note the break in scale.

relation between post-rest decay and previous exposure of the patient to Ca^{2+} antagonists was noted (6). Figure 3 shows the size of the first post-rest beat relative to steady state contraction (B1/SS) from individual myocytes following a 3 min rest interval. The arrow represents the decay in the presence of thapsigargin (non-SR-dependent condition) for comparison. Analysis of variance revealed that the between-patient variation was significantly (P = 0.001) greater than the within-patient (between cell): this indicates that myocytes from a given patient behaved in a similar way. Following thapsigargin treatment, variability was significantly reduced in both the non-failing and failing groups (variance ratio before:after thapsigargin P < 0.001 for both groups).

Isoprenaline on post-rest contraction

Concentrations of isoprenaline close to the EC_{50} value (10) were used; these ranged between 10^{-8} M and 10^{-7} M for failing and 3×10^{-11} M and 3×10^{-8} M for non-failing hearts. Stimulation by isoprenaline had little effect on post-rest decay in non-failing myocytes (Fig. 4) or in failing myocytes with pre-existing post-rest decay (n = 2, data not shown). However, post-rest potentiation in myocytes from failing heart was converted to decay in the presence of isoprenaline. B1/SS (3 min), following isoprenaline pretreatment, was no longer significantly different between myocytes from non-failing (49.7 ± 6.5 %, n = 4) and failing (68.0 ± 10.8, n = 5) hearts. Addition of equal inotropic concentrations of Ca^{2+} did not produce the same effect; in one experiment basal contraction amplitude in 1 mM Ca^{2+} (change in cell length with each beat) was less than 0.5 µm, and this was raised to 7.2 µm by either 3×10^{-8} M isoprenaline, or by 6 mM Ca^{2+}. In 6 mM Ca^{2+}, B1/SS was 118%, while in isoprenaline this was reduced to 54.2 %.

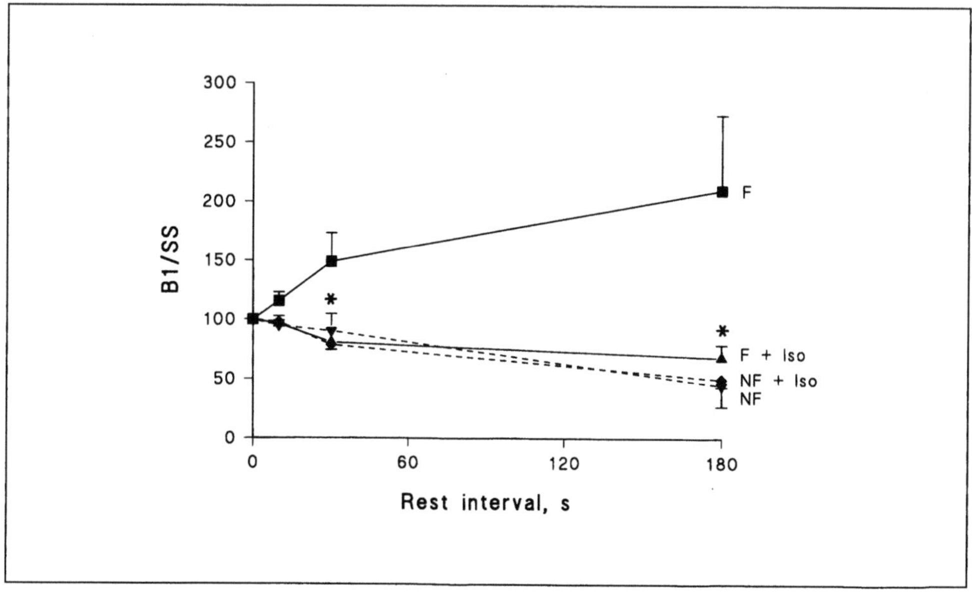

Fig. 4 First post-rest beat, as a percentage of steady state contraction (B1/SS) for increasing rest intervals in the presence and absence of isoprenaline in myocytes from failing (F, n = 5, solid lines) and non-failing hearts (NF, n = 4, dashed lines). Significantly different from failing *P< 0.05.

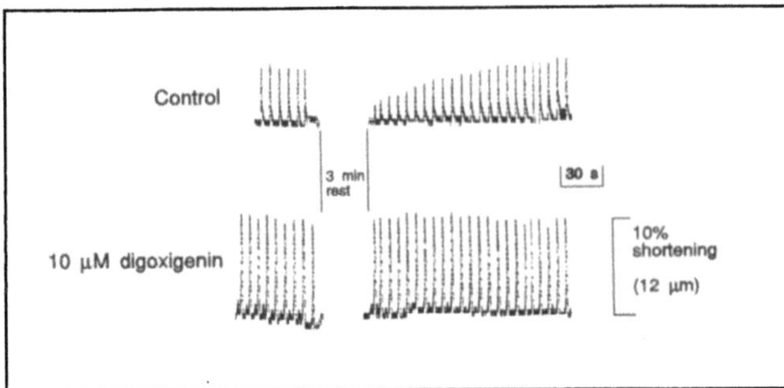

Fig. 5 Sample trace of the effects of digoxigenin on post-rest decay in a myocyte from failing human left ventricle. Steady state (0.2 Hz) contraction amplitude in this myocyte (cell length 127 µm) was 8.7 µm before 12.5 µm after digoxigenin.

Digoxigenin on post-rest contraction

The inotropic effects of digoxigenin started at 1 µM, and the average increase in contraction was $65.8 \pm 10.9\,\%$. The effect of digoxigenin was to minimise post-rest decay; a sample trace is shown in Fig. 5, and summarised data in Fig. 6. The effect was seen in cells from either failing or non-failing hearts which had originally shown post-rest decay. Once again, simply increasing Ca^{2+} did not produce the same effect as digoxigenin. In one experiment, B1/SS was initially 21.4 % after 3 min rest under basal conditions and exposure to 10^{-5} M digoxigenin increased B1/SS to 100 %. After washout of digoxigenin, B1/SS was 22.2 %, which indicates the stability of the measurement. Raising Ca^{2+} to 12 mM, a concentration which resulted in a decrease in diastolic length (a sign of Ca^{2+} overload) had little effect, with B1/SS remaining at 29 %.

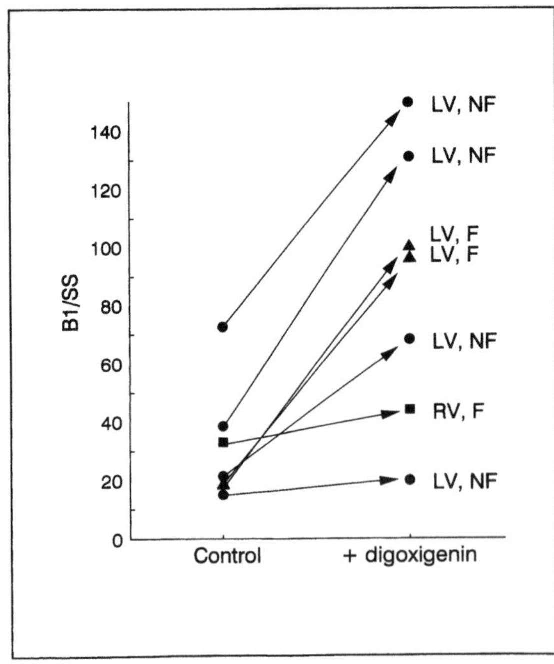

Fig. 6 Effect of digoxigenin on the first post-rest beat, as a percentage of steady state contraction (B1/SS) at 3 min in myocytes from failing (F) and non-failing (NF) left ventricle (LV) and failing right ventricle (RV).

Discussion

We have shown that myocytes from the failing heart are more variable in their post-rest behaviour, and more likely to exhibit post-rest potentiation of contraction than those from non-failing. This is due to accumulation of Ca^{2+} in the SR during rest: emptying of the SR stores by prolonged treatment with thapsigargin abolishes post-rest potentiation and significantly reduces variability between cells. The presence of thapsigargin reveals another rest-sensitive mechanism that is presumably non-SR dependent. Therefore, to decide whether Ca^{2+} has accumulated in the SR during rest under a given condition we compared the size of the first post-rest beat to that after thapsigargin.

The patient-to-patient differences were shown statistically to be greater than the cell-to-cell differences in a given preparation, but we have not yet identified any factors associated with the patient that would predispose to the appearance of post-rest potentiation. Neither patient age, nor etiology of disease, drug treatment or type of preparation (large sample v. biopsy) was significantly associated with large post-rest beats in the subsequently isolated myocyte (6). In the present study we describe preliminary experiments in which we have attempted to manipulate post-rest behaviour with digoxigenin or isoprenaline.

Digoxigenin was used in concentrations producing increases of contraction amplitude of around 50 %. Since this aglycone has no direct effect on SR Ca^{2+} release (12), the inotropic effect is mainly due to an increase in intracellular Na^+. At these concentrations, digoxigenin increased the size of the first post-rest beat in myocytes which had previously shown post-rest decay. Interestingly, the effect was much more marked in cells from failing or non-failing human heart than in those from guinea-pig, where digoxigenin concentrations with similar inotropic effects raised the post-rest contraction slightly after 30 s rest, but not after 3 min (Davia and Harding, unpublished observations). After digoxigenin, human myocytes behave more like those of rat, where post-rest potentiation is common (2). Rat myocardium has a naturally high intracellular Na^+ concentration, and it has been shown that Ca^{2+} is actively taken up by the rat myocyte at rest (19). It has been hypothesised that the Na^+/Ca^{2+} exchange runs in the direction of Na^+ extrusion and Ca^{2+} uptake at rest, because of this high intracellular Na^+. We suggest that during contraction in the failing myocyte the Na^+/Ca^{2+} exchanger is the main mechanism for Ca^{2+} removal, since SERCA levels are reduced (11, 14). Na^+ accumulates during contraction, and in the subsequent rest period either exchanges for Ca^{2+} or prevents effective Ca^{2+} extrusion.

Isoprenaline had the converse effect to digoxigenin, producing little change in post-rest behaviour in myocytes from non-failing heart, but reversing post-rest potentiation in those from failing heart. We hypothesize that the increase in intracellular cyclic AMP stimulates SERCA2a function through phosphorylation of phospholamban, thus, restoring some of the Ca^{2+} uptake function of the sarcoplasmic reticulum. This reduces the dependence on Na^+/Ca^{2+} exchange for Ca^{2+} removal, preventing the accumulation of intracellular Na^+ and reducing the probability of Ca^{2+} accumulation by the cell at rest. Stimulation of SERCA2a by cyclic AMP may also underlie the restoration of the positive staircase with increasing frequency by isoprenaline or forskolin (3, 16). Reductions in both SERCA2a protein levels and basal intracellular cyclic AMP have been reported for failing heart, and it is not yet known which makes the most contributions to the loss of SR Ca^{2+}-uptake function.

Increasing extracellular Ca^{2+} to match the inotropic effects of isoprenaline or digoxigenin did not alter the post-rest beat appreciably. This was unexpected; it might be predicted that high pre-rest intracellular Ca^{2+} combined with high extracellular Ca^{2+} during rest would delay full extrusion and predispose to SR Ca^{2+} accumulation. We have also noted in guinea-pig myocardium that increasing extracellular Ca^{2+} does not convert post-rest decay to potentiation (unpublished observations).

These preliminary findings must now be investigated further, for example, by manipulation of intracellular Na^+ levels using low Na^+ or Na^+/Ca^{2+} free media during rest and contraction in these myocytes. Measurement of intracellular Na^+ activities, their cyclic AMP-dependence, and their relation to post-rest and frequency-dependent changes in contraction will also be required to determine functional effects of the biochemical changes seen in failing human heart.

Acknowledgments   We would like to thank Pfizer for their generous support of Kerry Davia, and Professor Sir Magdi Yacoub, Mr John Pepper, Mr Graham Bennett and the immunologists of Harefield Hospital for help with supply of tissue.

References

1. Arai M, Alpert NR, MacLennan DH, Barton P, Periasamy M (1993) Alterations in sarcoplasmic reticulum gene expression in human heart failure. A possible mechanism for alterations in systolic and diastolic properties of the failing myocardium. Circ Res 72: 463–469
2. Bers DM (1985) Ca influx and sarcoplasmic reticulum Ca release in cardiac muscle activation during post rest recovery. Am J Physiol 248: H366–H381
3. Bohm M, La Rosee K, Schmidt U, Schulz C, Schwinger RH, Erdmann E (1992) Force-frequency relationship and inotropic stimulation in the nonfailing and failing human myocardium: implications for the medical treatment of heart failure. Clin Investig 70: 421–425
4. Bohm M, Reiger B, Schwinger RHG, Erdmann E (1994) cAMP concentrations, cAMP dependent protein kinase activity, and phospholamban in non-failing and failing myocardium. Cardiovasc Res 28: 1713–1719
5. Danielsen W, v der Leyen H, Meyer W et al. (1989) Basal and isoprenaline-stimulated cAMP content in failing versus nonfailing human cardiac preparations. J Cardiovasc Pharmacol 14: 171–173
6. Davia K, Davies CH, Harding SE (1996) Effects of inhibition of sarcoplasmic reticulum Ca uptake on contraction in myocytes isolated from failing human ventricle. Cardiovascular Research (in press)
7. Davia K, Wynne DG, Harding SE (1995) Control of relaxation in cardiac myocytes isolated from noradrenaline-treated guinea-pigs and patients with heart failure. Br J Pharmacol 114: 17P (Abstract)
8. Davies CH, Davia K, Bennett JG, Pepper JR, Poole-Wilson PA, Harding SE (1995) Reduced contraction and altered frequency response of isolated ventricular myocytes from patients with heart failure. Circulation 92: 2540–2549
9. Harding SE, Brown LA, Wynne DG, Davies CH, Poole-Wilson PA (1994) Mechanisms of beta-adrenoceptor desensitisation in the failing human heart. Cardiovasc Res 28: 1451–1460
10. Harding SE, Jones SM, O'Gara P, del Monte F, Vescovo G, Poole-Wilson PA (1992) Isolated ventricular myocytes from failing and non-failing human heart; the relation of age and clinical status of patients to isoproterenol response. J Mol Cell Cardiol 24: 549–564
11. Hasenfuss G, Reinecke H, Studer R et al. (1994) Relation between myocardial function and expression of sarcoplasmic reticulum Ca^{2+}-ATPase in failing and nonfailing human myocardium. Circ Res 75: 434–442
12. McGarry SJ, Williams AJ (1993) Digoxin activates sarcoplasmic reticulum Ca^{2+}-release channels: a possible role in cardiac inotropy. Br J Pharmacol 108: 1043–1050
13. Mercadier JJ, Lompre AM, Duc P et al. (1990) Altered sarcoplasmic reticulum Ca^{2+}-ATPase gene expression in the human ventricle during end-stage heart failure. J Clin Invest 85: 305–309
14. Meyer M, Schillinger W, Pieske B et al. (1995) Alterations of sarcoplasmic reticulum proteins in failing human dilated cardiomyopathy. Circulation 92: 778–784
15. Movsesian MA, Karimi M, Green K, Jones LR (1994) Ca^{2+}-transporting ATPase, phospholamban, and calsequestrin levels in nonfailing and failing human myocardium. Circulation 90: 653–657
16. Mulieri LA, Leavitt BJ, Martin BJ, Haeberle JR, Alpert NR (1993) Myocardial force-frequency defect in mitral regurgitation heart failure is reversed by forskolin. Circulation 88: 2700–2704
17. Schwinger RH, Bohm M, Schmidt U et al. (1995) Unchanged protein levels of SERCA II and phospholamban but reduced Ca^{2+} uptake and Ca^{2+}-ATPase activity of cardiac sarcoplasmic reticulum from dilated cardiomyopathy patients compared with patients with nonfailing hearts. Circulation 92: 3220–3228
18. Schwinger RHG, Bohm M, Muller-Ehmsen J et al. (1993) Effect of inotropic stimulation on the negative force-frequency relationship in the failing human heart. Circulation 88: 2267–2276
19. Shattock MJ, Bers DM (1989) Rat vs. rabbit ventricle: Ca flux and intracellular Na assessed by ion-selective microelectrodes. Am J Physiol 256: C813–C822

20. Terracciano CM, Naqvi RU, MacLeod KT (1995) Effect of rest interval on the release of calcium from the sarcoplasmic reticulum in isolated guinea pig ventricular myocytes. Circ Res 77: 354–360
21. von der Leyen H, Mende U, Meyer W et al. (1991) Mechanism underlying the reduced positive inotropic effects of the phosphodiesterase III inhibitors pimobendan, adibendan and saterinone in failing as compared to nonfailing human cardiac muscle peparations. Naunyn-Schmiedeberg's Arch Pharmacol 344: 90–100

Author's address:
Dr. S. E. Harding
Imperial College of Science
Technology and Medicine
Royal Brompton Campus (Heart and Circulation)
Dovehouse St, London SW3 6LY
UK

Influence of SR Ca²⁺-ATPase and Na⁺-Ca²⁺-exchanger on the force-frequency relation

W. Schillinger, S. E. Lehnart, J. Prestle, M. Preuss, B. Pieske, L. S. Maier,
M. Meyer, H. Just, G. Hasenfuss

Universitätsklinik Göttingen, Zentrum Innere Medizin, Kardiologie und Pneumologie

Abstract

The data presented indicate that altered systolic and diastolic function in failing human hearts may result from altered expression of calcium cycling proteins. Decreased systolic force production and inversion of the force-frequency relation seem to be related to reduced protein levels of SR Ca^{2+} ATPase and/or to increased protein levels of the Na^+-Ca^{2+} exchanger resulting in an increased ratio of Na^+-Ca^{2+} exchanger to SR Ca^{2+} ATPase. Impaired diastolic function may result from reduced SR Ca^{2+} ATPase and is most pronounced in failing hearts with lack of upregulation of the Na^+-Ca^{2+} exchanger. Thus, failing hearts with reduced SR Ca^{2+} ATPase protein levels and unchanged Na^+-Ca^{2+} exchanger protein levels exhibit severe impairment of both systolic and diastolic function.

Key words   Calcium channel – ryanodine receptor – sarcoplasmic reticulum – calcium pump – Na^+-Ca^{2+} exchanger

Introduction

Increased heart rate during exercise enhances cardiac output through an increased number of beats per minute as well as by its action on myocardial performance. The latter, termed force-frequency relation, strength-interval relation, or Treppe (staircase) phenomenon has first been observed by Bowditch in the isolated frog heart (3). Recent studies demonstrated that the force-frequency relation is also present in isolated myocardium from nonfailing human hearts. However, in failing human myocardium, the force-frequency relation is flattened or inversed (7, 11, 27). The altered force-frequency behavior in failing human myocardium has also been observed in clinical studies showing depressed frequency potentiation of hemodynamic parameters of myocardial performance (6, 13). A positive force-frequency relation was also observed in conscious dogs with and without autonomic blockade (9). This finding, however, is in contrast to other animal studies in which the force-frequency relation was flat during control conditions and not significantly altered in failure models (5, 15). Interestingly, frequency-potentiation of force can be significantly enhanced by adrenergic stimulation (17). For in vitro experiments in isolated myocardium, the term

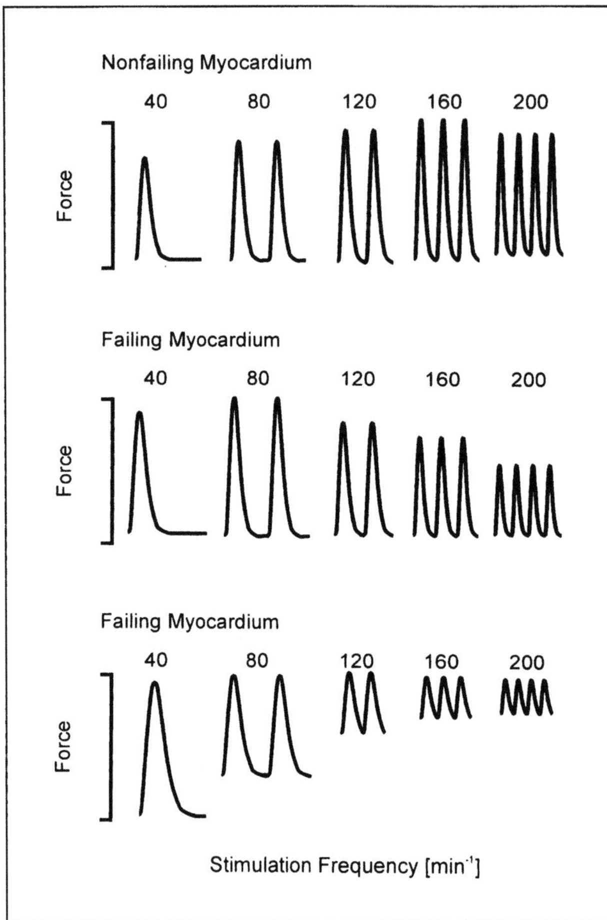

Fig. 1   Sketches of the force-frequency relation in electrically stimulated myocardial trabeculae from a nonfailing (upper panel) and two failing human hearts. Inversion of the force-frequency relation is defined as frequency-dependent decrease in developed force. This can result from a frequency-dependent decrease in systolic force (middle panel) or a frequency-dependent increase in diastolic force (lower panel) or from both mechanisms.

force-frequency relation generally is used to describe the relation between stimulation rate and developed force of the myocardium which represents the amplitude between diastolic force and peak systolic force. Accordingly, alterations of the force-frequency relation in failing human myocardium may result from altered systolic or altered diastolic function or from a combination of both (Fig. 1). In this manuscript we discuss recent findings of subcellular and molecular alterations which may underly the altered force-frequency relation of the failing human heart.

Functional and subcellular alterations

Altered force-frequency relation may result from disturbed frequency-dependent regulation of calcium transients or calcium sensitivity. To study this question, intracellular calcium

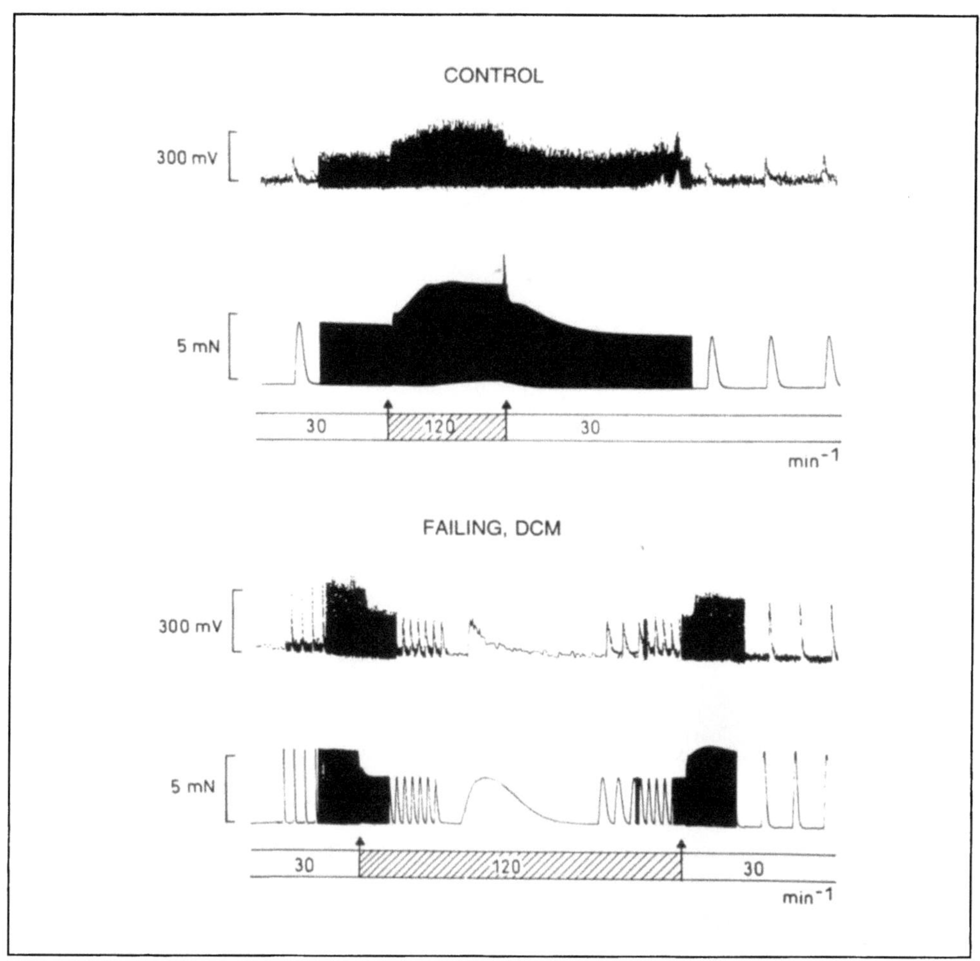

Fig. 2 Original recordings of aequorin light transients and isometric force signals in muscle strips from a non-failing (control) and a failing human heart with dilated cardiomyopathy (DCM). In both experiments, stimulation frequency was changed from 30 min⁻¹ to 120 min⁻¹ and aequorin light (upper panels) and isometric force (lower panels) were recorded. Reproduced with permission from Pieske et al. (30).

transients have been evaluated using the photoprotein aequorin (30). As is shown in Fig. 2, the frequency-dependent increase in isometric force observed in nonfailing human myocardium is associated with a parallel increase in aequorin light signal indicating frequency-dependent increase in intracellular calcium transients. In contrast, inversion of the force-frequency relation is associated with a frequency-dependent decline of the calcium transients, possibly indicating decreased calcium release from the sarcoplasmic reticulum at higher stimulation rates in the failing human heart. This in turn may result from altered calcium-induced calcium release despite normal calcium load of the sarcoplasmic reticulum (SR) or from alterations in the SR calcium content.

To investigate these possibilities, post-rest potentiation and rapid cooling contractures have been measured in nonfailing and failing human myocardium (31, 32); Fig. 3 shows post- rest contractile behavior of nonfailing and failing human myocardium. When

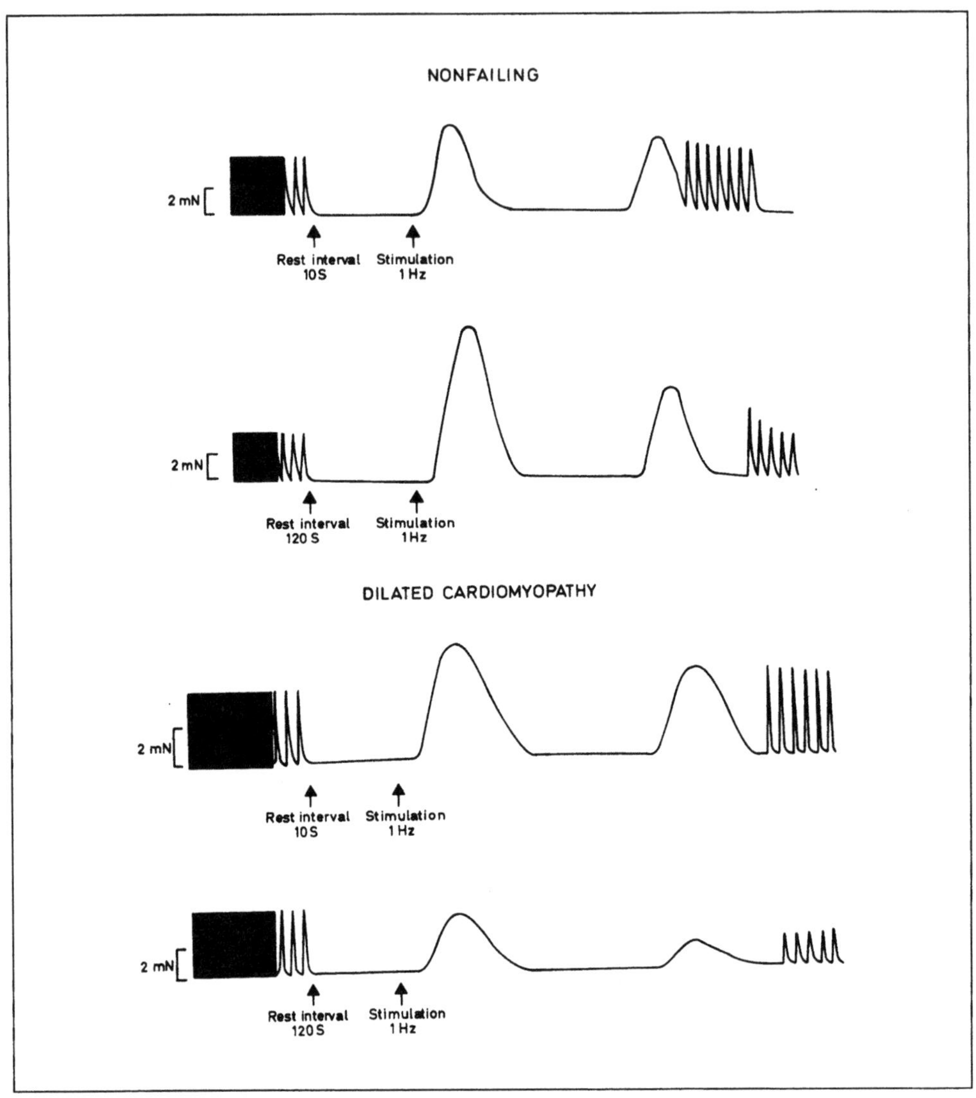

Fig. 3 Influence of rest intervals on post-rest contraction. Original recordings of post-rest behavior in a muscle strip preparation from a nonfailing heart (top) and an end-stage failing heart (bottom). Rest intervals were 10 s and 120 s. Basal stimulation frequency was 1 Hz. Reproduced with permission from Pieske et al. (32)

stimulation is stopped for a defined period of time, calcium is eliminated from the cytosol predominantly by calcium uptake into the SR and by calcium elimination across the sarcolemma by the Na^+-Ca^{2+} exchanger. Force development upon restimulation, thus, depends on the relative activity of these two transport mechanisms. As is obvious from the upper part of Fig. 3, post-rest potentiation of isometric force occurs in the nonfailing human myocardium indicating dominance of SR calcium uptake over transsarcolemmal calcium elimination. In contrast in a muscle strip from a failing human heart (lower 2 tracings) post-rest potentiation of force is attenuated after a rest period of 10 s and even converted to rest decay after a period of 120 s. This indicates increased transsarcolemmal calcium elimination relative to SR calcium uptake during the rest interval in the failing compared to the non-failing myocardium. Disturbed sarcoplasmic reticulum calcium handling as a dominant cause for the altered force-frequency relation was also suggested from rapid cooling contracture experiments. This technique is based on the fact that rapid cooling (within 1 s) of a muscle strip results in instantaneous release of all calcium stored in the SR with subsequent activation of contractile proteins and development of a contracture. The amplitude of the contracture is an index of the calcium content of the sarcoplasmic reticulum. There is a pronounced increase in cooling contractures with increasing stimulation rates of twitches preceeding the rapid cooling procedure in nonfailing myocardium (middle panel of Fig. 4). The frequency-dependent increase in cooling contractures is blunted in the failing human heart (lower panel of Fig. 4).

The alterations of post-rest potentiations and rapid cooling contractures observed in the failing human myocardium strongly suggest that sarcoplasmic reticulum calcium loading is disturbed in the failing human heart and that this is the dominant defect underlying blunting or inversion of the force-frequency relation. This does of course not exclude that alterations in calcium-induced calcium release at the level of the sarcolemmal L-type calcium channel or the SR calcium release channel (ryanodine receptor) are also involved.

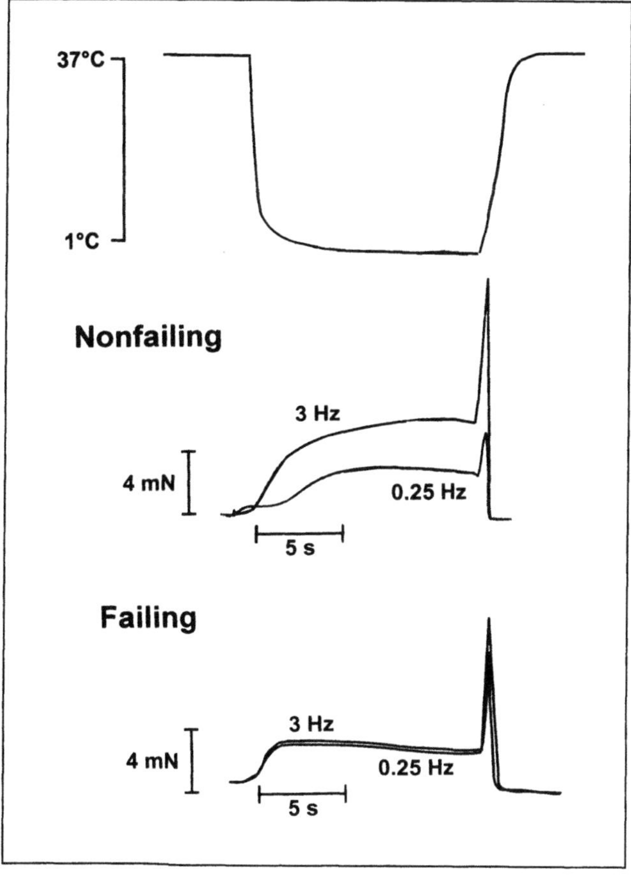

Fig. 4 Original recordings of isometric force during rapid cooling contractures in muscle strips from a nonfailing human heart (middle panel) and from an end-stage failing heart with idiopathic dilated cardiomyopathy (lower panel). Following steady state stimulation at 0.25 Hz temperature of the organ bath is rapidly decreased from 37°C to 1°C (upper panel) which results in complete SR calcium release and development of a contracture. Rewarming results in a rapid increase in force due to changes in calcium sensitivity (rewarming spike) followed by complete relaxation of the muscle. Thereafter, stimulation rate was increased to 3.0 Hz and the rapid cooling procedure was repeated during steady state force development. Cross-sectional areas of muscle strips were 0.28 mm² (nonfailing) and 0.24 mm² (failing).

Regarding L-type calcium channels, measurements in isolated myocytes indicated that calcium current densities, measured during basal conditions, were similar in myocytes from failing hearts with dilated cardiomyopathy and from nonfailing hearts (2, 22). However, measurements by Piot et al. recently suggested that function of L-type calcium channels may be altered in human heart failure (33). They observed that increasing stimulation frequencies augment calcium currents in myocytes from nonfailing hearts, whereas high frequency upregulation of calcium currents was lost or attenuated in myocytes from hearts with reduced left ventricular function. These findings may indicate that blunting of frequency-dependent upregulation of L-type calcium current and, thus, altered calcium-induced calcium release may contribute to the altered force-frequency relation in the failing human heart.

Regarding function of ryanodine receptors and interaction between L-type calcium channels and ryanodine receptors, a recent finding by Gomez et al. in failing rat hearts should be discussed (10). They observed that the relationship between calcium current density and the probability of evoking a calcium spark, i.e., opening of one or a few ryanodine receptors, is reduced in myocytes from failing hearts, indicating that calcium influx through L-type calcium channels is less effective in inducing SR calcium release in this rat model. The authors suggested that this may be the consequence of altered spatial orientation of L-type calcium channels and ryanodine receptors. Of note, one major difference between this study in failing rat hearts and findings in failing human hearts is that SR calcium accumulation and load were unaltered in the rat myocardium.

Altered function of ryanodine receptor was also suggested by D'Agnolo et al. (4). They found that caffeine threshold of the ryanodine receptor was increased, indicating impaired gating mechanism of the calcium release channel in dilated cardiomyopathy. Furthermore, Nimer et al. reported differences in response to ryanodine between failing and nonfailing human myocardium which may also reflect altered function of the ryanodine receptor (29). In contrast, Holmberg and Williams who studied activity of single ryanodine receptors under voltage-clamp conditions reported normal basal properties of the ryanodine receptor from failing human hearts (16). Thus, no conclusive data on possible alterations in function of ryanodine receptors or coupling between L-type calcium channels and ryanodine receptors are available. Such changes could contribute to the altered function of the failing human heart.

Molecular alterations

Under physiological conditions calcium release from the SR is the dominant regulatory mechanism for systolic activation of contractile proteins and force development. Assuming unaltered function of L-type calcium channels and ryanodine receptors and unaltered interaction between both, calcium release from the SR is determined by SR calcium load. The latter depends on SR calcium uptake by SR Ca^{2+} ATPase which is in competition with sarcolemmal calcium elimination by the Na^+-Ca^{2+} exchanger. Thus, regarding systolic function, the Na^+-Ca^{2+} exchanger opposes the action of SR Ca^{2+} ATPase. Although the Na^+-Ca^{2+} exchanger can work in both directions and can directly activate contractile proteins, the latter seems to occur only with unphysiological high experimental intracellular calcium concentrations (1). Regarding diastolic function of the myocardium, SR Ca^{2+} ATPase and Na^+-Ca^{2+} exchanger work in concert.

In the failing human heart SR calcium uptake was shown to be reduced and Na$^+$-Ca^{2+} exchange to be increased (14, 19, 34, 36). Reduced SR calcium uptake may result from decreased SR calcium ATPase protein levels and from decreased activity of the pump (24, 35–37), and increased Na$^+$-Ca^{2+} exchange may result from increased protein levels (8, 37, and for review see Ref. 12). Decreased SR Ca^{2+} ATPase and increased Na$^+$-Ca^{2+} exchanger favor decreased SR calcium load and, thus, decreased calcium available for release and systolic activation of contractile proteins in the failing human heart. In contrast, with respect to diastolic function, reduced SR Ca^{2+} ATPase protein levels and activity may be partly compensated by increased Na$^+$-Ca^{2+} exchanger protein levels. However, it should be mentioned that a previous study did not find an impairment of SR calcium uptake in failing human myocardium (25).

Relationship between altered force-frequency relation and SR Ca^{2+} ATPase protein levels

In order to test the hypothesis that altered force-frequency relation may be related to altered protein levels of SR Ca^{2+} ATPase, we plotted the relation between the frequency-dependent change in contractile force and protein levels of SR Ca^{2+} ATPase both measured in myocardium from the same hearts. As is shown in Fig. 5, there is a close positive correla-

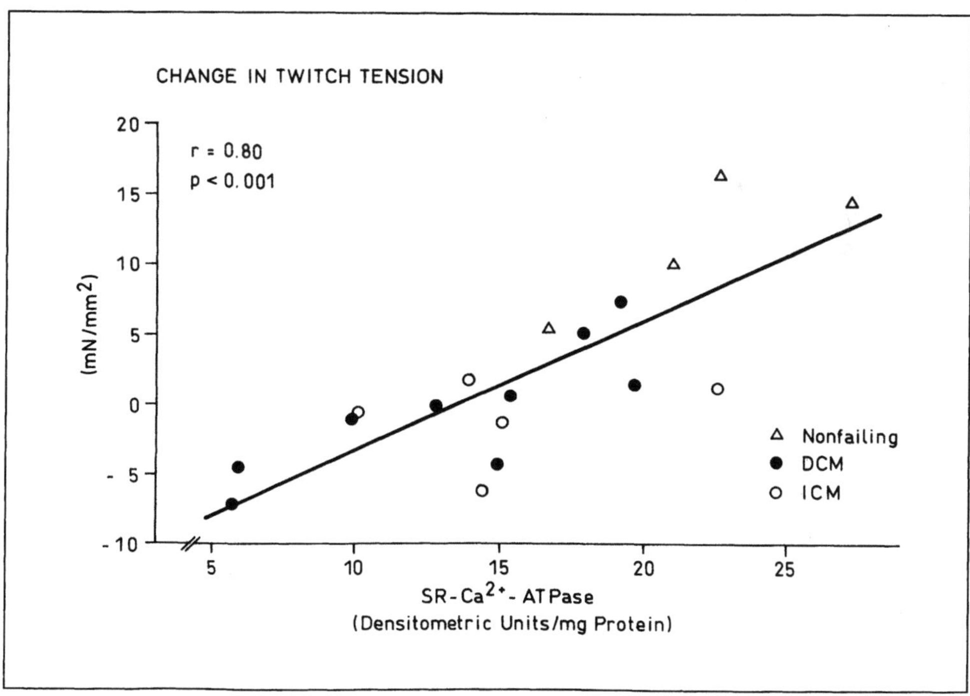

Fig. 5 Graph showing the relation between change in twitch force after an increase in the stimulation frequency from 30 to 120 min^{-1} and protein levels of sarcoplasmic reticulum (SR) Ca^{2+} ATPase normalized per total protein. DCM indicates dilated cardiomyopathy, ICM indicates ischemic cardiomyopathy. The correlation was also highly significant when the analysis was exclusively performed in failing myocardium (r = 0.66; p < 0.02). Reproduced with permission from Hasenfuss et al. (14).

tion between both parameters. Important to note, a significant correlation also exists when the regression analysis is performed from the data of failing human hearts exclusively. This may indicate that protein levels of SR Ca^{2+} ATPase and thereby activity of the pump system are a major determinant of frequency-dependent potentiation of contractile force. In this study, protein levels of the Na^+-Ca^{2+} exchanger as a potential covariant were not investigated.

Relationship between frequency-dependence of systolic and diastolic force and protein levels of SR Ca^{2+} ATPase and Na^+-Ca^{2+} exchanger

The relevance of SR Ca^{2+} ATPase and Na^+-Ca^{2+} exchanger protein levels on systolic and diastolic function was evaluated in a study which was primarily designed to test the hypothesis that in end-stage failing human hearts with blunted force-frequency relation and decreased sarcoplasmic reticulum calcium accumulation diastolic function would depend on protein levels of the Na^+-Ca^{2+} exchanger. Indeed, as is shown in Fig. 6, there is a significant inverse correlation between the rise of diastolic force following an increase in the stimulation rate from 30 to 180 min^{-1} and protein levels of the Na^+-Ca^{2+} exchanger. In a further analysis, hearts were divided into two groups depending on frequency-dependent behavior of diastolic function (Fig. 7). In those hearts exhibiting a frequency-dependent rise of diastolic force (group II), alteration of the force-frequency relation was more severe than in those hearts with normal diastolic function (group I) (Fig. 7). Na^+-Ca^{2+} exchanger levels were significantly higher in group I hearts as compared to group II and to nonfailing hearts

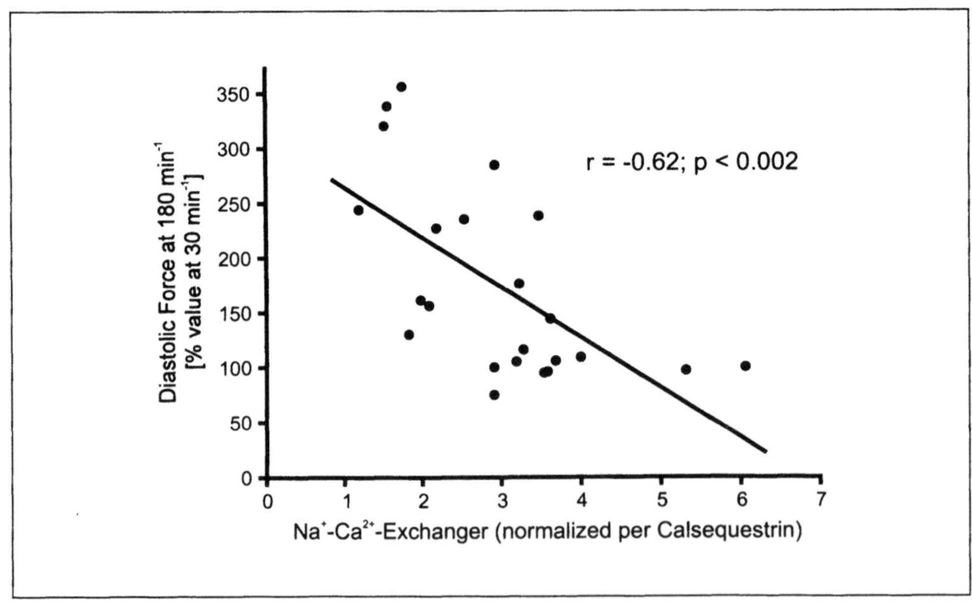

Fig. 6 Graph showing linear correlation between protein levels of the Na^+-Ca^{2+} exchanger and the change in diastolic force following an increase in the stimulation frequency from 30 to 180 min^{-1} given in percent of diastolic force value at 30 min^{-1}. Na^+-Ca^{2+} exchanger protein levels are normalized to calsequestrin protein levels, both in arbitrary densitometric units; therefore, the ratio has no unit.

Fig. 7 Graphs showing the influence of stimulation frequency on diastolic force (upper panel) and developed force (lower panel) in failing human myocardium. Group I (n = 6) includes myocardial trabeculae exhibiting no rise of diastolic force and group II (n = 17) includes trabeculae exhibiting a rise of diastolic force following an increase in the stimulation frequency above 30 min-1. Mean force values in both groups at different stimulation frequencies are given in percent of values at 30 min^{-1}. * = significantly different from the lowest stimulation frequency of 30 min^{-1}.

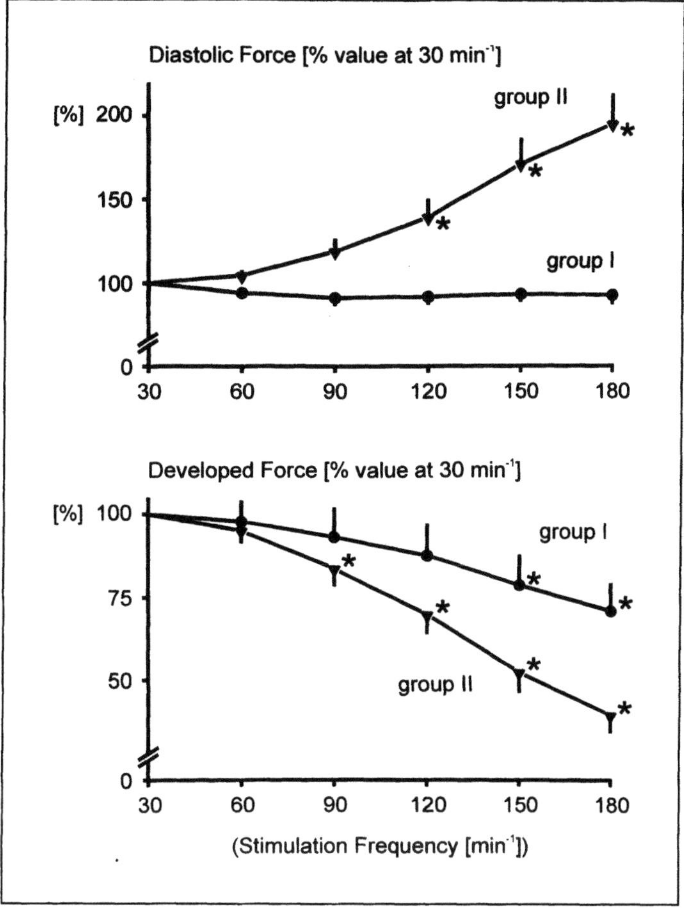

(Fig. 8). Moreover, SR Ca^{2+} ATPase protein levels in group II were significantly lower compared to nonfailing hearts (Fig. 8). Because Na^+-Ca^{2+} exchange opposes SR Ca^{2+} ATPase regarding SR calcium accumulation, we also calculated the ratio of Na^+-Ca^{2+} exchanger to SR Ca^{2+} ATPase. This ratio was significantly increased in both groups of failing hearts by a factor of about 3 relative to nonfailing hearts. In other words, by discriminating the hearts depending on their diastolic function, two subgroups of failing hearts are obtained: 1) hearts with normal diastolic function and moderately altered force-frequency relation (group I), and 2) hearts with impaired diastolic function and severely altered force-frequency relation (group II). In group II, SR Ca^{2+} ATPase was significantly decreased relative to nonfailing hearts and Na^+-Ca^{2+} exchanger was significantly lower than in group I hearts. This indicates reduced capacity of the SR to accumulate calcium for subsequent systolic release and severely reduced overall capacity to remove calcium from the cytosol to preserve diastolic function. In group I, SR Ca^{2+} ATPase is not significantly altered and Na^+-Ca^{2+} exchanger is increased compared to nonfailing myocardium. This may indicate that overall capacity for calcium removal from the cytosol is not impaired but rather increased. Important to note, although SR Ca^{2+} ATPase is not significantly reduced in group I compared to nonfailing hearts, blunting of the force-frequency could be explained by a

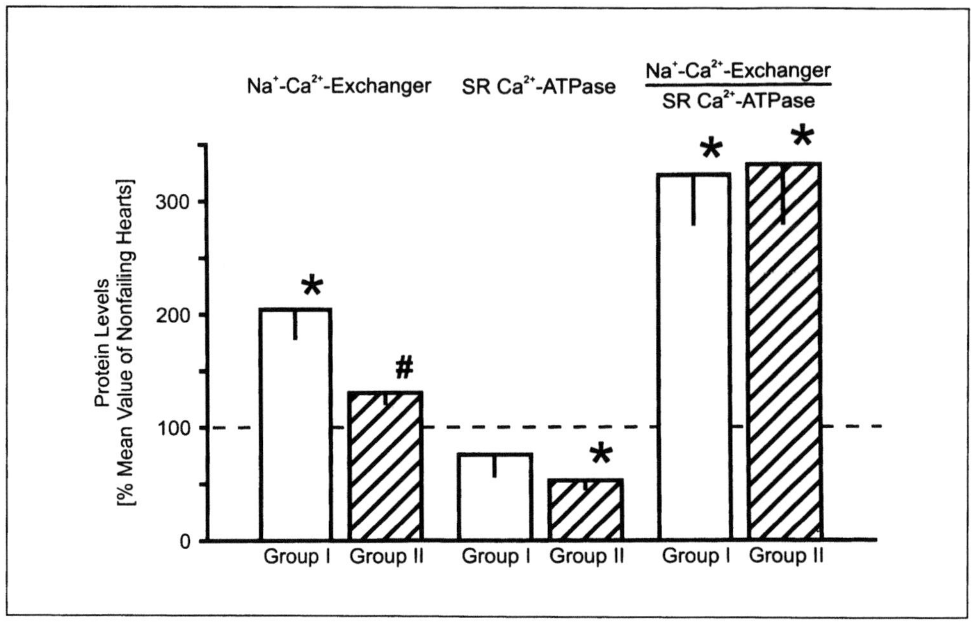

Fig. 8 Bar graph showing alterations in protein levels of SR Ca^{2+} ATPase and Na^+-Ca^{2+} exchanger in end-stage failing hearts with normal diastolic function (group I, n = 6) and with a frequency-dependent increase in diastolic force (group II, n = 17) relative to the situation in nonfailing human myocardium. Protein levels were determined in 5 nonfailing human hearts and average values were set 100%. Protein levels have been normalized to calsequestrin protein levels in order to compensate for changes in non-myocyte content of the myocardium. * p < 0.05 versus nonfailing hearts, # p < 0.05 versus group I hearts.

significant increase in the ratio of Na^+-Ca^{2+} exchanger to SR Ca^{2+} ATPase. This may indicate a relative shift of calcium transport by SR Ca^{2+} ATPase towards the Na^+-Ca^{2+} exchanger which may result in calcium loss across the sarcolemma and decreased SR calcium content. Of course, alterations in protein levels do not necessarily mean that overall function of these proteins is altered in the failing heart.

Besides alterations in protein expression of SR Ca^{2+} ATPase and Na^+-Ca^{2+} exchanger, levels of protein phosphorylation as well as intracellular sodium levels are critically important for transport activity into the SR or across the sarcolemma. Phosphorylation of phospholamban, the regulatory protein of SR Ca^{2+} ATPase, by protein kinase A and calcium/calmodulin – dependent protein kinase results in increased calcium sensitivity and activity of the pump (18, 38). Because the β-adrenoceptor-adenylyl cyclase system is downregulated in the failing human heart which may result in decreased protein kinase A activity, reduced phosphorylation of phospholamban may contribute to decreased sarcoplasmic reticulum calcium transport and altered force-frequency relation. Accordingly, Mulieri et al. (28) showed that stimulation of adenylyl cyclase with forskolin reverses the inverse force-frequency relation in failing human myocardium. Regarding the intracellular sodium concentration it is important to note that the electrochemical sodium gradient determines activity of the Na^+-Ca^{2+} exchanger which extrudes one calcium ion for three sodium ions. Differences in intracellular sodium concentration seem to be a major factor for species differences in force-frequency behavior. In this regard, high intracellular sodium in rat myocardium which exhibits an inverse force-frequency relation may favor calcium influx or decrease calcium efflux by the Na^+-Ca^{2+} exchanger resulting in high SR calcium load already at low stimulation frequencies (21). This may prevent significant increase in calcium load with higher stimulation rates as it occurs in rabbit myocardium which has a lower cytosolic sodium concentration and a positive force-frequency relation (26). Because intracellular sodium concentration was shown to be higher in failing compared to nonfailing human myocardium, this mechanism may additionally contribute to the altered force-frequency relation (20).

Energetic considerations

Because SR Ca^{2+} ATPase is sensitive to impaired energy supply, one may argue that altered systolic and diastolic function result from decreased SR calcium accumulation as a consequence of altered energetics. In order to study this possibility, frequency-dependent alterations of myocardial force and oxygen consumption were measured simultaneously (23). Figure 9 shows a graph relating myocardial oxygen consumption to force-time integral (calculated from developed and diastolic force). Both variables derive from the same muscle strip of an end-stage failing heart exhibiting a pronounced rise in diastolic force with increasing stimulation rate. As is obvious, there is a close linear correlation between both parameters over the whole frequency range investigated. If the rise in diastolic force would be the consequence of impaired energy supply to the calcium pump and the contractile machinery, this relation would no longer be linear. Therefore, the continuous increase in oxygen consumption in proportion with the increase in force-time integral strongly suggests

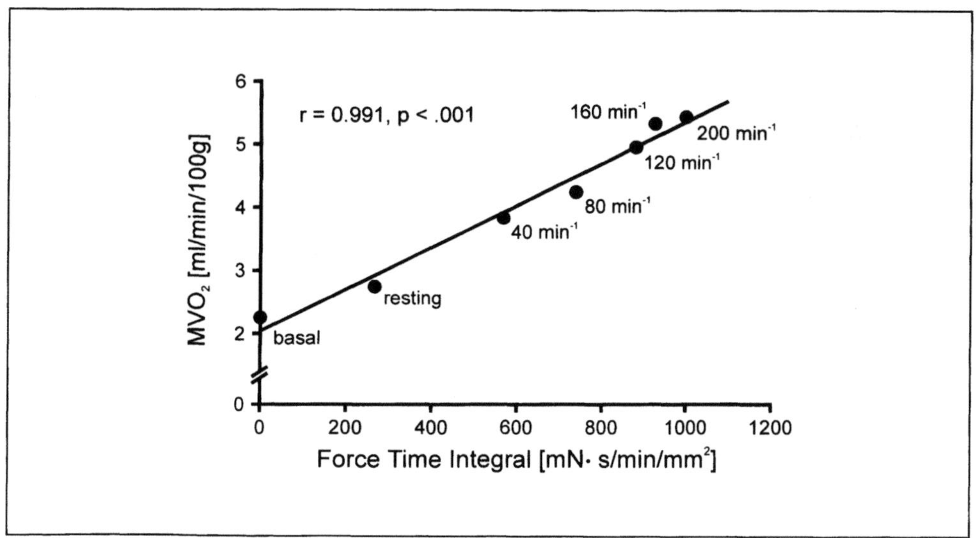

Fig. 9 Mechanical performance and frequency-dependence of myocardial oxygen consumption (MVO2) in a muscle strip from an end-stage failing human heart exhibiting a pronounced rise in diastolic force with increasing stimulation rate. Stimulation frequency was stepwise increased from 40 min⁻¹ to 200 min⁻¹ and force and MVO_2 were recorded. Resting force and MVO_2 were measured in the absence of stimulation. At the end of the experiment 30 mmol/l 2,3-butanedione monoxime was added to the unstimulated muscle to determine the basal force and MVO_2. MVO_2 was plotted versus total force-time integral and linear regression analysis was performed as shown.

that energy lack was absent in this muscle strip preparation and that increased diastolic force results from calcium induced crossbridge interaction with unaltered energetics.

References

1. Bers DM, Christensen DM, Nguyen TX (1988) Can Ca^{2+} entry via Na^+-Ca^{2+} exchange directly activate cardiac muscle contraction? J Mol Cell Cardiol 20: 405– 414
2. Beuckelmann DJ, Erdmann E (1992) Ca^{2+}-currents and intracellular $[Ca^{2+}]_i$-transients in single ventricular myocytes isolated from terminally failing human myocardium. Basic Res Cardiol 87 Suppl 1: 235– 243
3. Bowditch HP (1871) über die Eigenthümlichkeiten der Reizbarkeit, welche Muskelfasern des Herzens zeigen. Ber Sachs Ges Wiss 23: 652–689
4. D'Agnolo A, Luciani GB, Mazzucco A, Gallucci V, Salviati G (1992) Contractile properties and Ca^{2+} release activity of the sarcoplasmic reticulum in dilated cardiomyopathy. Circulation 85: 518–525
5. Eising GP, Hammond HK, Helmer GA, Gilpin E, Ross J Jr (1994) Force-frequency relations during heart failure in pigs. Am J Physiol 267: H2516–H2522
6. Feldman MD, Alderman JD, Aroesty JM, Royal HD, Ferguson JJ, Owen RM, Grossman W, McKay RG (1988) Depression of systolic and diastolic myocardial reserve during atrial pacing tachycardia in patients with dilated cardiomyopathy. J Clin Invest 82: 1661–1669
7. Feldman MD, Gwathmey JK, Phillips P, Schoen F, Morgan JP (1988) Reversal of the force-frequency relationship in working myocardium from patients with end-stage heart failure. J Appl Cardiol 3: 273–283
8. Flesch M, Schwinger RH, Schiffer F, Frank K, Sudkamp M, Kuhn-Regnier F, Arnold G, Bohm M (1996) Evidence for functional relevance of an enhanced expression of the Na^+-Ca^{2+} exchanger in failing human myocardium. Circulation 94: 992–1002
9. Freeman GL, Little WC, O'Rourke RA (1987) Influence of heart rate on left ventricular performance in conscious dogs. Circ Res 61: 455–464
10. Gomez AM, Valdivia HH, Cheng H, Lederer MR, Santana LF, Cannell MB, McCune SA, Altschuld RA, Lederer WJ (1997) Defective excitation-contraction coupling in experimental cardiac hypertrophy and heart failure. Science 276: 800–806
11. Gwathmey JK, Slawsky MT, Hajjar RJ, Briggs GM, Morgan JP (1990) Role of intracellular calcium handling in force-interval relationships of human ventricular myocardium. J Clin Invest 85: 1599–1613
12. Hasenfuss G (1998) Alterations of calcium-regulatory proteins in heart failure. Cardiovasc Res (in press)
13. Hasenfuss G, Holubarsch C, Hermann HP, Astheimer K, Pieske B, Just H (1994) Influence of the force-frequency relationship on haemodynamics and left ventricular function in patients with non-failing hearts and in patients with dilated cardiomyopathy. Eur Heart J 15: 164–170
14. Hasenfuss G, Reinecke H, Studer R, Meyer M, Pieske B, Holtz J, Holubarsch C, Posival H, Just H, Drexler H (1994) Relation between myocardial function and expression of sarcoplasmic reticulum Ca^{2+}-ATPase in failing and nonfailing human myocardium. Circ Res 75: 434–442
15. Higgins CB, Vatner SF, Franklin D, Braunwald E (1973) Extent of regulation of the heart's contractile state in the conscious dog by alteration in the frequency of contraction. J Clin Invest 52: 1187–1194
16. Holmberg SR, Williams AJ (1989) Single channel recordings from human cardiac sarcoplasmic reticulum. Circ Res 65: 1445–1449
17. Kambayashi M, Miura T, Oh BH, Rockman HA, Murata K, Ross J Jr (1992) Enhancement of the force-frequency effect on myocardial contractility by adrenergic stimulation in conscious dogs. Circulation 86: 572–580
18. Kranias EG, Garvey JL, Srivastava RD, Solaro RJ (1985) Phosphorylation and functional modifications of sarcoplasmic reticulum and myofibrils in isolated rabbit hearts stimulated with isoprenaline. Biochem J 226: 113–121
19. Limas CJ, Olivari MT, Goldenberg IF, Levine TB, Benditt DG, Simon A (1987) Calcium uptake by cardiac sarcoplasmic reticulum in human dilated cardiomyopathy. Cardiovasc Res 21: 601–605
20. Maier LS, Hasenfuss G, Pieske B (1997) Frequency-dependent changes in intracellular Na^+-concentration in isolated human myocardium. Circulation 96 Suppl 1: 178 (Abstract)
21. Maier LS, Pieske B, Allen DG (1997) Influence of stimulation frequency on $[Na^+]_i$ and contractile function in Langendorff-perfused rat heart. Am J Physiol 273: H1246–H1254
22. Mewes T, Ravens U (1994) L-type calcium currents of human myocytes from ventricle of non-failing and failing hearts and from atrium. J Mol Cell Cardiol 26: 1307–1320
23. Meyer M, Keweloh B, Güth K, Holmes J, Pieske B, Lehnart S, Just H, Hasenfuss G (1998) Frequency-dependence of myocardial energetics in failing human myocardium as quantified by a new method for the measurement of oxygen consumption in muscle strip preparations. J Mol Cell Cardiol (in press)
24. Meyer M, Schillinger W, Pieske B, Holubarsch C, Heilmann C, Posival H, Kuwajima G, Mikoshiba K, Just H, Hasenfuss G (1995) Alterations of sarcoplasmic reticulum proteins in failing human dilated cardiomyopathy. Circulation 92: 778–784

25. Movsesian MA, Karimi M, Green K, Jones LR (1994) Ca^{2+}-transporting ATPase, phospholamban, and calsequestrin levels in nonfailing and failing human myocardium. Circulation 90: 653–657
26. Mubagwa K, Lin W, Sipido K, Bosteels S, Flameng W (1997) Monensin-induced reversal of positive force-frequency relationship in cardiac muscle: role of intracellular sodium in rest-dependent potentiation of contraction. J Mol Cell Cardiol 29: 977–989
27. Mulieri LA, Hasenfuss G, Leavitt B, Allen PD, Alpert NR (1992) Altered myocardial force-frequency relation in human heart failure. Circulation 85: 1743–1750
28. Mulieri LA, Leavitt BJ, Martin BJ, Haeberle JR, Alpert NR (1993) Myocardial force-frequency defect in mitral regurgitation heart failure is reversed by forskolin. Circulation 88: 2700–2704
29. Nimer LR, Needleman DH, Hamilton SL, Krall J, Movsesian MA (1995) Effect of ryanodine on sarcoplasmic reticulum Ca^{2+} accumulation in nonfailing and failing human myocardium. Circulation 92: 2504–2510
30. Pieske B, Kretschmann B, Meyer M, Holubarsch C, Weirich J, Posival H, Minami K, Just H, Hasenfuss G (1995) Alterations in intracellular calcium handling associated with the inverse force-frequency relation in human dilated cardiomyopathy. Circulation 92: 1169–1178
31. Pieske B, Maier LS, Weber T, Bers DM, Hasenfuss G (1997) Alterations in sarcoplasmic reticulum Ca^{2+}-content in myocardium from patients with heart failure. Circulation 96 Suppl 1: 199 (Abstract)
32. Pieske B, Sütterlin M, Schmidt-Schweda S, Minami K, Meyer M, Olschewski M, Holubarsch C, Just H, Hasenfuss G (1996) Diminished post-rest potentiation of contractile force in human dilated cardiomyopathy. Functional evidence for alterations in intracellular Ca^{2+} handling. J Clin Invest 98: 764–776
33. Piot C, Lemaire S, Albat B, Seguin J, Nargeot J, Richard S (1996) High frequency-induced upregulation of human cardiac calcium currents. Circulation 93: 120–128
34. Reinecke H, Studer R, Vetter R, Holtz J, Drexler H (1996) Cardiac Na$^+$/Ca^{2+} exchange activity in patients with end-stage heart failure. Cardiovasc Res 31: 48–54
35. Schillinger W, Meyer M, Kuwajima G, Katsuhiko M, Just H, Hasenfuss G (1996) Unaltered ryanodine receptor protein levels in ischemic cardiomyopathy. Mol Cell Biochem 160/161: 297–302
36. Schwinger RH, Bohm M, Schmidt U, Karczewski P, Bavendiek U, Flesch M, Krause EG, Erdmann E (1995) Unchanged protein levels of SERCA II and phospholamban but reduced Ca^{2+} uptake and Ca^{2+}-ATPase activity of cardiac sarcoplasmic reticulum from dilated cardiomyopathy patients compared with patients with non-failing hearts. Circulation 92: 3220–3228
37. Studer R, Reinecke H, Bilger J, Eschenhagen T, Bohm M, Hasenfuss G, Just H, Holtz J, Drexler H (1994) Gene expression of the cardiac Na$^+$-Ca^{2+} exchanger in end-stage human heart failure. Circ Res 75: 443–453
38. Voss J, Jones LR, Thomas DD (1994) The physical mechanism of calcium pump regulation in the heart. Biophysical Journal 67: 190–196

Author's address:
G. Hasenfuss
Universitätsklinik Göttingen
Zentrum Innere Medizin
Kardiologie und Pneumologie
Robert-Koch-Str. 40
37075 Göttingen, Germany

Force-frequency relations in nonfailing and failing animal myocardium

B. Crozatier

Unité INSERM U400, Faculté de Médecine, Creteil, France

Abstract

This paper reviews the recent data concerning the force-frequency relations in experimental animals with heart failure. After a brief overview of the nature of these relations, which are induced by 2 opposite phenomena, the potentiation of force of contraction by heart rate and the restitution process, the paper reviews first the force-frequency relations in isolated failing myocardium. This is followed by a review of recent data obtained in the in situ failing heart. The cellular mechanisms of the force-frequency relations are then discussed.

Introduction

In most mammalian species, changes in stimulation frequency induce an increase in contractile force. This phenomenon (the treppe effect or positive staircase) was described more than a century ago by Bowdich. However, this relation is not always positive. In some species, particularly in rats, it is negative and, in humans where it is usually positive, it has been shown to be negative in heart failure (15, 17, 25, 27, 29).

Force-frequency relations can be interpreted in terms of 2 opposite phenomena: frequency potentiation and restitution, which coexist in the same preparation. In this review, we will first quickly consider the basic mechanisms responsible for the force-frequency relations and their cellular basis. We will then review the results of experiments performed in animals with heart failure.

Nature of the force-frequency relations

Frequency potentiation is the increase in force of contraction induced by an increased heart rate. This is the basis for the positive staircase (1, 2, 7, 9, 18, 20), which has been attributed to increased transsarcolemmal Ca entry and loading of intracellular stores due to an increased number of depolarizations per unit of time (11). The rate-dependent regulation of dihydropyridine-sensitive L-type Ca^{2+} current (I_{ca}) has been recently evaluated in isolated atrial cardiac myocytes using whole cell patch-clamp technique (30). I_{ca} was potentiated in a graded manner when the rate of stimulation was increased with an increase in peak amplitude and a slowing in current decay. Ca^{2+} influx was markedly increased within seconds. Isoproterenol potentiated this increase in I_{ca}. Other phenomena including reduced Ca^{2+} extrusion by the Na^{+}/ Ca^{2+} exchanger and lag of the Na^{+} pump function may also contribute to frequency potentiation.

In opposition with force potentiation, when the interval between beats is too short, the force of the following contraction may be decreased due to an incomplete restitution process. Restitution is the time necessary for Ca^{2+} to reach the releasable site by translocation in the sarcoplasmic reticulum after its uptake from the contractile apparatus (19, 38, Fig. 1). There is also evidence however that delayed recovery of the Ca^{2+} release channel also plays a role in the restitution process (32).

A method to analyze the restitution process is to introduce a test stimulus after varying time-intervals in isolated prerations previously paced at regular rates (28). With increased delays, the force of contraction increases until it reaches a plateau, describing a restitution curve. When the rate of regular stimulation is higher, the curve is shifted upwards, due to the potention induced by the increased pacing rate. Similar results have been found in the isolated heart with the measurement of dP/dtmax at fixed end-diastolic volume (6).

The addition of these two opposite phenomena (restitution and potentiation) may, thus, induce a positive staircase when the restitution process is close to its optimum or, conversely, a negative staircase when restitution is incomplete. The staircase is also negative in species such as rats in which the calcium avalaible for contraction originates principally from the sarcoplasmic reticulum. The mechanical restitution process has been studied in conscious dogs using the simple beat elastance analysis by Freeman and Colston (13).

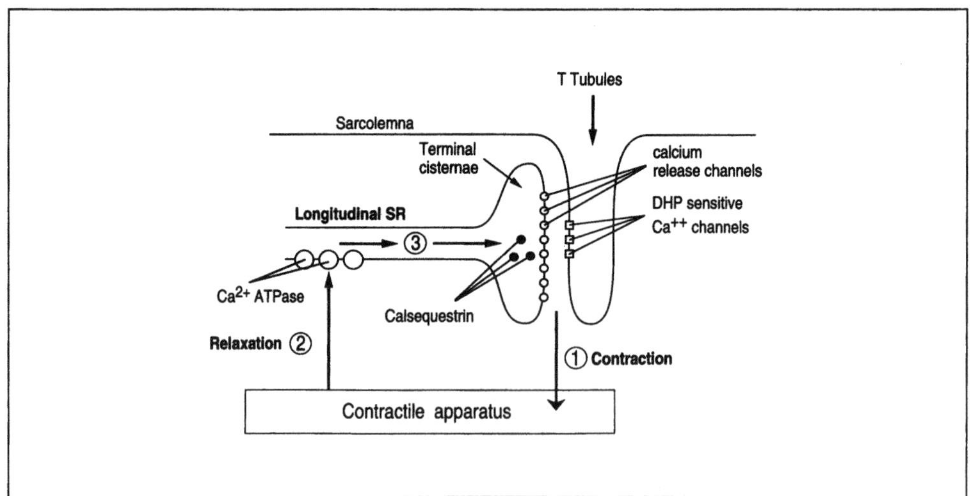

Fig. 1 Schematic representation of the cellular basis of the force-frequency relations. An increase in the rate of stimulation increases the calcium entry through the dihydropyridine (DHP) sensitive Ca^{2+} channels. This increases the calcium available for contraction and loads the calcium stores. This is the basis of the potentiation process. After a contraction (1), the calcium originating from the foot region (terminal cisternae of the sarcoplasmic reticulum and the T tubules) is again taken up by the Ca^{2+} ATPase located in the longitudinal sarcoplasmic reticulum (SR). The time necessary for calcium to reach the sites of release (3) is responsible, at least in part, for the restitution process.

Frequency potentiation and restitution are also the determinants of postextrasystolic potentiation, since the force of the postextrasystolic beat is related to the prematurity of the extrasystolic beat and the duration of the subsequent pause (5). The decrease of the potentiation of force has been shown in isolated hearts to be exponential, the time constant of this exponential being attributed to calcium recirculation (39).

Force-frequency relations in isolated failing myocardium

In contrast with human myocardium in which a number of studies analyzed the force-frequency relations of failing hearts (15, 17, 25, 27, 29), few studies were performed in experimental animals. Although studies performed in human myocardium can lead to important conclusions concerning the mechanisms of decompensation of the heart, they do not abolish the importance of experimental studies. The origin of calcium available for contraction is different among species (12): it mostly originates from transsarcolemmic movements in frogs, from the sarcoplasmic retitulum in rats and has both origins in most mammalian species such as rabbits, dogs or humans. The force-frequency relations are different among these species and their modifications induced by heart failure may suggest specific abnormalities induced by this syndrome.

The force-frequency relations were recently studied in the myocardium obtained from 2 species: cardiomyopathic syrian hamsters and dogs with pacing induced heart failure (21). In syrian hamsters, the force-frequency relation was biphasic in both normal and cardiomyopathic hamsters with an initial negative phase which was markedly attenuated in normal hamsters by increasing extracellular Ca^{2+} concentration. This phase was followed by a positive staircase in both strains of hamsters but the slope was significantly lower in myopathic syrian hamsters. In both strains, the addition of phenylephrine induced an uniphasic positive staircase. In contrast with the decrease of the positive staircase in syrian cardiomyopathic hamsters, in dogs with pacing-induced heart failure the tension-frequency relations were similar to those of control dogs and was not modulated by phenylephrine.

Besides the positive staircase and, thus, force potentiation by the increase of heart rate, the restitution phenomenon appears to play a major role in the abnormalities of the force-frequency relations in heart failure. In the study of Li and Rouleau (21), the initial negative staircase observed in syrian hamsters was attributed to a limitation of sarcoplasmic reticulum calcium handling since the negative staircase disappeared under ryanodine. We analyzed further the restitution phenomenon (10) in a model of heart failure produced in rabbits by the association of a pressure plus double overload. This leads to a marked (close to 100 %) left ventricular hypertrophy and a cardiac decompensation within one month (14). In this model, we previously described abnormalities of the beta-adrenergic system (4). We also analyzed in detail the force-frequency relations (10) in isolated hearts. The force-frequency relation was positive in normal hearts and was negative in failing hearts. Although the differences were statistically significant, they were small but major abnormalities were found when postextrasystolic potentiation (PESP) and poststimulation potentiation (PSP) were analyzed. PSP was clearly positive in normal hearts with an increased peak LV dP/dt in the beat following the regular pacing beats when heart rate was increased progressively from 100 to 200 beats/min. In contrast, contractility increased only slightly for heart rate increases up to 150 beats/min and decreased thereafter. This was associated with an increase in end-diastolic pressure, suggesting that there was a calcium overload of the cell. Such diastolic abnormalities have been demonstrated by Gwathmey et al. (16) in isolated preparations obtained from patients in end-stage heart failure.

The role of sarcoplasmic reticulum in the force-frequency relations was clearly shown in our study in rabbits (10) since both PESP and PSP were completely abolished by pretreatment by ryanodine in both normal and failing hearts. Our data strongly suggested that, since for the utilized doses, ryanodine blocks sarcoplasmic calcium release (23) and since abnormalities of the force-frequency disappeared in failing hearts under ryanodine, force-frequency relation abnormalities were due to abnormalities in sarcoplasmic reticulum. This could be due either by an abnormal calcium uptake which has been already shown in hypertrophy and heart failure (see (22) for review) and/or to an abnormal calcium circulation and/or release.

The relation between alterations in intracellular calcium handling and the force-frequency relation has been analyzed by Hasenfuss' group in human cardiac muscle strips obtained from patients with end-stage heart failure (29). The inverse force-frequency relation has been attributed to a decreased calcium uptake by the sarcoplasmic reticulum (29). This group also showed a decreased protein level of the sarcoplasmic reticulum calcium ATPase which decreased more than those of phospholamban while protein levels of ryanodine receptors, calsequestrine, and calreticulin were not different from the control (24). In contrast, the gene expression of the Na/Ca exchanger was increased (35).

The effect of cardiac overload and failure on ryanodine receptors is different in different species. A recent study by Rannou et al. (34) showed a decreased ryanodine receptor density in guinea-pig and in ferrets during the development of cardiac hypertrophy but not in rats while the density was decreased in all 3 species in heart failure. Similarly, a decrease in myocardial ryanodine receptors was found in dogs early in the development of heart failure induced by rapid ventricular pacing (37). Thus, besides a decrease in sarcoplasmic reticulum calcium uptake, abnormalities in calcium release exist in some models and species and may modify the force-frequency relation.

In our model of cardiac failure in rabbits, we recently studied sarcoplasmic reticulum calcium uptake, which was significantly but only slightly decreased (by 20 %) with an absence of change in ryanodine receptor density (3). It is unlikely that the small decrease in calcium uptake capacity of the sarcoplasmic reticulum is responsible for the abnormal force-frequency relations in this model. In our study (3), we also showed an abnormality of the ultrastructure of the heart with abnormally dilated T tubules. They appeared as a dilatation of normally present tubules rather than a proliferation of new T tubules along the hypertrophied contractile apparatus. A harmonious hypertrophy would have probably lead to a normal aspect of T tubules along hypertrophied myofibrils. Since T tubules correspond to the zone where sarcolemmal plasma membrane is closely related to sarcoplasmic reticulum, inducing the calcium induced-calcium release, it is possible to speculate that although sarcoplasmic reticulum itself was not directly observed in this study, an inadequate calcium release may occur in the failing heart even though the amount of ryanodine channel and membrane calcium channel is not modified. This hypothesis needs to be confirmed by cellular calcium imaging studies.

Another study in rat failing myocardium (26) recently showed an abnormal force-frequency relationship in which a decreased rate of calcium accumulation in the sarcoplasmic reticulum was not the primary cause. In this study, a pulsus alternans was produced in Langendorff perfused hearts obtained from a strain of rats with end-stage dilated cardiomyopathy (SHHF/Mcc-fa^T) during an increased ventricular pacing rate. This alternation was abolished by 1 mM caffeine, showing the role of the sarcoplasmic reticulum in its development but 50–500 nM thapsigargin, which blocks calcium uptake, did not induce alternans in normal myocardium. The intimate mechanism which induces mechanical alternans (an alternation of strong and weak beats) is not known but this study shows that although the sarcoplasmic reticulum is involved in its development, other mechanisms than abnormal calcium reuptake are its primary cuase. Similarly with our study (3), the authors concluded that the appearance of abnormal force-frequency relations may be due to a slow rate of calcium transport from the uptake sites (the longitudinal sarcoplasmic reticulum) to the release sites (the junctional and corbular sarcoplasmic reticulum) or that the ryanodine channels require a finite time to recover from inactivation.

Force-frequency relations in the hypertrophied and failing in situ heart

We recently evaluated the force-frequency relations in the conscious state in the model of heart failure in dogs (36). In contrast to the study of Li and Rouleau in which the force-frequency relations were not impared in isolated muscles obtained from dogs with the same pacing-induced heart failure (21), we found a smaller increase in left ventricular dP/dt max during regular pacing in failing dogs than in control dogs and a decreased poststimulation potentiation. The diffence between our in vivo study (36) and the in vitro study (21) in the same model of heart failure and in the same species may be due to a number of factors: temperature (29 °C in the bath), calcium concentration, rate of stimulation (1–60 beats/min in vitro, 120 to 240 beats/min in our study), etc. Our results can, however, be compared to those published some years ago by Pouleur et al. (31) who found, in the in situ heart, a decrease in poststimulation potentiation in dogs with cardiac volume overload. The results of the force-frequency relations were however different by other aspects since Pouleur et al. (31) found an increased stimulation potentiation but the models were different since, in this study (31), the phase during which the animals were studied was the initial phase of cardiac overload and no sign of heart failure was present.

Mechanical restitution has been studied by Prabhu and Freeman (3) by the analysis of postextrasystolic contraction in close-chest dogs with heart failure induced by rapid pacing which was prolongated. The authors (3) attributed this prolongation to an abnormal sarcoplasmic reticulum calcium kinetics.

In a recent study by Eising et al. (8), the force-frequency relations were further studied in a model of pacing-induced cardiomyopathy in a different species, the pig. Before heart failure, the force-frequency relation was flat but, importantly, it showed a significant positive slope during dobutamine infusion showing thus an amplification in the in situ heart of the force-frequency relation by beta-receptor stimulation. This can be compared with the study of Piot et al. (30) in isolated human cardiomyocytes where the increase in I_{Ca} induced by an increase in pacing rate was potentiated by isoproterenol. In contrast, in failing in situ hearts, beta-adrenergic stimulation did not amplify the force-frequency relation (8). Besides abnormalities of the force-frequency relations which have been described in vitro, this phenomenon may play an important role in the impaired response to excercise in patients with heart failure.

Conclusions

This brief review was focused on the recent results concerning the force-frequency relation in failing and nonfailing animal myocardium.

Although results were different depending upon the model, the species, and the experimental conditions, this review shows the physiological importance of these relationships. Obviously, they play a major role in the adaptation to exercise. Their analysis is, thus, most useful for the evaluation of the clinical status of patients with heart failure. Another important aspect of these relations is that they may help to suspect subcellular abnormalities by the study of potentiation and restitution which can be confirmed by direct cellular and biochemical studies.

References

1. Anderson PAW, Manring A, Serwer GA, Benson WK, Edwards SB, Armstrong BE, Sterba RJ, Floyd IV RD (1979) The force-interval relationship of the left ventricle. Circulation 60: 334–348
2. Arentzen CE, Rankin JS, Anderson PAW, Feezor MD, Anderson RW (1978) Force-frequency characteristics of the left ventricle in the conscious dog. Circ Res 42: 64–71
3. Bouanani NEH, Perennec J, Ezzaher A, Jdaiaa H, Crozatier B (1994) Sarcoplasmic reticulum function abnormalities in rabbit failing hearts. C R Acad Sci Paris, Sciences de la vie/Life sciences, 317: 825–831
4. Bouanani NEH, Corsin A, Gilson N, Crozatier B (1991) Beta-adrenoceptors and adenylate cyclase activity in hypertrophied and failing rabbit left ventricule. J Mol Cell Cardiol 23: 537–581
5. Braunwald E, Ross J Jr, Sonnenblick EH, Frommer PL, Braunwald NS, Morrow AG (1965) Slowing of heart rate, electroaugmentation of ventricular performance, and increase of myocardial oxygen consumption produced by paired electrical stimulation. Bull NY Acad Med 41: 481–497
6. Burkhoff D, Yue DT, Franz MR, Hunter WC, Sagawa K (1984) Mechanical restitution of isolated perfused canine left ventricles. Am J Physiol 246 (Heart Circ Physiol 15): H8–H16
7. Edman KAP, Johannsson M (1976) The contractile state of rabbit papillary muscle in relation to stimulation frequency. J Physiol (Lond) 254: 565–581
8. Eising GP, Hammond HK, Helmer GA, Gilpin E, Ross J Jr (1994) Force-frequency relations during heart failure in pigs. Am J Physiol 267 (Heart Circ Physiol 36): H2516–H2522
9. Elzinga G, Lab MJ, Noble MIM, Papadoyannis DE, Pidgeon J, Seed A, Wohlfart B (1981) The action-potential duration and contractile response of the intact heart related to the preceding interval and the preceding beat in the dog and cat. J Physiol (Lond) 314: 481–500
10. Ezzaher A, Bouanani NEH, Crozatier B (1992) Force-frequency relations and response to ryanodine in failing rabbit hearts. Am J Physiol 263 (Heart Circ Physiol (32): H1710–H1715
11. Fabiato A (1985) Simulated calcium current can both cause calcium loading in and trigger calcium release from the sarcoplasmic reticulum of a skinned canine cardiac Purkinje coll. J Gen Physiol 85: 291–320
12. Fabiato A, Fabiato F (1978) Calcium-induced release of calcium from the sarcoplasmic reticulum of skinned cells from adult human, dog, cat, rabbit, rat, and frog hearts and from fetal and new-born rat ventricles. Ann NY Acad Sci 307: 491–522
13. Freeman GL, Colston JI (1990) Evaluation of left ventricular mechanical restitution in closed-chest dogs based on single-beat elastance. Circ Res 67: 1437–1445
14. Gilson N, Bouanani NEH, Corsin A, Crozatier B (1990) Left Ventricular function and beta-adrenoceptors in rabbit failing heart. Am J Physiol 258 (Heart Circ Physiol 27): H634–H641
15. Gwathmey JK, Slawsky MT, Hajjar RJ, Briggs GM, Morgan JP (1990) Role of intracellular calcium handling in force-interval relationships of human ventricular myocardium. J Clin Invest 85: 1599–1613
16. Gwathmey JK, Warren SE, Briggs GM, Copelas L, Feldman MD, Phillip PJ, Callahan M, Schoen FJ, Grossman W, Morgan JP (1991) Diastolic dysfunction in hypertrophic cardiomyopathy. J Clin Invest 87: 1023–1031
17. Hasenfuss G, Reinecke H, Studer R, Meyer M, Pieske B, Holtz J, Holubarsch C, Posival H, Just H, Drexler H (1994) Relation between myocardial function and expression of sarcoplasmic reticulum Ca^{2+}-ATPase in failing and nonfailing human myocardium. Circ Res 75: 434–442
18. Higgins CB, Vatner SF, Franklin D, Braunwald E (1973) Extent of regulation of the heart's contractile state in the conscious dog by alteration in the frequency of contraction. J Clin Invest 52: 1187–1194

19. Hilgemann DW, Noble D (1987) Excitation-contraction coupling and extracellular calcium transients in rabbit atrium: reconstruction of basic cellular mechanisms. Proc R Soc Lond B Biol Sci 230: 163–205

20. Koch-Weser J, Blinks JR (1963) The influence of the interval between beats on myocardial contractility. Pharmacol Rev 15: 601–652

21. Li K, Rouleau JL (1995) Tension-frequency relationships in normal and cardiomyopathic dog and hamster myocardium. J Mol Cell Cardiol 27: 1251–1261

22. Lompré AM, Anger M, Levitsky D (1994) Sarco (endo) plasmic reticulum calcium pumps in the cardiovascular system: function and gene expression. J Mol Cell Cardiol 26: 1109–1121

23. Meissner G (1986) Ryanodine activation and inhibition of the Ca^{2+} release channel of sarcoplasmic reticulum. J Biol Chem 261: 6300–6306

24. Meyer M, Schillinger W, Pieske B, Holubarsch C, Heilmann C, Posival H, Kuwajima G, Mikoshiba K, Just H, Hasenfuss G (1995) Alterations of sarcoplasmic reticulum proteins in failing human dilated cardiomyopathy. Circulation 92: 778–784

25. Mulieri LA, Hasenfuss G, Leavitt B, Allen PD, Alpert NR (1992) Altered myocardial force-frequency relation in human heart failure. Circulation 85: 1743–1750

26. Narayan P, McCune SA, Robitaille PML, Hohl CM, Altschuld RA (1995) Mechanical alternans and the force-frequency relationship in failing rat hearts. J Mol Cell Cardiol 27: 523–530

27. Phillips PJ, Gwathmey JK, Feldman MD, Schoen FJ, Grossman W, Morgan JP (1990) Post-extrasystolic potentiation and the force-frequency relationship: differential augmentation of myocardial contractility in working myocardium from patients with endstage heart failure. J Mol Cell Cardiol 22: 99–110

28. Pidgeon J, Lab M, Seed A, Elzinga G, Papadoyannis D, Noble M (1980) The contractile state of cat and dog heart in relation to the interval between beats. Circ Res 47: 559–567

29. Pieske B, Kretschmann B, Meyer M, Holubarsch C, Weirich J, Posival H, Minami K, Just H, Hasenfuss G (1995) Alterations in intracellular calcium handling associated with the inverse force-frequency relation in human dilated cardiomyopathy. Circulation 92: 1169–1178

30. Piot C, Lemaire S, Albat B, Seguin J, Nargeot J, Richard S (1996) High frequency-induced upregulation of human cardiac calcium currents. Circulation 93: 120-128

31. Pouleur H, Rousseau MF, Petein H, Van Mechelen H, Charlier AA (1983) Effects of chronic volume overload on left ventricular response to tachycardia. Am J Physiol 245 (Heart Circ Physiol 14): H218–H228

32. Prabhu SD, Freeman GE (1992) Kinetics of restitution of left ventricular relaxation. Circ Res 70: 29–38

33. Prabhu SD, Freeman GL (1995) Postextrasystolic mechanical restitution in closed-chest dogs. Effect of heart failure. Circulation 92: 2652–2659

34. Rannou F, Sainte-Beuve C, Oliviero P, Do E, Trouvé P, Charlemagne D (1995) The effects of compensated cardiac hypertrophy on dihydropyridine and ryanodine receptors in rat, ferret and guinea-pig hearts. J Mol Cell Cardiol 27: 1225–1234

35. Studer R, Reinecke H, Bilger J, Eschenhagen T, Böhm M, Hasenfuss G, Just H, Holtz J, Drexler H (1994) Gene expression of the cardiac Na^{+}-Ca^{2+} exchanger in end-stage heart failure. Circ Res 75: 443–453

36. Su JB, Barbe F, Laplace M, Crozatier B, Hittinger L (1995) Regional alterations of left ventricular contraction and inotropic reserve in conscious dogs with heart failure. Cardiovasc Res 30: 848–856

37. Vatner DE, Sato N, Kiuchi K, Shannon RP, Vatner SF (1994) Decrease in myocardial ryanodine receptors and altered excitation-contraction coupling early in the development of heart failure. Circulation 90: 1423–1430

38. Wier WG, Yue DT (1986) Intracellular calcium transients underlying the short-term force-interval relationship in ferret ventricular myocardium. J Physiol (Lond) 376: 507–530

39. Yue DT, Burkhoff D, Franz MR, Hunter WC, Sagawa K (1985) Postextrasystolic potentiation of the isolated canine left ventricle. Relationship to mechanical restitution. Circ Res 56: 340–350

Author's address:
Bertrand Crozatier
Unité INSERM U400
Faculté de Médecine
8, rue du Général Sarrail
Creteil, France

Heart rate as a determinant of L-type Ca^{2+} channel activity: Mechanisms and implication in force-frequency relation

S. Lemaire, C. Piot, F. Leclercq, V. Leuranguer, J. Nargeot, S. Richard

Institut de Génétique Humaine, CNRS, UPR 1142, Montpellier, France

Abstract

Early studies in enzymatically isolated animal cardiomyocytes indicated that voltage-gated "L-type" Ca^{2+} currents (I$_{CaL}$) can be upregulated following an increase of the frequency of activation. Recently, we evidenced a similar regulation of I$_{CaL}$ in human cardiomyocytes from both left and right ventricles and atria over a physiopathological range of stimulations (between 0.5 and 5 Hz). This regulation, enhanced by the β-adrenergic stimulation, may be involved in the frequency-dependent potentiation of cardiac contractile force in the human healthy myocardium. We show here that the frequency-dependent regulation of I$_{CaL}$ is controled by the level of phosphorylation, as well as dephosphorylation, of the Ca^{2+} channels. It was enhanced following activation of the protein kinase A activated by intracellular cyclic AMP (cAMP). Therefore, we anticipate that all agents stimulating cAMP production will favor this process, which was demonstrated here by activating 5HT-4 receptors using serotonin. Alternatively, it was also enhanced by the phosphatase inhibitor okadaic acid which prevents Ca^{2+} channels dephosphorylation. Alteration or abnormal modulation by β-adrenergic receptor stimulation of the frequency-dependent facilitation of I$_{CaL}$ may partly explain the altered force-frequency relation described in heart failure.

Key words Human cardiomyocytes – Ca^{2+} channels – frequency-induced upregulation – force-frequency relation – β-adrenergic stimulation

Introduction

Heart rate has long been known as a determinant of cardiac performance. In many animal species, it has been shown that increasing the cardiac frequency induces a positive inotropic effect, known as the force-frequency relation or Bowditch "staircase" (4). Recent experiments showing amplification of the force-frequency relation by β-adrenergic receptor stimulation and by exercise in vivo have reemphasized the importance of this potent inotropic mechanism in the physiology of the normal heart (46). Various subcellular mechanisms have been proposed to be involved in the force-frequency relation. Curiously, a role of L-type Ca^{2+} channels, which constitute a major target of the β-adrenergic receptor stimulation, has been ignored or minimized. The aim of this paper is to show that the activity of

L- (but not T-) type Ca^{2+} channels is regulated by their frequency of activation and that they may, thereby, be involved in the regulation of the force frequency-relation.

Force-frequency relationship

The frequency-dependent potentiation of cardiac contractile force was first described by Bowditch in 1871 (4). Since then, numerous studies have shown that the positive force-frequency relation is present in vitro in most animal species (12, 22, 49), including humans (6). Moreover, increased contractility (positive inotropic effect) in response to rapid atrial pacing has been demonstrated in vivo in healthy patients with normal left ventricular function (16). Although the molecular events underlying the force-frequency effect on inotropic state are not perfectly understood, multiple mechanisms have been proposed. There is evidence to suggest that under basal conditions this phenomenon is related to increased Ca^{2+} availability for the myofilaments (29). Pieske et al., using the bioluminescent protein aequorin to measure intracellular Ca^{2+} cycling, also showed recently that the force-frequency relation of human nonfailing myocardium results from frequency-dependent increases in the intracellular Ca^{2+} transients (39). An increased amount of Ca^{2+} released from the sarcoplasmic reticulum at higher rates of stimulation was suggested to result from both enhanced transsarcolemmal Ca^{2+} influx through the L-type Ca^{2+} channels per unit of time and reduced time available for diastolic Ca^{2+} efflux through the Na^{+}/Ca^{2+} exchanger leading to greater filling of the sarcoplasmic reticulum (2).

Frequency-dependent potentiation of cardiac contractile force appears to be a major physiological mechanism for the regulation of myocardial performance in the normal heart in vivo. In physiological conditions, increased reflex norepinephrine release and circulating catecholamines during exercise induce both positive inotropic and chronotropic effects, so that heart rate changes are always coupled with contractility changes. To study the effects of heart rate alone during exercise in conscious dogs, Miura et al. controlled the atrial rate by atrial pacing after pharmacologically slowing the spontaneous sinus rate (28). They showed a pronounced negative inotropic influence after slowing the heart rate, supporting the conclusion that heart rate per se influences myocardial contractility during exercise. Using the same experimental canine model, Kambayashi et al. demonstrated that β-adrenergic stimulation with graded perfusion of dobutamine under resting conditions causes a dose-dependent increase of the force-frequency potentiation (19). In addition to the direct myocardial effect of β-adrenergic receptor stimulation and the basal force-frequency relation at rest, these results suggest that the amplification of the force-frequency effect during β-adrenergic stimulation is an important indirect mechanism regulating myocardial contractility in vivo (46). Both phosphorylation of L-type Ca^{2+} channels by cAMP-dependent protein kinase A, which enhances transsarcolemmal Ca^{2+} entry, and phosphorylation of phospholamban, which increases sarcoplasmic reticulum Ca^{2+} loading via regulation of Ca^{2+} pump ATPase, may theoretically be involved in the amplification by β-adrenergic stimulation of the force-frequency effect on myocardial contraction.

Recent experiments in isolated myocardium from patients with heart failure demonstrated that the high frequency-induced potentiation of cardiac contractile force was significantly impaired or absent, depending on stages of heart failure (30, 38, 47). Similar findings were demonstrated by increasing pacing rates during atrial or ventricular stimulation in human hearts with low left ventricular function (10, 16). Pieske et al. observed that the decline in contractility at higher rates of stimulation was associated with a decrease in the free intracellular Ca^{2+} concentration in failing human myocardium (39). These data indicate that the altered force-frequency relation in failing human myocardium may result from decreased intracellular Ca^{2+} transients at higher stimulation frequencies. A reduced amount of Ca^{2+} entering the cell through L-type Ca^{2+} channel, a reduced sarcoplasmic reticulum Ca^{2+} uptake capacity or a defect of the sarcoplasmic reticulum Ca^{2+} release channels may contribute to explain these findings. In contrast, changes in Ca^{2+} sensitivity or changes in the behavior of the contractile proteins appear to be unlikely. Moreover, it was shown recently that β-adrenergic amplification of the force-frequency effect on myocardial contractility was impaired in pigs with cardiac failure (8). Since a number of steps in the β-adrenergic stimulation pathway have been described as abnormal in human failing heart, loss of β-adrenergic control of the force-frequency relation may have a major functional significance in patients with heart failure (46).

Transmembrane Ca^{2+} channels in cardiac cells

Voltage-gated Ca^{2+} channels are the main route for Ca^{2+} entry into cardiac myocytes and, thereby, have a major role in the development and control of both heart contractility and pacemaking activity (15, 25, 55). These proteins can transduce an electrical signal (membrane depolarization) into a chemical signal (transarcolemmal Ca^{2+} influx) during the transient action potential. Cardiac cells express only two types of transmembrane Ca^{2+} currents (I_{Ca}): the L-type I_{Ca} (I_{CaL}; L for "long lasting"), which corresponds to the "slow inward current" originally observed in multicellular preparations 30 years ago (25, 42, 45), and the T-type I_{Ca} (I_{CaT}; T for "transient") discovered a decade ago using patch-clamp experiments (1, 25). The L- and T-type Ca^{2+} channels have clearly distinct electrophysiological and pharmacological properties. Overall, they are distinguished commonly by their activation threshold and their sensitivity to sustained depolarization. I_{CaL} is activated by strong depolarizations (> −40 mV). I_{CaT} is low-voltage-activated (> −60 mV). I_{CaL} is fully available at the resting membrane potentials of −50 mV whereas I_{CaT} requires more negative voltages (< −50 mV). I_{CaL} is the target of different exogenous synthetic ligands, termed "Ca^{2+} channels modulators", such as dihydropyridines (DHPs), phenylalkylamines, and benzothiazepines. In contrast, there is a deficit of specific ligands for I_{CaT} though the new I_{CaT}-selective compound Ro 40-5967 (mibefradil) opens interesting perspectives.

The structural characterization of L-type Ca^{2+} channels has been performed in two steps: purification of the Ca^{2+} channel provided the subunit composition of this multimeric protein and molecular cloning identified several genes encoding the different subunits. Specific ligands such as DHPs and the discovery of a rich source of high affinity DHP-receptors in skeletal muscle T-tubules (11) has allowed demonstration that skeletal muscle L-type Ca^{2+} channels are formed of several associated subunits: the pore-forming subunit α1 which bears pharmacological binding sites for Ca^{2+} channel modulators, the α2 subunit associated via a disulfide bridge to the δ subunit, a cytoplasmic β subunit, and a γ subunit. It is believed that cardiac L-type Ca^{2+} channels are also formed by the association of an α1 subunit with α2-δ and β subunits related to that from skeletal muscle (Fig. 1A). Molecular cloning and structure-function studies in heterologous expression systems have provided insights in the molecular basis of α1 subunit of the cardiac L-type Ca^{2+} channel. It is encoded by the Class C gene and exhibits alternative splicing variants that are able to carry

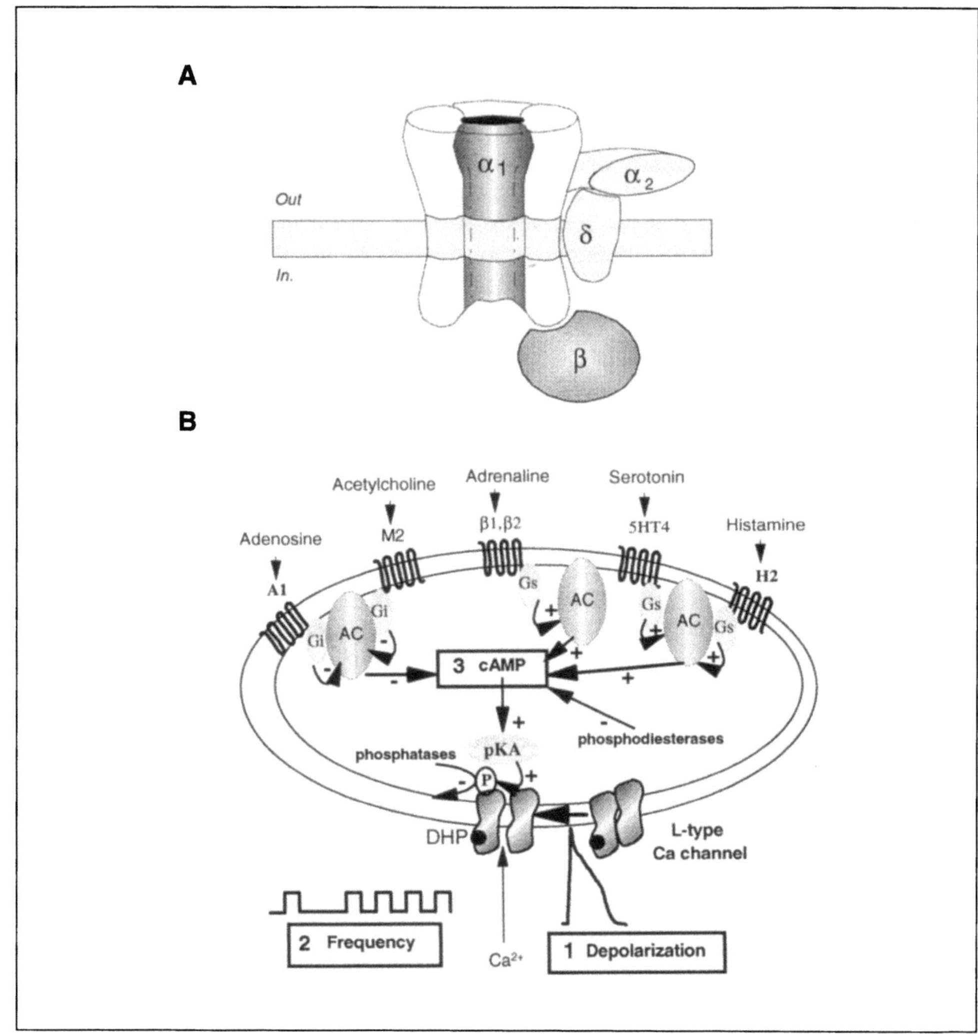

Fig. 1 Structure and major regulations of the cardiac L-type Ca^{2+} channel. (A) The cardiac L-type Ca^{2+} channel is composed of three subunits: the transmembrane $\alpha1$ and $\alpha2$-γ subunits and the cytoplasmic β-subunit. (B) Regulation of the cardiac L-type Ca^{2+} channel. Membrane depolarization during the action potential is the primary effector (1). Frequency of activation (i.e., time-dependent gating properties during the diastolic interval between action potentials) is also an important determinant of Ca^{2+} channel activity (2). Intracellular cAMP, augmented or, alternatively, decreased by various hormones and transmitter systems, modulates protein kinase A and, thereby, Ca^{2+} channel activity (3).

specific pharmacological profiles (51). Taken together, these results indicate that a first degree of diversity in L-type Ca^{2+} channels is provided by $\alpha1$ subunit(s). A second degree of diversity may be brought about by the variety of combinations with different β subunits (four genes identified). Of major interest, the β subunits are to be considered as endogenous modulators of Ca^{2+} channel activity ($\alpha1$ subunit) influencing their electrical as well as their pharmacological properties. In contrast, one must realize that the gene(s) encoding the T-type Ca^{2+} channels has (have) not yet been identified, owed to the lack of specific ligands which has impaired their structural and functional characterization.

I_{CaL} is the trigger of the cardiac excitation-contraction coupling. The influx of Ca^{2+} through L-type Ca^{2+} channels is responsible for the action potential plateau and induces a release of Ca^{2+} ions from sarcoplasmic reticulum, a process named "Ca^{2+} induced-Ca^{2+} release" which evokes the contraction (2). The function of the T-type Ca^{2+} channel is largely unknown but because of its low threshold of activation or its high expression in sino-atrial node cells, a role in pacemaking activity has been suggested (14). I_{CaT} is not detected electrophysiologically in adult rat ventricular and human atrial cells (24, 34, 43, 44).

Regulation of L-type Ca^{2+} channels activity

Ca^{2+} channels are closed at the normal membrane resting potentials. During the fast upstroke of the action potential, they are gated into open state by membrane depolarization (Fig. 1B). Although voltage is the primary effector, modulation of Ca^{2+} channels activity by a variety of neurotransmitters, hormones, drugs, and intracellular second messengers is also fundamental (15, 25, 55). Best known is the regulation of I_{CaL} by β-adrenergic receptors stimulation via a protein kinase A-dependent phosphorylation pathway. Activation of β1 as well as β2 adrenergic receptors stimulates the production of intracellular second messenger cAMP via Gs protein and adenylate-cyclase cascade (Fig. 1B). Liberation of catalytic subunits of protein kinase A by cAMP increases both the availability and the opening probability of Ca^{2+} channels via the phosphorylation of either the Ca^{2+} channel protein itself or another closely associated protein (25, 32, 55). The large increase in I_{CaL} peak amplitude explains in part the positive inotropic effect observed on cardiac myocytes in the presence of β-adrenergic agonists.

Frequency-dependent regulation of I$_{CaL}$

In addition to membrane depolarization and Ca^{2+} channel phosphorylation, modulation of I_{CaL} by frequency of Ca^{2+} channel activation is also probably of major importance for heart physiology (Fig. 1B). Early studies suggested that an increase in the rate of cell stimulation can up-regulate Ca^{2+} channel activity in cardiac cells. Noble and Shimoni (33) were the first to report this regulation in frog atrial fibers which was confirmed later at the single cell level (48). Despite differences in terms of kinetics and underlying mechanisms, similar effects were described in enzymatically dissociated mammalian heart cells (9, 23, 37, 43, 44, 54, 56). Although these effects were not always consistent among studies (20), it is now clear that an increase in the rate of cell stimulation induces two opposite effects depending on the experimental recording conditions used. Decrease of I_{CaL} occurs when cells are stimulated from depolarized membrane holding potentials, reflecting a reduction of Ca^{2+} channel availability for opening because of incomplete voltage-dependent reactivation (9, 18, 26, 37, 44). Indeed, full recovery from inactivation requires more negative membrane potentials. Alternatively, an increase in the rate of stimulation can produce a potentiation of I_{CaL} only when cells are stimulated from negative holding potentials (9, 23, 27, 33, 37,

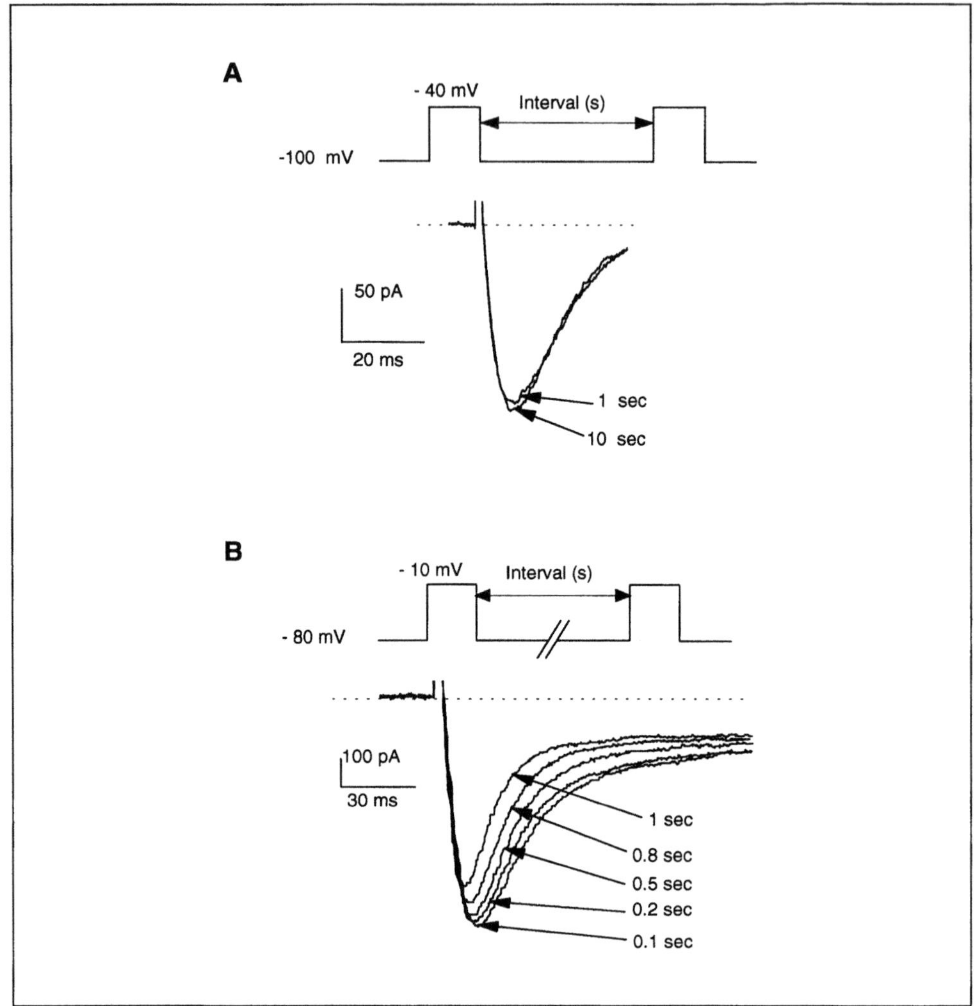

Fig. 2 Effect of the frequency of stimulation on I_{CaT} and I_{CaL} in cardiomyocytes. (A) Waveform of I_{CaT} evoked at –40 mV from HP –100 mV using stimulation frequencies of, respectively, 0.1 Hz and 1 Hz in a freshly isolated neonatal rat ventricular cell. There is no change of current waveform. A similar result was observed in all of 7 cells tested. (B) Different waveforms of I_{CaL} evoked at –10 mV from HP –80 mV using various frequencies of stimulation, i.e., various durations of the diastolic interval between stimulations: 0.1, 0.2, 0.5, 0.8, and 1 seconds interpulses (as quoted) in a human atrial myocyte. Note the graded slowing of I_{Ca} decay with shortening intervals.
Methods: Human cardiomyocytes were obtained and enzymatically (0.5 mg/ml protease, type 14, Sigma; 0.6 mg/ml collagenase, type 1, clostridium histolyticum and 0.2 mg/ml elastase, Boehringer Mannheim) isolated as described before (34–36, 41). Neonatal rat ventricular cells were prepared from 1 day old animals using a similar enzymatic procedure. In both cases, I_{Ca} were recorded and measured as described previously (41, 43, 44, 52, 53). Bath solution contained (mmol/l): TEACl (140), $CaCl_2$ (2), $MgCl_2$ (1.1), 4-AP (4), HEPES (25); adjusted to pH 7.4 with TEAOH. Recording pipettes contained (in mmol/l): CsCl (130), EGTA (10), HEPES (25), (Mg) ATP (3), (Mg) GTP (0.4); adjusted to pH = 7.4 with CsOH. The waveforms of I_{Ca} were measured at room temperature 2 to 10 hours after cell dispersion using the whole-cell patch-clamp technique (amplifier Biologic model RK-300, Grenoble, France) as described before (44). Use-dependent facilitation of I_{Ca} was examined using trains of stimulation at various rates (41).

43, 44, 48, 53, 54). In mammalian cardiomyocytes, the high frequency-induced potentiation of I_{CaL} consists of both a moderate increase of peak current amplitude and a marked slowing of the inactivation kinetics. The increase of peak I_{CaL} is only a consequence of the slowing of current decay which has been proposed to reflect a time-, voltage-, and Ca^{2+}-dependent overshoot in the reactivation of I_{CaL} (37, 44, 54). It should be noted that another type of voltage-dependent facilitation, which is independent of the rate of stimulation, has been described (40, 52). It is also worth noting that, in cardiac cells, T-type Ca^{2+} channels are not subject to modulation by the rate of activation as illustrated in Fig. 2A.

We have revently shown that I_{CaL} can also be up-regulated by the rate of activation in human cardioymocytes (41). This regulation was observed in myocytes from both right and left atria and ventricles. Therefore, frequency-dependent facilitation of I_{CaL} seems to be a general feature of human cardiomyocytes, i.e., irrespective of their topological origin. As illustrated in the right atrial human cardiomyocyte (Fig. 2B), I_{CaL} peak amplitude is augmented and its decay is slowed when the rate of activation of Ca^{2+} channels is increased from 0.1 Hz to 1 Hz. This change of I_{CaL} waveform, which contributes to increased Ca^{2+} influx during depolarization, occurs at all voltages activating an inward I_{CaL} (41). Interestingly, I_{CaL} is potentiated in a graded manner with increasing rates of stimulation (between 0.5 Hz and 5 Hz), i.e., with decreasing diastolic interval between two stimulations (Fig. 2B). As in animal cardiomyocytes, a negative membrane resting potential is required. There is no frequency-dependent potentiation when I_{CaL} is evoked from resting membrane potentials positive to -50 mV (41). Rather, no effect or a decrease in effect is observed with voltage-dependent inactivation of Ca^{2+} channels. Interestingly and in contrast with results obtained from hundreds of rat ventricular cells in our laboratory, this regulation was not found in all human cardiomyocytes. In particular, we determined that it was altered in cardiomyocytes of patients with end-stage heart failure (ejection fraction < 40 %) and in those of patients treated with Ca^{2+} channel antagonists or/and β-adrenergic blockers (41). Therefore, the ability of L-type Ca^{2+} channels to be regulated by the frequency of activation may be a feature of the healthy heart.

Regulation by cAMP-dependent phosphorylation of Ca^{2+} channels

We have shown that β-adrenergic receptor stimulation enhances the high frequency-induced upregulation of I_{CaL} in human cardiomyocytes (41). As illustrated in Fig. 3A, and in addition to its well-known potentiating effect on peak current, isoproterenol induced the frequency-dependent facilitation of I_{CaL} which was absent in control conditions. Therefore, a higher rate of activation, which is expected from the positive chronotropic effect of the β-adrenergic stimulation, is likely to amplify the direct effect of the β-adrenergic stimulation on L-type Ca^{2+} channels activity contributing to further increase of Ca^{2+} entry during the depolarization. This effect is related to changes in the gating properties rather than an increase in the number of activable Ca^{2+} channels (43, 44).

Enhancement of the frequency-dependent facilitation of I_{CaL} by β-adrenergic stimulation involves cAMP-dependent phosphorylation of the L-type Ca^{2+} channels in rat ventricular cells (53). Fig. 3B shows that the permeable analogue dibutyryl cAMP, by

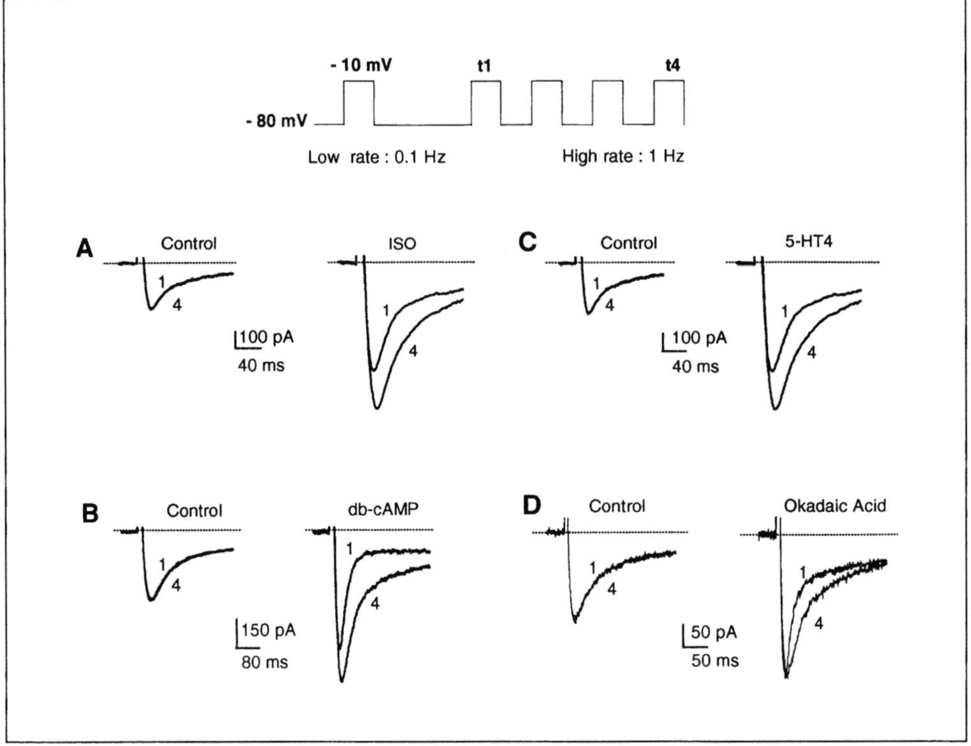

Fig. 3 Modulation by cAMP-dependent phosphorylation in human atrial cells. Waveforms of I_{CaL} recorded at, respectively, 0.1 Hz and 1 Hz in the absence and presence of 1 µM Isoproterenol (A), 100 µM dibutyryl-cAMP (B), 1 µM serotonine (C) or 1 µM okadaic acid (D).

Methods: Cells were prepared and stimulated as described in Fig. 2. Drugs (Sigma) were prepared as concentrated stock solutions which were diluted at the desired working concentrations in the test solution. Control and test solutions were applied to the exterior of each cell tested using a multiple capillary perfusion system placed in the vicinity of the cell (41, 52). Each capillary is fed by a reservoir 50 cm above the bath. Rapid (at most seconds) and complete solution changes can be made by switching from the opening from one capillary to the next.

directly activating the intracellular protein kinase A, can also promote the high frequency-induced upregulation of I_{CaL} in human cardiomyocytes, mimicking β-adrenergic receptors stimulation. Therefore, one would expect such a modulation for all factors stimulating intracellular cAMP production. To further test this hypothesis, we assessed the effect of serotonin which stimulates 5-HT$_4$ receptors in human atrial myocytes and, thereby, increases I_{CaL} by activating cAMP cascade (35). Fig. 3C shows that stimulation of 5-HT$_4$ receptors by serotonin first increases peak I_{CaL}, but also can result in the promotion of the high frequency-induced upregulation of I_{CaL}.

These data suggest that cAMP-dependent phosphorylation of L-type Ca^{2+} channels is a key event modulating the forcefrequency regulation of I_{CaL} in human cardiomyocytes. Therefore, we hypothesized that preventing dephosphorylation of L-type Ca^{2+} channels is also an alternative to enhance the frequency-dependent facilitation of I_{CaL}. Indeed, the phosphorylated state of Ca^{2+} channels, and thereby current amplitude, is the product of a dynamic equilibrium between phosphorylation and dephosphorylation processes. To assess this hypothesis, we exposed the cardiac cells to the phosphatase inhibitor okadaic acid known to increase I_{CaL} in absence of β-adrenergic receptors stimulation (17, 21). Fig. 3D shows that okadaic acid increases I_{CaL} peak amplitude and can promote the frequency-dependent facilitation of I_{CaL}. Therefore, frequency-dependent regulation of L-type Ca^{2+} channels can be modulated by both phosphorylation and dephosphorylation.

Physiological significance of the frequency-dependent facilitation of I_{CaL}

In addition to other intracellular mechanisms, the high frequency-induced upregulation of L-type Ca^{2+} channels has been suggested to be involved in the frequency-dependent potentiation of cardiac contractile force in the human healthy myocardium by Piot et al. (41). Indeed, this sophisticated and short term regulatory system which ensures a fine graded augmentation of transmembrane Ca^{2+} entry at higher rates of stimulation, allows a sudden adjustment of intracellular Ca^{2+} loading and, as a natural consequence, of myocardial contractility. Of major interest, it occurs over a range of frequencies corresponding to heart rates frequently encountered in human physiopathology. This process, which is highly sensitive to β-adrenergic receptors stimulation via a cAMP pathway, may be also a major mechanism involved in the amplification by β-adrenergic stimulation of the force-frequency effect on myocardial contraction (Fig. 4). Moreover, it would confer a key role to L-type Ca^{2+} channels in the notion of myocardic reserve. Persons, such as athletes, provided with a low heart beating rate (e.g., 40/50 beats per min) would be expected to have more reserve in terms of increased transmembrane Ca^{2+} entry during severe exercise (e.g., 180 beats per

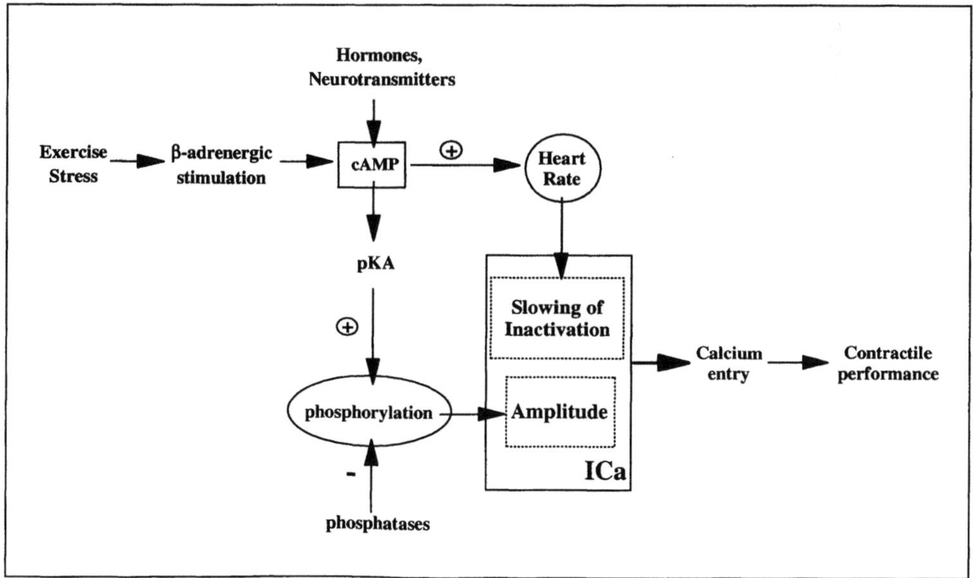

Fig. 4 Hypothetical scheme of the role and regulation of the frequency-dependent modulation of I_{CaL} in the human heart.

min) than those who have an already high heart beating rate (e.g., 80–100 beat per min) at rest. Thus, we anticipate that this regulation of transmembrane Ca^{2+} influx may be crucial in the adaptation of the nonfailing human heart to stress and exervise (Fig. 4).

Of major interest, many neurotransmitters and hormones receptors are also positively or negatively coupled to adenylate cyclase, modulating protein kinase A-dependent regulation and, thereby, modulating frequency-dependent facilitation of Ca^{2+} channel activity (Fig. 4). A variety of drugs acting at different levels of the β-adrenergic cascade, such as β-adrenergic agonists or antagonists and phosphodiesterases inhibitors, are used clinically to modulate cardiac inotropism via cAMP-dependent phosphorylation of L-type Ca^{2+} channels. According to this mechanism, heart rate needs to be considered in order to better understand inotropic effect of these drugs.

Frequency-dependent facilitation of I_{CaL} in failing heart

In addition to abnormal intracellular $[Ca^{2+}]_i$ handling (3, 13, 22), both high frequency-induced upregulation and β-adrenergic stimulation of I_{CaL} have been described as abnormal in failing human myocardium (36, 41). An alteration of transarcolemmal Ca^{2+} signaling via L-type voltage-gated Ca^{2+} channels may partly explain the altered force-frequency relation described in heart failure (10, 16, 30, 38, 39, 47). Moreover, an abnormal modulation of the frequency-dependent facilitation of I_{CaL} by β-adrenergic receptor stimulation may partly explain the loss of β-adrenergic control of the force-frequency relation in these patients (46). Indeed, stimulation by isoprenaline preserves the positive force-frequency in the non-failing myocardium but fails to restore it in the failing human heart (50). It is possible that this observation reflects simply a down regulation of β-adrenergic receptors in the failing hearts (5, 31), which leads to lower intracellular cAMP. However, it is also possible that Ca^{2+} channels themselves are altered in terms of structure (nature or stoichiometry of associated subunits) or of regulation by second messengers and phosphorylating-dephos-phorylating agents.

The frequency-dependent facilitation of I_{CaL} was also altered in patients pretreated with Ca^{2+} antagonists and/or β-blockers (i.e., classes IV and II of Vaughan-Williams) (41). Very interestingly, it can be partly restored in presence of isoproterenol both in nonfailing and failing patients but not in failing hearts that were not pretreated (41). These observations suggest two ideas: (i) that the regulation is altered by the disease itself in those patients that are not protected from Ca^{2+} overload at high rates of stimulation, and (ii) that agents that minimize Ca^{2+} overload preserve cell integrity and, thereby, prevent complete alteration of the regulation of Ca^{2+} channel activity by high rates of stimulation.

Concluding remarks and perspectives

The activity of cardiac L-type Ca^{2+} channels is expected to depend markedly on the heart rate which finely controls the duration and amount of Ca^{2+} influx and, thereby, the amplitude of the contraction. The frequency-dependent facilitation of I_{CaL} may explain, at least in part, both the frequency-dependent potentiation of cardiac contractile force and its amplification by β-adrenergic receptors stimulation in the human healthy myocardium. Such a rapid regulation might also be a major adaptive mechanism of the healthy human heart to exercise or stress. Alteration of this mechanism and its implication in failing hearts needs to be confirmed.

At the molecular level, it will be important to explore the mechanisms involved in the frequency-dependent facilitation of Ca^{2+} channels and the reason for its potential alteration in heart failure. Existence of multiple α1C isoforms and differential regulation by distinct β-subunits are expected to generate Ca^{2+} influx with various waveforms and regulatory profiles by voltage and phosphorylation. For example, the strong predepolarization-dependent facilitation of I_{CaL} expressed from the class C channel is abolished when coexpressed in Xenopus laevis oocytes with the β2 subunit (instead of the β1, β3 or β4 subunits) (7). There is also a real possibility of close interaction between Ca^{2+} channels and other systems which may control its activity (e.g., Ca^{2+} coming from the sarcoplasmic reticulum may exerts local influence on the gating of I_{CaL}) It will also be important to understand how Ca^{2+} channel activity is altered in heart failure and the mechanisms underlying the cardioprotective effects of agents targeting Ca^{2+} channels.

Acknowledgments We thank Stuart Hutchison for helpful comments on the manuscript. This work was supported by grants of the Association "Recherche et Partage" (to SR), the "Association Française contre les Myopathies", and the french MENESR (ACCSV9).

References

1. Bean BP (1985) Two kinds of calcium channels in canine atrial cells. Differences in kinetics, selectivity, and pharmacology. J Gen Physiol 86: 1–30
2. Bers DM (1991) Ca regulation in cardiac muscle. Med Sci Sports Exerc 23 (10): 1157–1162
3. Beuckelmann DJ, Näbauer M, Erdmann E (1992) Intracellular calcium handling in isolated ventricular myocytes from patients with terminal heart failure. Circulation 85: 1046–1055
4. Bowditch HP (1871) Uber die Eigenthûmlichkeiten der Reizbarkeit, welche die Muskelfarsen des Herzens zeigen. Arb Physiol Anst Leipzig 6: 139–176
5. Bristow MR, Ginsburg R, Minobe W, Cubiciotti RS, Sageman V, Lurie K, Billingham ME, Harrison DC, Stinson EB (1982) Decreased catecholamine sensitivity and beta-adrenergic-receptor density in failing human hearts. N Engl J Med 307: 205–211
6. Buckley NM, Penefsky ZJ, Litwak RS (1972) Comparative force-frequency relationships in human and other mammalian ventricular myocardium. Pflügers Arch 332: 259–270
7. Cens T, Mangoni M, Richard S, Nargeot J, Charnet (1996) Coexpression of the β2 subunit does not induce voltage-dependent facilitation of the class C 1-type calcium channel. Pflügers Archiv 431: 771–774
8. Eising GP, Hammond HK, Helmer GA, Gilpin E, Ross J Jr (1994) Force-frequency relations during heart failure in the pig. Am J Physiol 267: H2516–H2522
9. Fedida D, Noble D, Spindler AJ (1988) Use-dependent reduction and facilitation of Ca^{2+} current in guinea pig myocytes. J Physiol 405: 439–460
10. Feldman MD, Gwathmey JK, Phillips P, Schoen F, Morgan JP (1988) Reversal of the force-frequency-relationship in working myocardium from patients with endstage heart failure. J Appl Cardiol 3: 273–283
11. Fosset M, Jaimovich E, Delpont E, Lazdunski M (1983) [3H]nitrendipine receptors in skeletal muscle. J Biol Chem 258: 6086–6092
12. Frampton JE, Orchard CH, Boyett MR (1991) Diastolic, systolic and sarcoplasmic reticulum (calcium) during inotropic interventions in isolated rat myocytes. J Physiol 437: 351–375
13. Gwathmey JK, Slawsky MT, Hajjar RJ, Briggs GM, Morgan JP (1990) Role of intracellular calcium handling in force-interval relation-ship of human ventricular myocardium. J Clin Invest 85: 1599–1613
14. Hagiwara N, Irisawa H, Kameyama M (1988) Contribution of two types of calcium currents to the pacemaker potentials of rabbit sino-atrial node cells. J Physiol 395: 233–253
15. Hartzell HC (1988) Regulation of cardiac ion channels by catecholamines, acetylcholine and second messenger system. Prog Biophys Mol Biol 52: 165–247

16. Hasenfuss G, Holubarsch C, Hermann HP, Astheimer K, Pieske B, Just H (1994) Influence of the force-frequency relation on hemodynamics and left ventricular function in patients with nonfailing hearts and in patients with dilated cardiomyopathy. Eur Heart J 15: 164–170

17. Hescheler J, Mieskes G, Ruegg JC, Takai A, Trautwein W (1988) Effects of a protein phosphatase inhibitor, okadaic acid, on membrane currents of isolated guinea pig cardiac myocytes. Pflügers Archiv 412: 248–252

18. Hryshko LV, Bers DM (1990) Calcium current facilitation during postrest recovery depends on calcium entry. Am J Physiol 259: H951–H961

19. Kambayashi M, Miura T, Oh BH, Rockman HA, Murata K, Ross J Jr (1992) Enhancement of the force-frequency effect on myocardial contractility by adrenergic stimulation in conscious dogs. Circulation 86: 572–580

20. Kaspar S, Pelzer DJ (1995) Modulation by stimulation rate of basal and cAMP-elevated Ca^{2+} channel current in guinea pig ventricular cardiomyocytes. J Physiol 106: 175–201

21. Katsushige O, Fozzard HA (1993) Two phosphatase sites on the Ca^{2+} channel affecting different kinetic functions. J Physiol 470: 73–84

22. Koch-Weser J, Blinks JR (1963) The influence of the interval between beats on myocardial contractility. Pharmacol Rev 15: 601–652

23. Lee KS (1987) Potentiation of the calcium-channel currents of internally perfused mammalian heart cells by repetitive depolarisation. Proc Natl Acad Sci USA 84: 3941–3945

24. Le Grand B, Hatem S, Deroubaix E, Couetil JP, Coraboeuf E (1991) Calcium current depression in isolated human atrial myocytes after cessation of chronic treatment with calcium antagonists. Circ Res 69: 292–300

25. McDonald TF, Pelzer S, Trautwein W, Pelzer D (1994) Regulation and modulation of calcium channels in cardiac, skeletal, and smooth muscle cells. Physiol Rev 74 (2): 365–507

26. Mitchell MR, Powell T, Terrar DA, Twist VW (1985) Influence of a change in stimulation rate on action potentials, currents and contraction in rat ventricular cells. J Physiol 364: 113–130

27. Mitra R, Morad M (1986) Two types of calcium channels in guinea-pig ventricular myocytes. Proc Natl Acad Sci USA 83: 5340–5344

28. Miura T, Miyazaki S, Guth SD, Kambayashi M, Ross J Jr (1992) Influence of the force-frequency relation on left ventricular function during exercise in conscious dogs. Circulation 86: 563–571

29. Morgan JP, Blinks JR (1982) Intracellular calcium transients in the cat papillary muscle. Can J Physiol Pharmacol 60: 524–528

30. Mulieri LA, Hasenfuss G, Leavitt B, Allen PD, Alpert NR (1992) Altered myocardial force-frequency relation in human heart. Circulation 85: 1743–1750

31. Muntz KH, Zhao M, Miller, JC (1994) Downregulation of myocardial β-adrenergic receptors. Receptor subtype selectivity. Circ Res 74: 369–375

32. Nerbonne JM, Richard S, Nargeot J, Lester HA (1984) New photoactivable cyclic nucleotides produce intracellular jumps in cyclic AMP and cyclic GMP concentrations. Nature 310: 74–76

33. Noble S, Shimoni Y (1981) The calcium and frequency dependence of the slow inward current "staircase" in frog atrium. J Physiol 310: 57–75

34. Ouadid H, Seguin J, Richard S, Chaptal PA, Nargeot J (1991) Properties and modulation of calcium channels in adult human atrial cells. J Mol Cell Cardiol 23: 41–54

35. Ouadid H, Seguin J, Dumuis A, Bockaert, Nargeot J (1992) Serotonin increases calcium current in human atrial myocytes via the newly described 5-hydroxytryptamine receptors. Mol Pharmacol 25: 282– 291

36. Ouadid H, Albat, B, Nargeot, J (1995) Calcium currents in diseased human cardiac cells. J Cardiovasc Pharmacol 25: 282–291

37. Peineau N, Garnier D, Argibay JA (1992) Rate dependence of action potential duration and calcium current in isolated guinea pig cardiocytes. Exp Physiol 77: 615–625

38. Pieske B, Hasenfuss G, Holubarsch R, Shwinger R, Bôhm M, Just H (1992) Alteration of the force-frequency relationship in the failing human heart depend on the underlying cardiac disease. Basic Res Cardiol 87: 213–221

39. Pieske B, Kretschmann B, Meyer M, Holubarsch C, Weirich J, Posival H, Minami K, Just H, Hasenfuss G (1995) Alterations in intracellular calcium handling associated with the inverse force-frequency relation in human dilated cardiomyopathy. Circulation 92: 1169–1178

40. Pietrobon D, Hess P (1990) Novel mechanism of voltage-dependent gating in L-type calcium channels. Nature 346: 192–193

41. Piot C, Lemaire S, Albat B, Seguin J, Nargeot J, Richard S (1996) High frequency-induced upregulation of human cardiac calcium currents. Circulation 93: 120–128

42. Reuter H (1967) The dependence of slow inward current in Purkinje fibers on the extracellular calcium concentration. J Physiol 192: 479–492

43. Richard S, Tiaho F, Charnet P, Nargeot J, Nerbonne JM (1990) Two pathways for Ca^{2+} channel gating differentially modulated by physiological stimuli. Am J Physiol 258: H1872–1881

44. Richard S, Charnet P, Nerbonne JM (1993) Voltage- and time-dependent interconversion between distinct gating pathways of the high threshold cardiac calcium channel. J Physiol 462: 197–228

45. Rougier O, Vassort G, Garnier D, Gargouil YM, Coraboeuf E (1969) Existence and role of a slow inward current during the frog atrial potential. Pflügers Arch 308: 91–110
46. Ross J Jr, Miura T, Kambayashi M, Eising GP, Ryu K (1995) Adrenergic control of the force-frequency relation. Circulation 92: 2327–2332
47. Schmidt U, Schwinger RH, Bôhm M, Erdmann E (1994) Alterations of the force-frequency relation depending on stages of heart failure in humans. Am J Cardiol 74: 1066–1068
48. Schouten VJ, Morad M (1989) Regulation of Ca^{2+} current in frog ventricular myocytes by the holding potential, cAMP and frequency. Pflügers Arch 415: 1–11
49. Schouten VJ, Ter Keurs H (1991) Role of calcium current and Na/Ca exchange in the force-frequency relationship of rat heart muscle. J Moll Cell Cardiol 23: 1039–1050
50. Schwinger RHG, Bôhm M, Muller-Ehmensen J, Uhlman R, Schmidt U, Stablein A, Uberfuhr P, Kreuzer E, Reichart B, Eissner HJ, Erdman E (1993) Effect of inotropic stimulation of the negative force-frequency relationship in the failing human heart. Circulation 88: 2267–2276
51. Soldatov NM, Bouron A, Reuter H (1995) Different voltage-dependent inhibition by dihydropyridines of human Ca^{2+} channel splice variants. J Biol Chem 270: 10540– 10543
52. Tiaho F, Nargeot J, Richard S (1991) Voltage-dependent regulation of L-type cardiac calcium channels by isoproterenol. Pflügers Arch 419: 586–602
53. Tiaho F, Piot C, Nargeot J, Richard S (1994) Regulation of the frequency-dependent facilitation of L-type calcium currents in rat ventricular cells. J Physiol 477: 237–252
54. Tseng GN (1988) Calcium current restitution in mammalian ventricular myocytes is modulated by intracellular calcium. Circ Res 63: 468–482
55. Tsien RW, Bean BP, Hess P, Lansman JB, Nilius B, Nowycky MC (1986) Mechanisms of calcium channel modulation by β-adrenergic agents and dihydropyridine calcium agonists. J Mol Cell Cardiol 18: 691–710
56. Zygmundt AC, Maylie J (1990) Stimulation-dependent facilitation of the high threshold calcium current in guinea-pig ventricular myocytes. J Physiol 428: 653–671

Author's address:
S. Richard
Institut de Génétique Humaine,
CNRS, UPR 1142
141 Rue de la Cardonille
34296 Montpellier Cedex 5
France

Electrophysiological aspects of changes in heart rate

U. Ravens, E. Wettwer

Institut für Pharmakologie und Toxikologie, Universitätsklinikum Carl-Gustav-Carus,
Technische Universität Dresden

Abstract

Cardiac action potentials undergo characteristic changes in response to increasing pacing
frequency, i.e., the resting potential becomes less negative (depolarization), the amplitude
decreases, and the action potential duration (APD) shortens. The electrophysiological
properties of the major cardiac inward and outward currents are discussed with respect to
their possible contribution to rate-dependent changes in AP shape. Short diastolic intervals
may not allow sufficient time for channel recovery. Incomplete recovery from inactivation
will reduce both inward (I_{Na}, I_{Ca}) and outward (I_{to}) currents and hence lead to APD
shortening or prolongation, respectively. Incomplete deactivation during diastole will
increase current and, in the case of the delayed rectifier I_{Ks}, produces rate-dependent APD
shortening. Heterogeneity in current density of myocytes from various regions within the
ventricular wall complicates the direct translation of rate-dependent changes in APD into
changes of the QT interval of the ECG.

With increasing rates of stimulation, K^+ accumulates within the tubular system. Membrane depolarization may be attributed to this frequency-dependent increase in $[K^+]_o$,
whereas APD shortening is not mimicked by high $[K^+]_o$. Nevertheless, the various cardiac
K^+ channels differ in their sensitivity to extracellular $[K^+]_o$. Some of the frequency-dependent effects of drugs with class III action may be related to an influence of $[K^+]_o$ on drug
potency to block K^+ channels.

Key words Heart rate – action potentials – membrane currents – K^+ currents –
K^+ accumulation – antiarrhythmic drugs with class III action

Introduction

The relationship between the QT interval of the electrocardiogram and heart rate was
discovered by Bazett in 1920 (5). In later years, the microelectrode technique was adapted
for application in isolated heart muscle (10) and provided a direct approach for investigating the relationship between intracellular action potentials (AP) and stimulation frequency
in isolated heart muscle (30).

Factors influencing the cardiac action potential

The shape of the action potential (AP) is determined by current flow across the sarcolemma [(29) for references]. Electric current is carried by Na^+, K^+, Ca^{2+}, and Cl^- ions as they move along their transmembrane concentration gradient passing through specific ion channels (37). The influx of Na^+ is responsible for the upstroke of the action potential, the influx of Ca^{2+} maintains the plateau phase, and the efflux of K^+ leads to repolarization. For an in-depth discussion of the particularly large diversity in electrophysiological and molecular properties of K^+ channels, the reader is referred to the excellent review by Barry and Nerbonne (4). Influx of Cl^- also produces repolarizing outward current (16). Additional currents contributing to the action potential are Na^+/Ca^{2+} exchanger and Na^+ pump currents.

Sarcolemmal ion channels open and close in a time- and potential-dependent manner ("gating"), the resulting current flow can be studied with the voltage clamp technique. Upon changes in membrane potential, ion channels are activated by undergoing conformational changes from a closed, non-conducting into an open, conducting state. With maintained depolarization, some ion channels may pass from the open into another non-conducting (inactivated) state, which is different from the resting state and from which they will recover and become available again only after repolarization. This process of "recovery from inactivation" requires time to complete and is an important factor for frequency-dependent modulation.

As current flows, changes in ion concentrations occur on both sides of the sarcolemma. For maintenance of ionic homeostasis, these must be compensated by active transport. If compensation is incomplete, the resulting changes in intra- and extracellular ion concentrations may on their own account influence membrane currents. Accumulation of K^+ ions in the extracellular space with a sudden increase in stimulation frequency has in fact been measured with K^+-sensitive electrodes (21).

Sodium ions are supposed to accumulate in the hypothetical "fuzzy space", a space of restricted diffusion in the close vicinity of the plasma membrane (22), but this so far escaped experimental detection.

Effects of stimulation rate

Frequency-dependent AP changes typically observed in a guinea-pig papillary muscle are illustrated in Fig. 1. With increasing rates of stimulation, the resting potential becomes less negative (depolarization), the action potential amplitude decreases and the action potential duration (APD) is shortened [for early reviews see (7, 8)]. In the example shown, electrical and mechanical alternans develop at 7.5 Hz and above. The concomitant changes in force of contraction, i.e., force-frequency relations, are described elsewhere in this volume. Since the shape of the action potential is determined by the net current flow at any one instant, several individual currents contribute to rate-dependent changes. The putative roles of the major inward and outward currents are going to be discussed in the following sections.

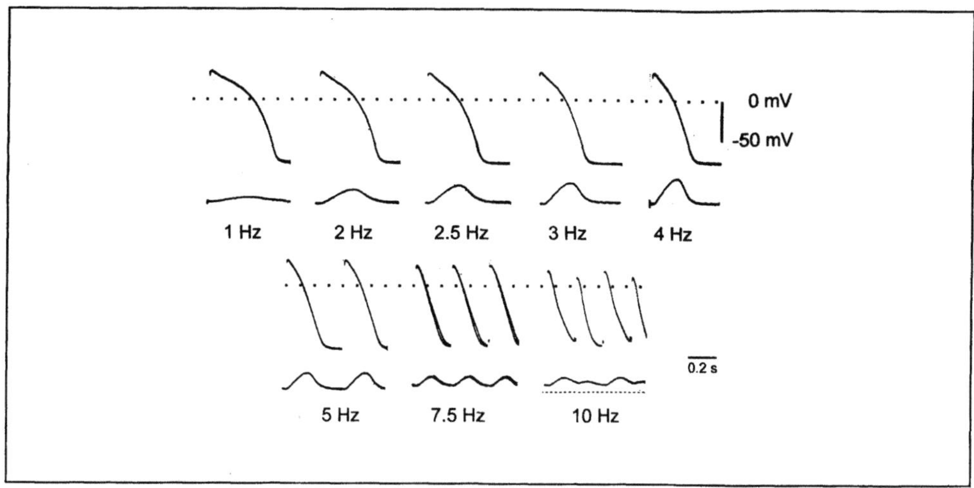

Fig. 1 Frequency-dependence of action potentials in guinea pig right ventricular papillary muscle. The muscle was superfused with oxygenated Tyrode's solution at 32 °C and allowed to equilibrate for at least 1.5 h (stimulation rate 1 Hz) before a stable microelectrode tracing (upper tracings) was recorded together with force of contraction (lower tracings). The frequency was then changed to successively higher values and another recording was taken once the shape of the action potential had stabilized (3–5 min). Dotted horizontal line: level of zero potential; dashed line, passive resting tension. For frequencies of 1–4 Hz force of contraction returned to the level of resting tension between successive beats. Note that electrical and mechanical alternans developed at 7.5 and 10 Hz.

Inward currents I_{Na} and I_{Ca}

I_{Na} In human ventricular myocytes, I_{Na} peaks within 1–2 ms upon a step clamp pulse to the potential of maximum activation (–30 mV); the time course of inactivation is best described by the sum of two exponentials, where 92 % of the current inactivates rapidly (τ_{fast} 2.8 ms) and the rest more slowly [τ_{slow} 16 ms (33)]. Recovery from inactivation is potential dependent; at –100 mV the fast and rapid time constants are 120 ms for τ_{fast} and 461 ms for τ_{slow} (33). These time constants were, however, measured at room temperature and should be much smaller at physiological temperature where the recovery process is faster. Using the maximum depolarization velocity of the action potential upstroke as a surrogate for I_{Na}, recovery from inactivation at resting membrane potential is in the order of 10–30 ms (7). Thus, complete I_{Na} recovery from inactivation is expected to be attained between two successive action potentials as long as increase in frequency does not depolarize the membrane. In that case, the upstroke may decline because Na^+ channel availability is reduced.

I_{Ca} In earlier experiments with the sucrose gap voltage clamp method, the activation and inactivation of I_{Ca} were found to be slow (6). During a train of clamp steps after rest, I_{Ca} decreases from pulse to pulse (31). However, frequency- and time-dependent properties of L-type calcium current have been revised with introduction of the whole cell patch clamp technique. Thus, I_{Ca} kinetics are much faster than originally estimated (17). Details of frequency-dependence of I_{Ca}, and in particular high frequency-induced up-regulation of I_{Ca} are discussed by Richard in this volume (32).

Outward currents I$_{K1}$, I$_K$, and I$_{to}$

The inward rectifier current I$_{K1}$ The major role of the inward rectifier I$_{K1}$, is to stabilize the resting membrane potential. At voltages negative to its reversal potential, the channel passes a large inward current, whereas at more positive potentials, it passes a small outward current. Because of the negative slope in the current-voltage relation of this latter component between -70 and -40 mV, I$_{K1}$ contributes to the fast rate of final repolarization. I$_{K1}$ is almost time-independent and hence governed by membrane potential only. Little is known about direct frequency-dependent changes in current amplitude; however, due to its dependence on extracellular [K$^+$], it may contribute indirectly to frequency related changes in AP configuration. Increasing [K$^+$]$_o$ enhances the outward branch of I$_{K1}$ in addition to shifting the equilibrium potential to more positive voltage [feline myocytes: (11)].

The delayed rectifier current I$_K$ Following voltage-dependent activation, channels for I$_K$ do not inactivate but stay open and deactivate only upon repolarization. Incomplete deactivation of channels before the next action potential arrives will add a background of increasing K$^+$ current that may contribute to the APD shortening at high rates of stimulation.

Recently, two components of I$_K$ have been characterized, which can be distinguished on the basis of their time- and voltage-dependent properties and pharmacological sensitivities (35). The slowly activating current called I$_{Ks}$ (for slowly activating) shows rate dependency (Fig. 2). Current amplitude increases by approximately 25 % with a change in frequency from 30 to 240/min. This increase in outward current contributes to rate-dependent abbreviation of APD (18) .

I$_K$ has recently received much attention as a target for drugs with class III action. Analysis of the drug effect revealed that I$_K$ contains a second component I$_{Kr}$ (for rapid acti-

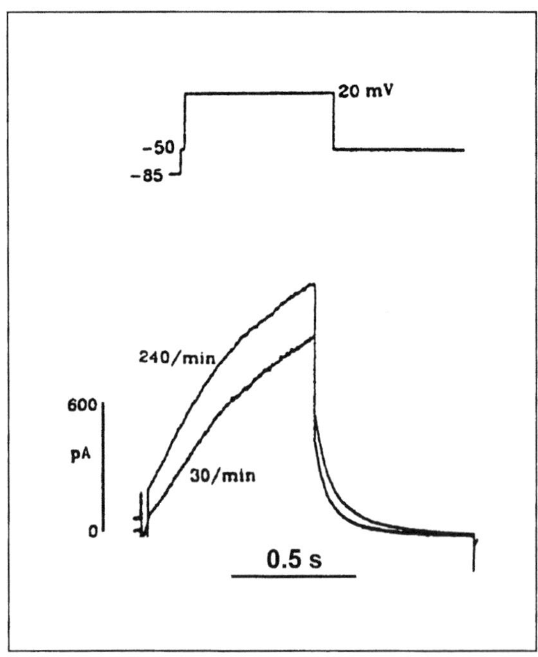

Fig. 2 Rate-dependent increase in the slowly activating delayed rectifier K$^+$ current (I$_{Ks}$) in a guinea pig ventricular myocyte. Top: clamp pulse protocol, bottom: currents measured at a test pulse to + 20 mV, either at 0.5 or 4 Hz, as indicated. Rate dependent increase in I$_{Ks}$ was 24 %. From (18), with permission of the publisher.

vation). In fact, I_{Kr} activates much more rapidly than I_{Ks}, shows strong inward rectification at potentials positive to 10 mV, and can be selectively blocked by methane-sulfonanilide derivatives as for instance E-4031 (35).

The transient outward current I_{to}   Mammalian myocardium contains two components of transient outward current. They can be distinguished by their sensitivity towards Ca^{2+} and 4-aminopyridine (4-AP): I_{to1} is blocked by 4-AP and is insensitive to Ca^{2+}, whereas I_{to2} is 4-AP insensitive and depends on Ca^{2+} (9, 20). The latter current is probably a chloride current (40) and is not measured under voltage-clamp conditions where high Ca^{2+} buffering concentrations of EGTA in the pipette are used. Hence in the following section, I_{to} refers to the Ca^{2+} insensitive component.

There is general agreement that I_{to} is responsible for the prominent "notch" between the upstroke and the plateau phase of human and dog ventricular action potentials (13, 23). I_{to} activates rapidly at the positive potential range of the notch, but is also rapidly inactivated. Because of the rapid kinetics of I_{to} it is not immediately obvious that the current should also account for later phases of repolarization. Nevertheless, several experimental findings suggest an important influence of I_{to} on action potential duration: (i) In failing myocardium, APD is prolonged as compared to nonfailing controls (14) and I_{to} of myocytes from failing hearts is significantly downregulated (19, 25). (ii) In the canine pacing-induced tachycardia model of heart failure, the main electrophysiological features of myocytes were loss of the prominent AP notch and APD prolongation. These characteristics could be reproduced in myocytes from control hearts by blocking I_{to} with 4-aminopyridine (4-AP). Furthermore, 4-AP produced dramatic APD prolongations in myocytes from failing hearts suggesting that these cells depend on the residual I_{to} for timely repolarization (19). (iii) In the same study, APD prolongation could be reversed by artificially recreating the phase-1 notch with an 8 ms repolarizing current pulse delivered shortly after the upstroke of the AP (19). These findings provide evidence that I_{to} may indeed influence late repolarization phases.

Inactivation of I_{to} in human ventricular myocytes is rapid: the time constant of inactivation is 59 ± 4 ms at room temperature and decreases to 25 ± 4 ms at the more physiological temperature of 35 °C (1). After repolarization, inactivated I_{to} channels must recover from inactivation before they can open once more. The recovery process depends on membrane potential. At -100 mV we estimated a time constant of I_{to} recovery from inactivation for the rapid initial phase of 24.0 ± 1.6 ms and this time constant increases at less negative potentials [room temperature (1)]. Therefore, at short intervals between action potentials I_{to} may not completely recover from inactivation; however, as outlined above, reduced I_{to} amplitude at high frequency of stimulation is expected to prolong rather than shorten APD. One important role of I_{to} current could be to set the plateau potential for activation of I_{Ca}.

Heterogeneity of channel distribution
within the ventricular wall

Analysis of rate-dependent changes in APs is complicated by marked variations in shapes of APs that exist within the ventricular wall (24, 26, 38). While APs of epicardial myocytes have a pronounced "spike-and-dome" configuration, APs in endocardial cells show hardly any separation between the early rapid repolarization and the plateau phase (Fig. 3), suggesting smaller I_{to} current amplitude in endo- than in epicardial cells. This variation is

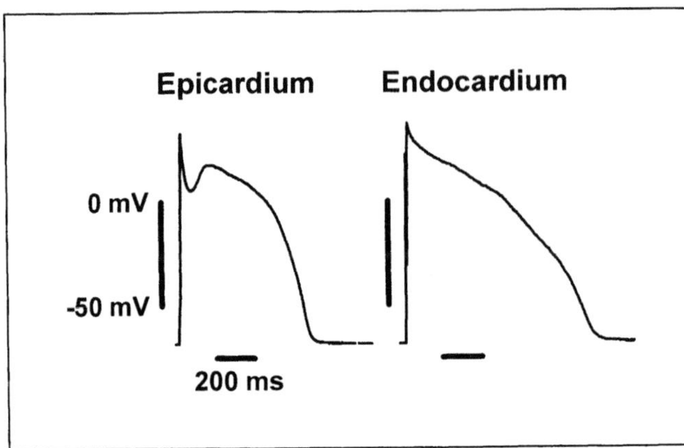

Fig. 3 Transmembrane potentials from human ventricular myocytes of epicardial (left) and endocardial (right) origin. Whole cell patch clamp technique in current clamp mode was used (15). Measurements were made at room temperature with a stimulation frequency of 0.2 Hz. Myocytes were obtained from a healthy donor heart. See (38) for experimental details.

parallelled by significantly lower I_{to} current density in endo- versus epicardial myocytes (38). Furthermore, I_{to} of endo- and epicardial myocytes can be distinguished by a much slower rate of recovery from inactivation in the former (38). As a consequence, I_{to} of endocardial cells recovers incompletely after short intervals and should exhibit marked "use-dependency". In a very recent study, Näbauer et al. (1996) actually measured strong "use-dependency" of I_{to} in endocardial and much less in epicardial myocytes from the human heart.

In addition to heterogeneity of I_{to}, regional differences in I_K have been reported for dog heart with larger I_{Ks} current density in epi- than midmyocardial myocytes, explaining the longer APD in midmyocardial cells. No differences were observed for I_{Kr} (12). I_{K1} appears to have a larger outward current region in feline endo- than in epicardial myocytes (11). Our own preliminary results from dog hearts did not reveal any regional differences for I_{Ca}, but I_{Na} gating appears to be significantly different in endo- and epicardial myocytes (Ravens et al., unpublished results). Taken together, heterogenity in current density of myocytes from various regions within the ventricular wall complicates the direct translation of rate-dependent changes in APD into changes of the QT interval of the ECG.

Intra- and extracellular ion concentrations

In the last part of this paper, the contribution of changes in ion concentrations to the rate-dependence of APs is going to be discussed.

As mentioned before, resting membrane potential is affected by stimulation rate as illustrated in Fig. 4 with microelectrode recordings from human papillary muscle. Resumption of regular stimulation following 90 s of quiescence leads to depolarization of the membrane, but this effect is transient. When stimulation is turned off again, a transient hyperpolarization is observed. The depolarization is explained by frequency-induced cumulation of K^+ in the extracellular space, and the effect is counterbalanced by the $(Na^+ + K^+)$-ATPase which activates with a certain time lag. Restraint of diffusion in multicellular preparations has been postulated particularly in the "narrow clefts" between cells. Even single myocytes possess

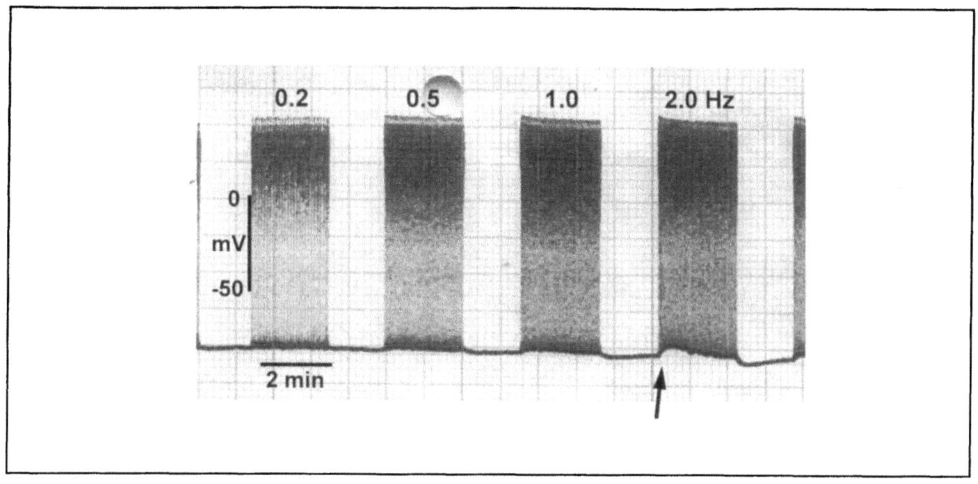

Fig. 4 Frequency dependence of action potential amplitude and resting membrane potential in a right ventricular papillary muscle obtained from the explanted heart of a cardiac transplant recipient (ischemic cardiomyopathy). Please note the characteristic biphasic change in membrane potential after an abrupt change in stimulation rate. Frequencies as indicated. Taken from (27) with kind permission of the author.

some extracellular space of restricted ion exchange with the bulk bath solution because of their T-tubular system. The technique of computer-assisted image tilting allows the construction of a three dimensional view of a mammalian myocyte, in which the extensive ramification of long, irregular tubules is readily appreciated (2). If it is assumed that ion channels are similarly distributed in tubular as in superficial sarcolemma, inhomogeneities of ion concentrations could occur in the depth of the tubules.

Increasing the extracellular K^+ concentration in the superfusion solution of an isolated papillary muscle shifts the resting potential to less negative values but does not mimick rate-dependent AP shortening (3). Thus cumulation of K^+ during high frequency pacing can account only for the observed depolarization but cannot explain AP shortening, suggesting that high rates of stimulation directly modulate kinetics or gating of ion currents.

Some outward currents are directly affected by high $[K^+]_o$. Current density of I_{to} in human ventricular myocytes is decreased by one third in zero $[K^+]_o$, despite the increase in driving force (Wettwer, unpublished results). However, little increase in I_{to} is observed with elevated $[K^+]_o$ suggesting that $[K^+]_o$ is not a main regulatory determinant at physiological or pathophysiological conditions. I_{Kr} and I_{Ks} are regulated in opposite directions by $[K^+]_o$. While I_{Ks} is enhanced, I_{Kr} is diminished in the absence of extracellular K^+ (36). Conversely, I_{Kr} increases with elevated $[K^+]_o$ (34).

Although the different sensitivities of K^+ currents to $[K^+]_o$ do not provide a sufficient explanation for rate-dependent changes in APD, these properties may contribute to the long known frequency-dependent effect of antiarrhythmic drugs with class III actions. E-4031 and other selective I_{Kr}-blockers prolong the action potential duration in a rate-dependent manner (Fig. 5). Under control conditions, the APD of guinea pig papillary muscles decreases with frequencies increasing between 0.5 and 2 Hz. E-4031 (1 µM) does indeed prolong APD, but the effect becomes smaller at fast stimulation rates (28). This "reverse frequency dependency" of action is characteristic for I_{Kr} blockers. The slowly activating component I_{Ks} is not affected by E-4031 and cumulates at high rates due to incomplete de-activation, elevating background level of repolarizing K^+ current. Therefore, at high rates

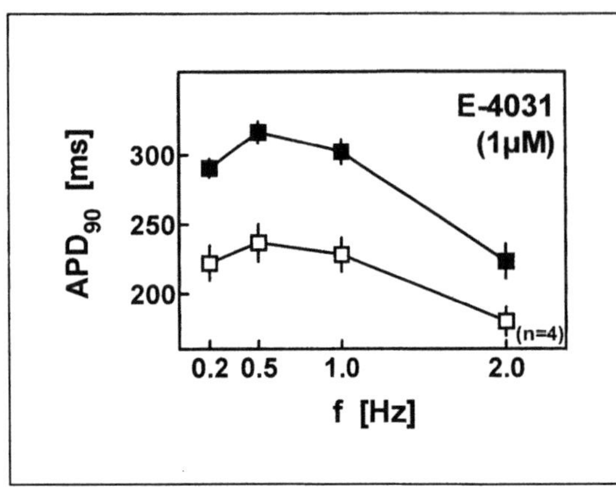

Fig. 5 Frequency dependence of action potential duration before (open squares) and after addition of 1 µM of E-4031 (filled squares). Ordinate: action potential duration at 90 % of repolarization (APD_{90}) in ms; abscissa, frequency f in Hz. mean values from n = 4 right ventricular papillary muscles of guinea pig hearts.

of stimulation, contribution of I_{Kr} to the total potassium conductance is reduced against an elevated level of I_{Ks}. Hence, blocking of a smaller fraction of total I_K by I_{Kr} blockers produces less APD prolongation. Recently, another mechanism contributing to reverse frequency dependence of I_{Kr} blockers has been reported. The potency of the agents is decreased at high $[K^+]_o$. Since rapid pacing causes elevation of $[K^+]_o$ (see above), the block becomes smaller at high frequencies (39).

Conclusions

Rate-dependence of shapes of cardiac action potentials appears to be a multifactorial phenomenon. Increase of extracellular $[K^+]_o$ alone is not sufficient to explain APD shortening at high rates, suggesting that ion channels must also be directly affected. Cumulation or respective depletion of cations close to either side of the plasmalemma may further modulate channel behavior. Marked heterogeneity of electrophysiological properties of myocytes derived from different regions within the ventricular wall further complicates the issue. Comprehensive data on all ion conducting processes are required for a thorough understanding of rate-dependent APD shortening.

References

1. Amos GJ, Wettwer E, Metzger F, Li Q, Himmel HM, Ravens U (1996) Differences between outward currents of human atrial and subepicardial ventricular myocytes. J Physiol (London) 491: 31–50
2. Amsellem J, Delorme R, Souchier C, Ojeda C (1995) Transverse-axial tubular system in guinea pig ventricular cardiomyocyte: 3D reconstruction, quantification and its possible role in K⁺ accumulation-depletion phenomenon in single cells. Biol Cell 85: 43–54
3. Attwell D, Cohen I, Eisner DA (1981) The effects of heart rate on the action potential of guinea-pig and human ventricular muscle. J Physiol (London) 313: 439–461
4. Barry DM, Nerbonne JM (1996) Myocardial potassium channels: Electrophysiological and molecular diversity. Annu Rev Physiol 58: 363–394
5. Bazett HD (1920) An analysis of the time relationship of electrocardiography. Heart 7: 353–370

6. Beeler GW, Reuter H (1972) Membrane calcium current in ventricular myocardial fibres. J Physiol (London) 207: 191–209

7. Boyett MR, Jewell BR (1980) Analysis of the effects of changes in rate and rhythm upon electrical activity in the heart. Progr Biophys Mol Biol 36: 1–52

8. Carmeliet E (1977) Repolarization and frequency in cardiac cells. J Physiol (Paris) 73: 903–923

9. Coraboeuf E, Carmeliet E (1982) Existence of two transient outward currents in sheep cardiac Purkinje fibres. Pflügers Arch 392: 352–359

10. Draper MH, Weidmann S (1951) Cardiac resting action potentials recorded with an intracellular electrode. J Physiol (London) 115: 74–94

11. Furukawa T, Kimura S, Furukawa N, Bassett AL, Myerburg RJ (1992) Potassium rectifier currents differ in myocytes of endocardial and epicardial origin. Circ Res 70: 91–103

12. Gintant GA (1995) Regional differences in I_K density in canine left ventricle: role of $I_{K,s}$ in electrical heterogeneity. Am J Physiol 268: H604–H613

13. Gross GJ, Burke RP, Castle NA (1995) Characterization of transient outward current in young human myocytes. Cardiovasc Res 29: 112–117

14. Gwathmey JK, Slawsky MT, Hajjar RJ, Briggs GM, Morgan JP (1990) Role of intracellular calcium handling in force-interval relationships of human ventricular myocardium. J Clin Invest 85: 1599–1613

15. Hamill OP, Marty A, Neher E, Sakmann B, Sigworth FJ (1981) Improved patchclamp techniques for high-resolution current recording from cells and cell-free membrane patches. Pflügers Arch 391: 85–100

16. Harvey RD (1996) Cardiac chloride channels. News Physiol Sci 11: 175–181

17. Isenberg G, Klöckner U (1982) Calcium currents in isolated bovine ventricular myocytes are fast and of large amplitude. Pflügers Arch 395: 30–41

18. Jurkiewicz NK, Sanguinetti MC (1993) Rate-dependent prolongation of cardiac action potentials by a methanesulfonanilide class III antiarrhythmic agent. Specific block of rapidly activating delayed rectifier K^+ current by dofetilide. Circ Res 72: 75–83

19. Kääb S, Nuss HB, Chiamvimonvat N, O'Rourke B, Pak PH, Kass DA, Marban E, Tomaselli GF (1996) Ionic mechanism of action potential prolongation in ventricular myocytes from dogs with pacing-induced heart failure. Circ Res 78: 262–273

20. Kenyon JL, Gibbons WR (1979) 4-Aminopyridine and the early outward current of sheep cardiac Purkinje fibers. J Gen Physiol 73: 139–157

21. Kunze DL (1977) Rate-dependent changes in extracellular potassium in the rabbit atrium. Circ Res 41: 122–127

22. Lederer WJ, Niggli H, Hadley RW (1990) Sodium-calcium exchange in excitable cells. Science 248: 283

23. Litovsky SH, Antzelevitch C (1988) Transient outward current prominent in canine ventricular epicardium but not endocardium. Circ Res 72: 1092–1103

24. Liu D-W, Antzelevitch C (1995) Characteristics of the delayed rectifier current (I_{Kr} and I_{Ks}) in canine ventricular epicardial, midmyocardial, and endocardial myocytes. A weaker I_{Ks} contributes to the longer action potential of the M cell. Circ Res 76: 351–365

25. Näbauer M, Beuckelmann DJ, Erdmann E (1993) Characteristics of transient outward current in human ventricular myocytes from patients with terminal heart failure. Circ Res 73: 386–394

26. Näbauer M, Beuckelmann DJ, Überfuhr P, Steinbeck G (1996) Regional differences in current density and rate-dependent properties of the transient outward current in subepicardial and subendocardial myocytes of human left ventricle. Circulation 93: 168–177

27. Ohler A (1996) Die Wirkung der neuen Klasse III-Antiarrhythmika E4031, Dofetilide, Almokalant und Tedisamil auf das Aktionspotential und den Kaliumstrom am menschlichen Herzen und am Meerschweinchenherzen. Thesis: Medical Doctor's degree, Medical Faculty, University of Essen

28. Ohler A, Amos GJ, Wettwer E, Ravens U (1994) Frequency-dependent effects of E-4031, almokalant, dofetilide and tedisamil on action potential duration: no evidence for "reverse use dependent" block. Naunyn-Schmiedeberg's Arch Pharmacol 349: 602–610

29. Ravens U, Wettwer E, Ohler A, Amos GJ, Mewes T (1996) Electrophysiology of ion channels of the heart. Fund Clin Pharmacol 10: 321–328

30. Reiter M, Stickel FJ (1968) Der Einfluß der Kontraktionsfrequenz auf das Aktionspotential des Meerschweinchen-Papillarmuskels. Naunyn-Schmiedeberg's Arch Pharmacol 260: 342–365

31. Reuter H (1973) Time- and voltage-dependent contractile responses in mammalian cardiac muscle. Eur J Cardiol 1/2: 177–181

32. Richard S (1998) Influence of stimulation frequency on Ca^{2+}-currents in human myocytes. [This volume]

33. Sakakibara Y, Furukawa T, Singer DH, Jia H, Backer CL, Arentzen CE, Wasserstrom JA (1993) Sodium current in isolated human ventricular myocytes. Am J Physiol 265: H1301–H1309

34. Sanguinetti MC, Jiang CG, Curran ME, Keating MT (1995) A mechanistic link between an inherited and an acquired cardiac arrhythmia. Cell 81: 299–307

35. Sanguinetti MC, Jurkiewicz NK (1990) Two components of cardiac delayed rectifier K^+ current. J Gen Physiol 96: 195–215

36. Sanguinetti MC, Jurkiewicz NK (1992) Role of external Ca^{2+} and K^+ in gating of cardiac delayed rectifier K^+ currents. Pflügers Arch 420: 180–186
37. Task force of the working group on arrhythmias of the European Society of Cardiology (1991) The Sicilian Gambit. A new approach to the classification of antiarrhythmic drugs based on their actions on arrhythmogenic mechanisms. Circulation 84: 1831–1851
38. Wettwer E, Amos GJ, Posival H, Ravens U (1994) Transient outward current in human ventricular myocytes of subepicardial and subendocardial origin. Circ Res 75: 473– 482
39. Yang T, Roden DM (1996) Extracellular potassium modulation of drug block of I_{Kr}. Implications for torsade de pointes and reverse use-dependence. Circulation 93: 407–411
40. Zygmunt AC (1994) Intracellular calcium activates a chloride current in canine ventricular myocytes. Am J Physiol 267: H1984–H1995

Author's address:
Prof. Dr. med. U. Ravens
Institut für Pharmakologie und Toxikologie
Universitätsklinikum Carl-Gustav-Carus
Technische Universität Dresden
Karl-Marx-Str. 3
01109 Dresden
Germany

Influence of Forskolin on the force-frequency behavior in nonfailing and end-stage failing human myocardium

B. Pieske[1], S. Trost[1], K. Schütt[3], K. Minami[3], H. Just[2], G. Hasenfuss[1]

[1] Zentrum Innere Medizin, Abteilung Kardiologie und Pneumologie, Georg-August-Universität Göttingen
[2] Medizinische Klinik III, Abteilung Kardiologie und Angiologie, Albert-Ludwigs-Universität Freiburg
[3] Klinik für Thorax- und Kardiovaskularchirurgie, Herzzentrum Nordrhein-Westfalen, Bad Oeynhausen

Abstract

End-stage failing human myocardium is characterized by a negative force-frequency relationship (FFR), possibly as a result of reduced SR Ca^{2+} uptake capacity. We investigated the effects of the direct adenylate cyclase stimulator, forskolin, on force of contraction and FFR in isolated human myocardium from 7 nonfailing hearts (NF) and end-stage failing hearts (NYHA IV) due to either ischemic (ICM; n = 13) or dilated cardiomyopathy (DCM; n = 16).

Methods: Isolated left ventricular muscle strips, isometric contraction, electrical stimulation at a basal stimulation rate of 1 Hz (37 °C). Inotropic responses: Cumulative concentration-response curves for forskolin (0.01–10 µM) and for Ca^{2+} (2.5–15 mM). Force-frequency experiments: stepwise increase in stimulation rate from 0.5 to 3.0 Hz without and in the presence of 0.3, 1.0 or 3.0 µM forskolin.

Results: Forskolin concentration – dependently increased force of contraction to 386 ± 28 % (n = 5) in NF, to 256 ± 48 % (n = 7) in ICM, and to 212 ± 13 % (n = 14) in DCM. The effectiveness of forskolin was significantly reduced in failing myocardium. Ca^{2+} increased force of contraction to maximally 438 ± 108 % in NF, to 267 ± 15 % in ICM, and to 292 ± 20 % in DCM. Again, the effectiveness of Ca^{2+} was significantly reduced in failing myocardium. Forskolin activated contractile reserve to similar extents in all types of myocardium (90 %, 95 %, and 82 %, respectively). Force of contraction continuously increased with increasing stimulation rates in nonfailing myocardium (positive FFR), but was blunted or inversed in ICM and DCM. Prestimulation with forskolin (0.3 µM) further enhanced frequency-potentiation in nonfailing, and normalized the slope and optimum stimulation frequency in ICM and DCM. However, at higher concentrations of forskolin, FFR was blunted or inversed in nonfailing myocardium, and further impaired in failing myocardium.

Conclusion: Low concentrations of forskolin with only marginal inotropic effects may partially normalize the inverse force-frequency relation in end-stage failing human myocardium. Reduced cAMP levels in conjunction with reduced expression of SR Ca^{2+} ATPase may be the underlying cause for altered excitation-contraction coupling in diseased human hearts.

Key words Force-frequency relation – human myocardium – forskolin – cyclic adenosine-
monophosphate – SR Ca^{2+} ATPase

Introduction

Frequency potentiation of contractile force represents a potent inotropic mechanism. Under physiological conditions, intrinsic contractility of most mammalian hearts increases with increasing heart rates. This positive force-frequency relationship can also be observed in isolated human nonfailing myocardium (18, 23, 30, 31) and in patients with normal left ventricular function (17). The frequency-potentiation of force of contraction has been attributed to a parallel increase in intracellular Ca^{2+} transients (31), probably as a result of increased transsarcolemmal Ca^{2+} influx (35) and enhanced consecutive loading of the sarcoplasmic reticulum (SR) with Ca^{2+} (32).

In patients with heart failure, the positive force-frequency relationship is altered. While it is flattened in patients with short-term or moderately failing hearts (27, 30, 38), it may even be inversed in end-stage heart failure due to either dilated or ischemic cardiomyopathy (17, 18, 23, 30, 31). This blunted or inversed force-frequency relationship has been related to substantial alterations in intracellular Ca^{2+} handling. We could recently demonstrate that, in end-stage failing human myocardium, the decline in force of contraction at higher stimulation rates is due to a parallel decline in intracellular Ca^{2+} transients with increasing stimulation rates (31). This frequency-dependent reduction in intracellular activator Ca^{2+} has been related to a reduced Ca^{2+} uptake capacity of the sarcoplasmic reticulum (20, 31, 40), probably due to reduced expression of the Ca^{2+} pump proteins of the sarcoplasmic reticulum on mRNA and protein levels (18, 21, 22). In addition, the expression and activity of the sarcolemmal Na^+/Ca^{2+} exchanger is increased in failing human myocardium (36, 41).

These molecular alterations in Ca^{2+} handling proteins result in exhaustion of the SR Ca^{2+} uptake processes at higher stimulation rates and increased sarcolemmal vs. intracellular Ca^{2+} elimination from the cytosol. As a consequence, an increased amount of Ca^{2+} may be extruded from the myocytes at higher stimulation rates and can not further contribute to activation of the contractile proteins.

The activity of the SR Ca^{2+} pumps may be increased by phosphorylation of the inhibitory protein phospholamban and possibly of the Ca^{2+} pump itself (44). Phosphorylation of phospholamban may occur by cAMP dependent protein kinase A. However, a major defect in the failing human myocardium is a deficient production of cAMP, possibly as a result of downregulation of β_1-adrenoceptors (1, 4, 7), and an increase in the inhibitory G-proteins ($G_{i\alpha}$; 9, 11), without changes of the catalytic subunit of the adenylate cyclase. As a consequence, basal and guanine nucleotide-stimulated adenylate cyclase activity and intracellular cAMP concentrations are significantly reduced in failing human myocardium (2, 3, 8, 11). Direct stimulation of the catalytic subunit of adenylate cyclase with forskolin in failing myocardium results in normal cAMP generation (2).

It has recently been demonstrated that the direct stimulation of adenylate cyclase activity with forskolin may partly normalize the flattened force-frequency relationship in moderately failing human myocardium (26). The subcellular alterations leading to reversal of the force-frequency relationship are even more pronounced in end-stage failing myocardium. Therefore, the goal of the present study was to assess the effect of direct stimulation of adenylate cyclase with forskolin on the force-frequency behavior in human end-stage failing myocardium from hearts with ischemic or dilated cardiomyopathy in comparison to nonfailing human myocardium. Emphasis was led on comparing the effects of different concentrations of forskolin.

Materials and methods

Myocardial tissue

Experiments have been performed in isolated left ventricular muscle strips from 7 nonfailing human hearts, 16 hearts with end-stage failing dilated cardiomyopathy, and 13 hearts with end-stage failing ischemic cardiomyopathy. None of the nonfailing donors displayed any signs of heart failure. End-stage failing hearts, obtained at the point of cardiac transplantation, had a significantly reduced ejection fraction (dilated cardiomyopathy: 22 ± 2 %, ischemic cardiomyopathy: 23 ± 3 %). The mean age in the donor group was 44 ± 5 years, 53 ± 6 years in patients with dilated cardiomyopathy, and 61 ± 5 years in patients with ischemic cardiomyopathy.

Muscle strip preparation

Left ventricular muscle strips were prepared and mounted to an isometric force transducer as described elsewhere (30). Briefly, small strips of papillary muscle or trabeculae were excised immediately after explantation and stored in a special cardioplegic solution containing 30 mM of 2,3-butanedione monoxime, bubbled with carbogen (95 % O_2, 5 % CO_2, pH of 7.4) at room temperature. Upon arrival in the laboratory, small (cross sectional area < 0.6 mm^2) muscle strips were dissected exactly along fiber orientation with the help of a stereomicroscope and specially designed preparation chambers. All preparation steps were carried out in the presence of the cardioprotective solution, which minimizes cutting injury (25). The muscle strips were then mounted horizontally in an organ bath (Hugo Sachs Electronics, March-Hugstetten, Germany) and connected to an isometric force transducer. Signals were recorded using a strip chart recorder (Graphtec Lineacorder, Yokohoma, Japan). Muscles were superfused with a carbogen-bubbled (pH of 7.4) modified Krebs-Henseleit solution of the following composition (in mM): Na$^+$, 152; K$^+$, 3.6; Cl$^-$, 135; Ca^{2+}, 2.5; Mg, 0.6; HCO^{3-}, 25; H$_2$PO^{4-}, 1.3; SO^{4-}, 0.6; glucose, 11.2; and insulin, 10 IU/L at 37 °C. After initially prestretching the muscle strips with 1 mN, they were stimulated by field stimulation using a voltage 20 % above threshold, at a frequency of 1 Hz. After equilibration and complete washout of the cardioprotective solution, the muscles were stretched along their length-tension curve in 0.05 mm steps until force of contraction was maximal. At the end of the experiment, muscle length and wet weight were measured and cross sectional area was determined by dividing wet weight by muscle length.

Concentration-response curves for forskolin and [Ca^{2+}]$_o$

In the first part of the study, concentration-response curves for forskolin and [Ca^{2+}]$_o$ were obtained in nonfailing and end-stage failing myocardium. To increase the solubility of forskolin, 2 vol % of dimethylformamide were added to the organ bath prior to the experiments. Then, cumulative concentration-response curves for forskolin (0.01–10 μM) were obtained. To assess the inotropic response to forskolin, force of contraction and time parameters of the isometric twitch were obtained at steady-state conditions at each concentration of forskolin. To test the contractile reserve of the myocardium, cumulative concentration-response curves for $[Ca^{2+}]_o$ (2.5–15 mM) were established in isolated muscle strips from the same hearts. Assuming that Ca^{2+} activates maximal contractile force, the fraction of contractile reserve obtained with forskolin can be obtained by dividing the maximal inotropic response after Ca^{2+} by the maximal inotropic response after forskolin.

Force-frequency relationship

To investigate the influence of forskolin on the force-frequency relationship, stimulation rates of isolated muscle strips from nonfailing and end-stage failing myocardium were step-wise increased from 0.5 to 3.0 Hz (0.5; 0.75; 1.0; 1.25; 1.5; 1.75; 2.0; 2.5; 3.0 Hz) before and after addition of forskolin. The effects of forskolin on force-frequency behavior were tested either within the same muscle strip preparation (force-frequency before and after forskolin) or in parallel in 2 muscle strips from one region of the same heart (one force-frequency relationship without, one with forskolin). Both methods yielded similar results. Three concentrations of forskolin for pre-stimulating muscle strips were derived from the concentration-response curves: a minimal effective concentration (0.3 μM) with only a marginal increase in force of contraction, an intermediate concentration (1.0 μM) with a half maximal activation of contractile force, and a submaximal concentration (3.0 μM) with a pronounced increase in contractile strength.

Forskolin was prepared as a stock solution (1 mM) in dimethylformamide. For experiments, appropriate concentrations of forskolin were prepared in aqua bidest. Forskolin was obtained from Sigma Chemicals (Deisenhofen, FRG). Ca^{2+} was prepared as a stock solution of 1 M in aqua bidest.

Statistical analysis

Average values are given as mean ± standard error of the mean. Comparisons between the different groups was performed by unpaired t-test. For comparison within one group of myocardium, the paired t-test, followed by the Bonferroni-Holms procedure, was applied. Differences were considered significant if p was < 0.05.

Results

Positive inotropic effects of forskolin

Forskolin exerted significant positive inotropic effects in both nonfailing and end-stage failing myocardium from ischemic or dilated cardiomyopathy. Figure 1 shows in original registrations the typical effects of forskolin in an intermediate concentration in a muscle strip from a nonfailing heart (upper panel), an end-stage failing heart due to ischemic

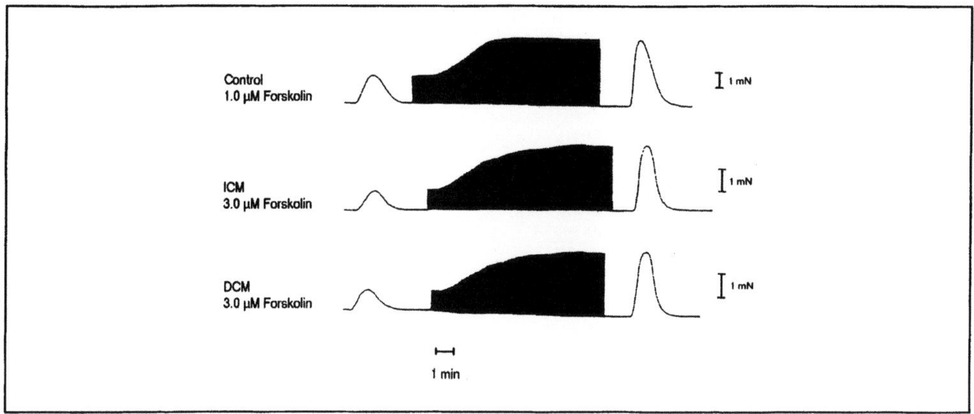

Fig. 1 Influence of forskolin on force of contraction. Original registration in a muscle strip from a nonfailing heart (control; 1.0 µM), an end-stage failing heart due to ischemic cardiomyopathy (ICM; 3.0 µM), and an end-stage failing heart due to dilated cardiomyopathy (DCM; 3.0 µM). Equieffectve concentrations of forskolin have been used, resulting in the lower concentration of forskolin in nonfailing myocardium. The pronounced inotropic effect in all three preparations developed over a time course of several minutes. Enhanced relaxation with forskolin becomes obvious by comparing the isometric twitch at higher registration speed before and after forskolin.

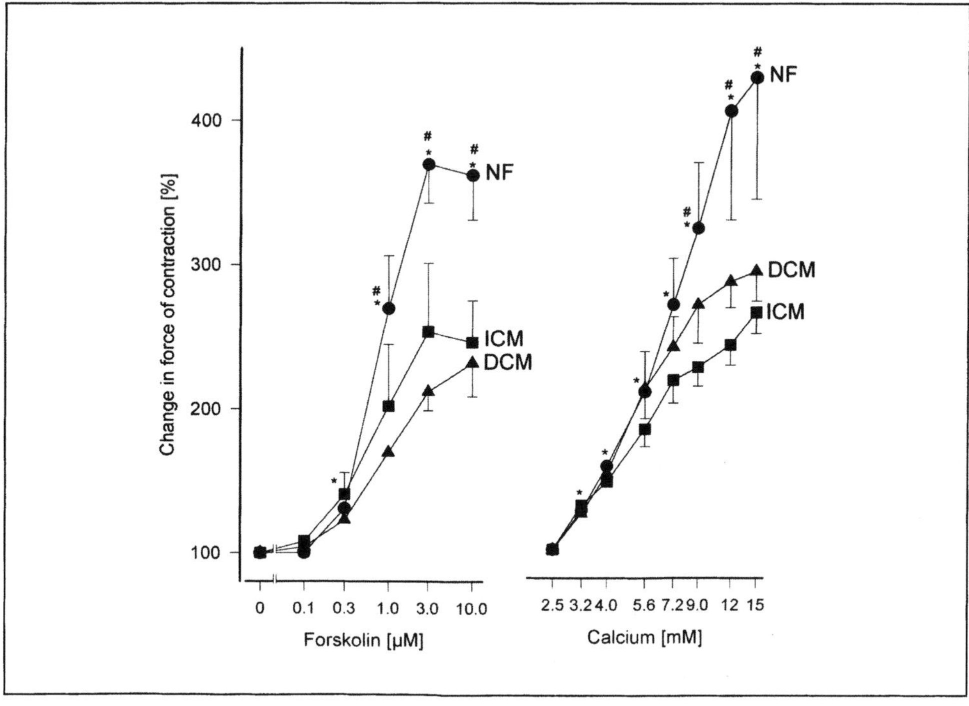

Fig. 2 Cumulative concentration-response curves for forskolin (0.1–10 µM; left) and Ca^{2+} (2.5–15 mM; right). For forskolin, experiments were performed in 5 muscle strips from 5 nonfailing hearts, 7 muscle strips from 7 ICM hearts, and 14 muscle strips from 14 DCM hearts. Ca^{2+} response curves were established in 4 muscle strips from the same nonfailing hearts, 7 muscle strips from the same ICM hearts, and 5 muscle strips from the same DCM hearts. * = $p < 0.05$ vs. basal value for NF, ICM and DCM at the respective concentration. # = $p < 0.05$ vs. ICM, DCM.

Table 1 Time parameters of the isometric twitch with forskolin

Forskolin	base	0.3 µM	1.0 µM	3.0 µM
TPT	NF	168 ± 10	161 ± 13	159 ± 8*	130 ± 3*
	ICM	180 ± 9	180 ± 7	164 ± 7*	147 ± 6*
	DCM	146 ± 5	145 ± 5	141 ± 3	140 ± 6*
RT_{50}	NF	123 ± 11	117 ± 10	110 ± 8*	92 ± 4*
	ICM	109 ± 4	106 ± 5	98 ± 5*	86 ± 4*
	DCM	110 ± 5	106 ± 5	96 ± 5*	86 ± 4*
TT	NF	576 ± 49	564 ± 46	517 ± 38*	446 ± 23*
	ICM	526 ± 16	530 ± 13	469 ± 22*	437 ± 22*
	DCM	515 ± 31	493 ± 33	454 ± 26*	428 ± 24*

base: basal value before forskolin; NF, ICM, DCM: nonfailing myocardium, ischemic cardiomyopathy, dilated cardiomyopathy; TPT: time to peak tension (ms); RT_{50}: time to 50 % relaxation (ms); TT: total time of the isometric twitch (ms); * $p < 0.05$ vs. basal value

cardiomyopathy (ICM; middle panel), and an end-stage failing heart due to dilated cardiomyopathy (DCM; lower panel). The inotropic effect after addition of forskolin developed gradually over a time course of several minutes and was maximal after 10.7 ± 1.3 min in nonfailing (n = 5), 13.7 ± 1.2 in ICM (n = 7), and 12.6 ± 1.2 min in DCM (n = 14). Furthermore, from the single twitch tracings before and after forskolin, the shortening of the total duration of the twitch after forskolin due to reduced time to peak tension and enhanced relaxation becomes obvious.

The cumulative concentration-response curves for forskolin are shown in Fig. 2 (left). In nonfailing myocardium, the positive inotropic effect of forskolin started at a concentration of 0.3 µM and was maximum at 3.0 µM (increase to 386 ± 28 %, $p < 0.05$ vs. basal value; n = 5). In ischemic cardiomyopathy, the inotropic effect started again at 0.3 µM and was maximum at 3.0 µM (increase to 256 ± 48 %, $p < 0.05$ vs. basal value; n = 7). In dilated cardiomyopathy, the inotropic effect also started at 0.3 µM and was maximum at 10 µM (increase to 212 ± 13 %, $p < 0.05$ vs. basal value; n = 14). The positive inotropic effect of forskolin was significantly smaller in end-stage failing as compared to nonfailing myocardium ($p < 0.05$ for NF vs. DCM and ICM). There were no differences in the inotropic response between ischemic and dilated cardiomyopathy. In addition to its inotropic effect, forskolin increased time to peak tension and shortened relaxation time, resulting in an abbreviation of the isometric twitch. Time parameters of isometric contractions after forskolin are given in Table 1.

Ca^{2+} concentration-response curves

On the right hand of Fig. 2, the corresponding Ca^{2+} response curves obtained in muscle strips from the same nonfailing or failing hearts are shown. It can be seen that the cumulative increase in the Ca^{2+} concentration in the organ bath from 2.5–15 mM significantly increased force of contraction to maximally 438 ± 108 % in nonfailing, to 267 ± 15 % in ICM, and to 292 ± 20 % in DCM ($p < 0.05$ vs. basal values for all groups). As with forskolin, the maximal inotropic response to Ca^{2+} was significantly reduced in end-stage failing myocardium with no differences between ICM and DCM.

To assess whether or not forskolin can fully activate the contractile reserve of the muscle strip (as assessed with Ca^{2+}), the maximal inotropic response of forskolin was related to the maximal inotropic response of Ca^{2+} in each group. Forskolin achieved 90 % of the maximal inotropic effect of Ca^{2+} in nonfailing myocardium, 95 % in ICM, and 82 % in DCM (differences not significant). Therefore, forskolin activates a large fraction of the maximal contractile reserve of the muscle strips in both nonfailing and failing myocardium. This is in contrast to β-adrenoceptor stimulation, where only a fraction of the maximal Ca^{2+} response can be activated in failing human myocardium due to defective signal transduction (1).

Influence of stimulation rates on isometric force

Figure 3 shows the influence of stimulation rate on isometric force of contraction in human nonfailing and end-stage failing myocardium due to ischemic or dilated cardiomyopathy. In nonfailing myocardium, force of contraction continuously increased with increasing stimulation rates and was maximum at 3.0 Hz (increase to 152 ± 12 % of the basal value at

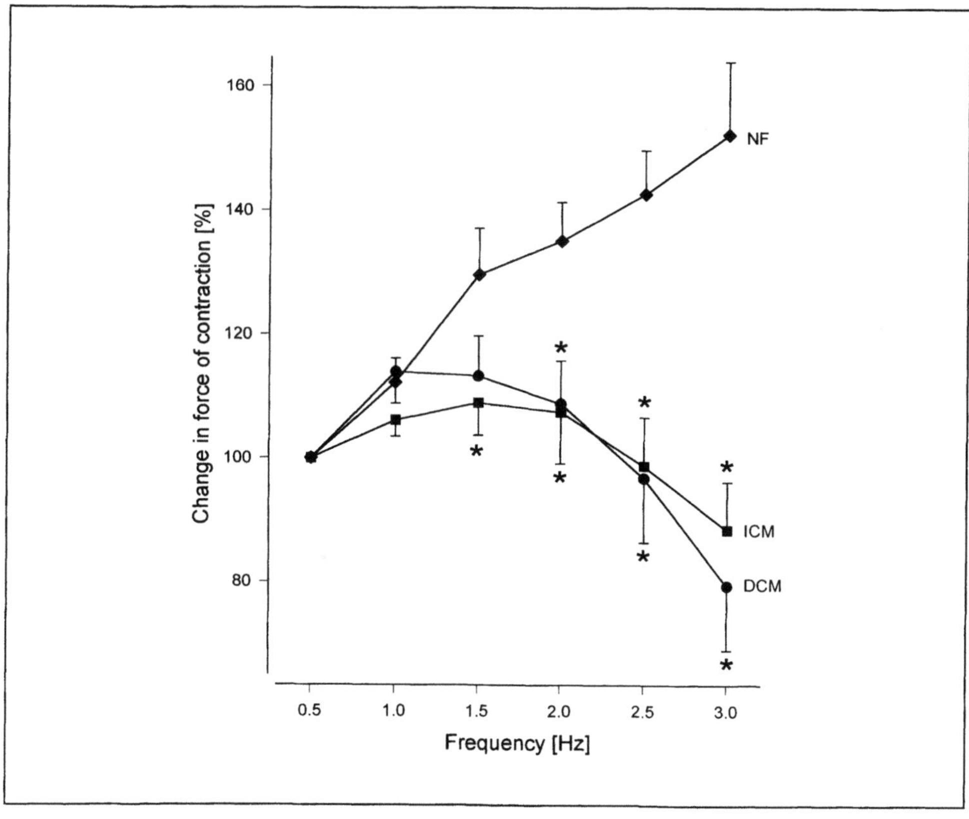

Fig. 3 Force-frequency behavior in isolated nonfailing and end-stage failing myocardium. Experiments were performed in 11 muscle strips from 5 nonfailing hearts, in 15 muscle strips from 13 end-stage failing hearts due to ischemic cardiomyopathy (ICM), and in 8 muscle strips from 8 end-stage failing hearts due to dilated cardiomyopathy. * = p < 0.05 vs. nonfailing.

0.5 Hz; p < 0.05; n = 11). This positive force-frequency relationship was blunted and converted to a negative force-frequency relationship in end-stage failing myocardium. In ICM, force of contraction slightly increased at slow stimulation rates, and continuously declined at higher stimulation rates (to 88 ± 7 % of the basal value at 3.0 Hz; p < 0.05; n = 15). Similarly, in DCM force of contractions slightly increased at low stimulation rates, but significantly declined at higher stimulation rates to 81 ± 12 % of the basal value at 3.0 Hz (p < 0.05; n = 8).

Influence of forskolin on the force-frequency relationship

The influence of forskolin on the force-frequency relationship was tested by pre-stimulating muscle strips with either 0.3, 1.0, or 3.0 µM forskolin. In nonfailing myocardium, these concentrations increased force of contraction by 36 ± 18 %, 153 ± 24 %, and 252 ± 28 %, respectively (p < 0.05 for all values). The results are summarized in Fig. 4. As can be seen, forskolin in a low concentration (left) slightly, albeit not significantly, enhanced the positive force-frequency relationship. After the intermediate concentration of forskolin, the force-frequency relationship was unaffected up to a stimulation rate of 1.75 Hz, but was converted to a negative force-frequency relationship at high stimulation rates. At the high concentration of forskolin, the positive force-frequency relationship without forskolin was converted to a negative force-frequency relationship (right).

The influence of forskolin on the force-frequency relationship in end-stage failing ischemic cardiomyopathy is shown in Fig. 5. Again, forskolin was applied at 0.3, 1.0, and 3.0 µM (increase in force of contraction by 20 ± 5 %, 60 ± 8 % and 154 ± 9 %, p < 0.05 for all concentrations). After forskolin in the low concentration (left), the negative force-

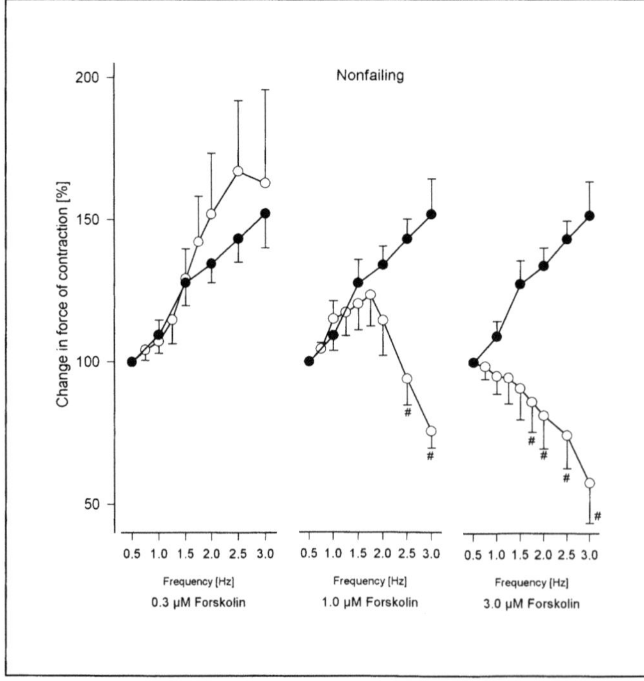

Fig. 4 Influence of forskolin (0.3 µM, left; 1.0 µM, middle; 3.0 µM, right) on force-frequency behavior in nonfailing human myocardium. ● = force-frequency without forskolin. ○ = force-frequency in the presence of forskolin. Changes in force of contraction are given in % change from the basal value at 0.5 Hz. Experiments were performed in 11 muscle strips without forskolin (same reference data for the three parts of the figure), in 4 muscle strips after 0.3 µM forskolin, in 5 muscle strips after 1.0 µM forskolin, and in 6 muscle strips after 3.0 µM forskolin. # = p < 0.05 vs. value without forskolin.

Fig. 5 Influence of forskolin (0.3 µM, left; 1.0 µM, middle; 3.0 mM, right) on force-frequency behavior in ischemic cardiomyopathy. • = force-frequency without forskolin. ○ = force-frequency in the presence of forskolin. Changes in force of contraction are given in % change from the basal value at 0.5 Hz. Experiments were performed in n = 7, n = 8, and n = 7 muscle strips before, and n = 8, n = 8, and n = 10 muscle strips with 3.0, 1.0, or 3.0 µM forskolin, respectively, # = p < 0.05 vs. value without forskolin.

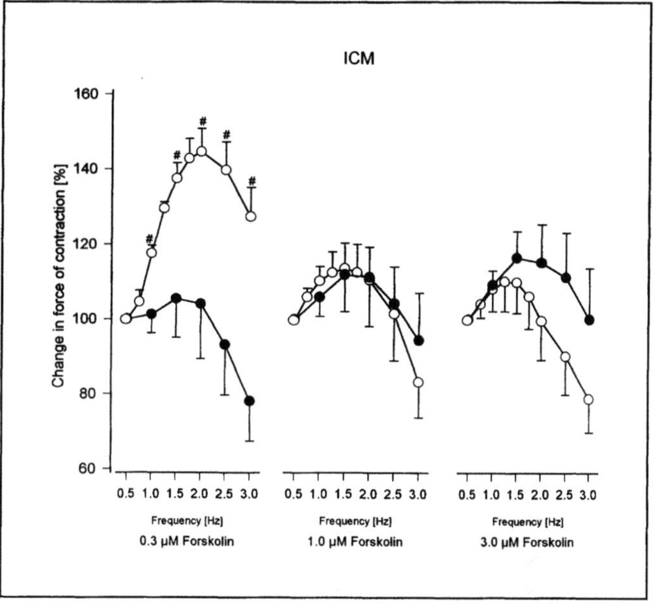

frequency relationship was converted to a positive force-frequency relationship: without forskolin, force of contraction did not change at heart rates up to 2 Hz, and then significantly declined to 79 ± 10 % of the basal value at 3 Hz. In the presence of 0.3 µM forskolin, however, force of contraction continuously increased with increasing stimulation rates up to a stimulation rate of 2 Hz (increase to 144 ± 5 %, p < 0.05), and force still remained significantly elevated at the highest stimulation rates. However, forskolin did not influence the shape of the force-frequency relationship in the intermediate concentration (middle) and further impaired the altered force-frequency relationship at the highest concentration (right). Increasing stimulation rates abbreviated relaxation times both without and after forskolin. Frequency-dependent relaxation times at 0.3 µM forskolin are shown in Table 2. For comparison, relaxation parameters for nonfailing myocardium are shown. As can be seen, relaxation times at each stimulation rate were significantly shorter in ICM in the presence of 0.3 µM forskolin as compared to untreated nonfailing myocardium.

Table 2 Relaxation parameters of the isometric twitch

Stimulation rate (Hz)		0.5	1.0	2.0	3.0
RT_{50}	NF	131 ± 6	121 ± 5	102 ± 4	85 ± 2
	DCM+F	116 ± 3*	106 ± 3*	89 ± 2*	79 ± 2*
	ICM+F	107 ± 7*	103 ± 6*	89 ± 5*	79 ± 3*
RT_{95}	NF	338 ± 27	303 ± 20	240 ± 9	180 ± 4*
	DCM+F	302 ± 13*	270 ± 11*	205 ± 10*	147 ± 4*
	ICM+F	295 ± 19*	268 ± 20*	206 ± 10*	145 ± 5*

RT_{50}, RT_{95}: Time to 50 %, 95 % relaxation (ms); DCM+F: dilated cardiomyopathy with 0.3 µM forskolin; ICM+F: ischemic cardiomyopathy with 0.3 µM forskolin; * p < 0.05 vs. NF

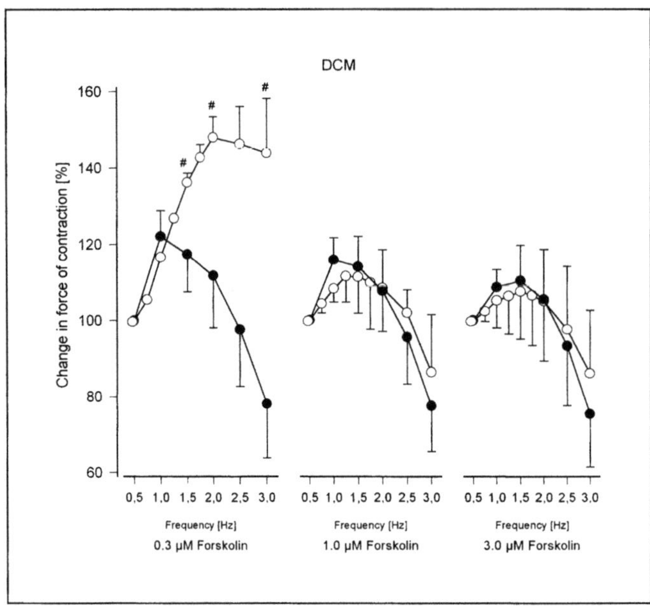

Fig. 6 Influence of forskolin (0.3 µM, left; 1.0 µM, middle; 3.0 µM, right) on force-frequency behavior in dilated cardiomyopathy. ● = force-frequency without forskolin. ○ = force-frequency in the presence of forskolin. Changes in force of contraction are given in % change from the basal value at 0.5 Hz. Experiments were performed in n = 4, n = 6, and n = 7 muscle strips before, and n = 7, n = 9, and n = 5 muscle strips with 3.0 µM, 1.0 µM, or 3.0 µM forskolin, respectively, # = p < 0.05 vs. value without forskolin.

Figure 6 summarizes the effects of forskolin on force-frequency behavior in dilated cardiomyopathy. In these experiments, forskolin increased force of contraction by $15 \pm 3\,\%$, $67 \pm 9\,\%$, and $164 \pm 27\,\%$ at 0.3, 1.0, or 3.0 µM, respectively (p < 0.05 for all values). With

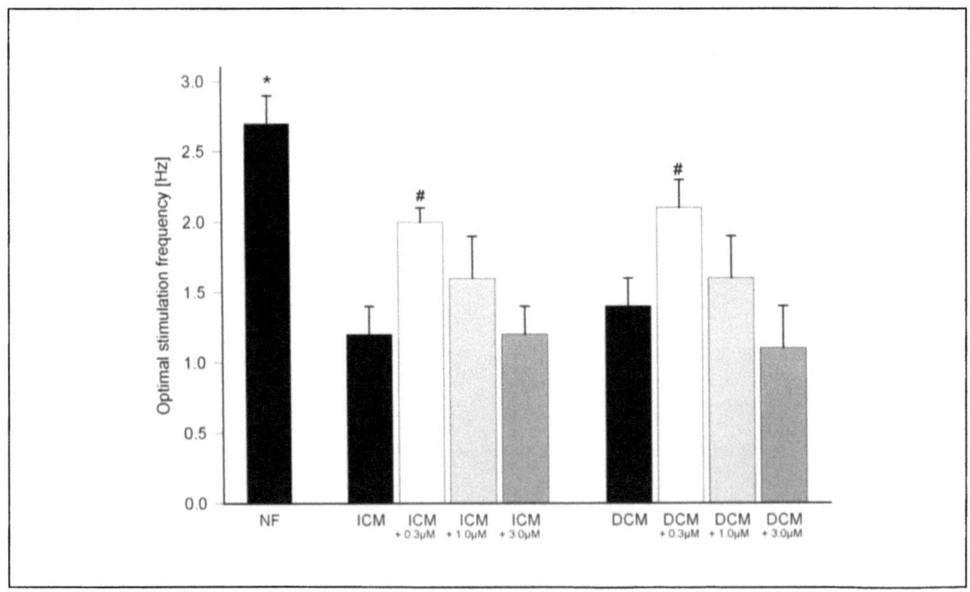

Fig. 7 Average optimal stimulation frequency in nonfailing human myocardium and in end-stage failing myocardium due to ICM or DCM without (black columns) or in the presence of 0.3, 1.0, or 3.0 µM forskolin. Data are derived from the experiments shown in Figs. 4–6. * = p < 0.05 vs. ICM, DCM without intervention. # = p < 0.05 vs. corresponding value without intervention.

0.3 µM forskolin (left), the negative force-frequency relationship in untreated muscle strips was converted to a positive force-frequency relationship. Force of contraction in the presence of 0.3 µM forskolin continuously increased up to a stimulation rate of 2.0 Hz (increase to $149 \pm 8\ \%$; $p < 0.05$; $n = 7$), and remained stable at the highest stimulation rates. Again, relaxation times were significantly shorter at each stimulation rate with 0.3 µM forskolin as compared to nonfailing myocardium (Table 2). In contrast, despite its large inotropic effect, forskolin in the intermediate (middle) and the high concentration (right) did not significantly alter the shape of the blunted and inverse force-frequency relationship in failing dilated cardiomyopathy.

Figure 7 summarizes the effects of forskolin on the optimal stimulation frequency, i.e., the frequency at which maximum inotropic response was obtained. Data are calculated from the experiments depicted in Figs. 4–6. In the untreated nonfailing myocardium, optimal stimulation frequency was 2.7 ± 0.2 Hz, in ischemic cardiomyopathy 1.2 ± 0.2 Hz ($p < 0.05$ vs. nonfailing), and 1.4 ± 0.2 Hz ($p < 0.05$ vs. nonfailing) in dilated cardiomyopathy. Pre-stimulation with 0.3 µM forskolin shifted the optimal stimulation frequency to 2.0 ± 0.1 Hz ($p < 0.05$ vs. untreated) and to 2.1 ± 0.2 Hz ($p < 0.05$ vs. untreated) in ischemic and dilated cardiomyopathy, respectively. With 1.0 µM forskolin, optimal stimulation frequency was 1.60 ± 0.3 Hz in ischemic (n.s. vs. untreated) and 1.63 ± 0.3 Hz (n.s. vs. untreated) in dilated cardiomyopathy. In the presence of 3.0 µM forskolin, the optimum average stimulation frequency was 1.20 ± 0.2 Hz (n.s. vs. untreated) in ischemic, and 1.13 ± 0.3 Hz (n.s. vs. untreated) in dilated cardiomyopathy.

Discussion

The main results of the present study were that 1) the maximal inotropic response to forskolin and $[Ca^{2+}]_o$ is significantly reduced in end-stage failing ischemic and dilated cardiomyopathy. 2) Forskolin completely activates the contractile reserve in both nonfailing and end-stage failing myocardium. 3) Forskolin in a low concentration partially normalizes the negative force-frequency relationship in end-stage failing myocardium, and 4) forskolin in a high concentration impairs the force-frequency response in nonfailing myocardium and does not significantly affect the negative force-frequency relationship in end-stage failing myocardium.

Force-frequency relations in human myocardium

Isometric twitch force continously increased with increasing stimulation rates in nonfailing human myocardium (this study, Fig. 3). This positive force-frequency behavior has previously been observed in isolated nonfailing human myocardium (18, 23, 30, 31, 33, 39) and was also observed under in vivo conditions (10, 17). It was related to a frequency-dependent increase in transsarcolemmal Ca^{2+} influx (35, 43) with subsequent enhanced loading of the SR with Ca^{2+} (1). In failing human myocardium, the positive force-frequency relationship increased only slightly at low stimulation rates, and twitch force even decreased at higher stimulation rates (Fig. 3). Again, the blunted or inverse force-frequency relationship in failing myocardium had previously been observed (18, 23, 30, 33, 39) and was related to disturbed intracellular Ca handling (31). The extent of alterations of the force-frequency response depend on the severity, time course, and underlying etiology of the disease (15, 27, 30, 38). There is a progressive lowering of the optimum stimulation frequency as the severity of heart disease increases (27). In end-stage failing myocardium, average optimum stimulation frequency was 1 Hz in DCM and 1.5 Hz in ICM (this study). This is consistent with early investigations showing an increase in force of contraction if stimulation rate was increased from 0.01 to 0.33 Hz in end-stage failing human myocardium (13). In the present study, the alterations in force-frequency behavior did not differ significantly between ischemic and dilated cardiomyopathy.

Which subcellular defects underly the negative force-frequency relationship in failing human myocardium?

Frequency potentiation of contractile force in nonfailing human myocardium has been attributed to an increased Ca^{2+} load and release at the level of the sarcoplasmic reticulum. The source of this increased activator Ca^{2+} ultimately originates from enhanced trans-sarcolemmal Ca^{2+} influx due to an increase in the depolarized time of the sarcolemmal membrane (which results in enhanced Ca^{2+} entry through the L-type Ca^{2+} channels) and a direct rate-dependent increase in single Ca^{2+} channel Ca^{2+} currents (35). While frequency inotropism in nonfailing myocardium critically depends on the intact function of subcellular organelles involved in intracellular Ca^{2+} handling, substantial alterations of these mechanisms occur in end-stage failing ischemic and dilated cardiomyopathy. A significant reduction in the Ca^{2+} uptake capacity of the sarcoplasmic reticulum has been observed in end-stage failing human myocardium (20, 31, 40) and was attributed to reduced expression of the SR Ca^{2+} pumps on the mRNA level (21, 40). Accordingly, most authors could also demonstrate a reduced protein expression of the SR Ca^{2+} pumps (18, 22). In addition, the protein expression (14, 41) and activity (36) of the Na^+/Ca^{2+} exchanger is significantly increased in failing human myocardium. These alterations in Ca^{2+} transporting proteins may result in a shift from intracellular Ca^{2+} cycling to transsarcolemmal Ca^{2+} cycling in the failing heart, which becomes more prominent at higher heart rates where diastole, i.e., the time for Ca^{2+} re-uptake to the sarcoplasmic reticulum, shortens. Accordingly, we could recently demonstrate a decrease in intracellular Ca^{2+} transients (31) and sarcoplasmic reticulum Ca^{2+} load (32) at higher stimulation rates in failing myocardium.

The activity of the SR Ca^{2+} pump proteins are regulated by the inhibitory action of phospholamban. This inhibitory action can be relieved by cAMP-protein kinase A-dependent or Ca^{2+}-calmodulin-dependent phosphorylation of phospholamban. Since decreased intracellular cAMP levels have been consistently observed in end-stage failing human myocardium (3, 8), phospholamban may predominate in its unphosphorylated inhibitory form in the failing tissue. In addition, by directly comparing protein expression of SR Ca^{2+} ATPase and phospholamban, a relative increase in phospholamban vs. Ca^{2+} ATPase expression has been demonstrated in failing human myocardium (22). This can further contribute to an enhanced inhibitory action of phospholamban on SR Ca^{2+} uptake. As a consequence, reduced expression of a functional intact SR Ca^{2+} pump and the unchanged expression of the inhibitory protein phospholamban as well as reduced cAMP-dependent phosphorylation of phospholamban may all contribute to the observed alterations in intracellular Ca^{2+} homeostasis responsible for the inverse force-frequency relationship.

The diterpene-derivative forskolin directly stimulates the catalytic subunit of the adenylate cyclase. It is independent from the β-adrenoceptor G-protein signal transduction pathway, and alterations in the β-adrenergic receptor system do not influence the effectiveness of forskolin. Accordingly, it has been demonstrated that forskolin increases adenylate cyclase activity and cAMP production in nonfailing and end-stage failing myocardium to a similar extent (5). In accordance with these data, forskolin activated contractile reserve (as assessed as the maximal inotropic response to Ca^{2+}) nearly completely in both nonfailing and end-stage failing myocardium in this study and in prior investigations (12). In contrast, both the increase in adenylate cyclase activity and cAMP production as well as the increase in force of contraction after β-adrenoceptor stimulation is significantly reduced in failing human myocardium (1, 6, 12).

Influence of forskolin on the force-frequency relation

Feldman et al. (13) were the first to describe a beneficial effect of forskolin on the force-frequency behavior in isolated human myocardium from failing hearts. However, these experiments were performed at low temperature (30 °C) and low stimulation rates (increase from 0.33 to 1.0 Hz). Subsequently, Mulieri et al. (26) tested the influence of forskolin (0.5 µM) on the force-frequency behavior in moderately failing myocardium from patients with mitral regurgitation. In their study, force of contraction increased only slightly with increasing stimulation rates before forskolin, but frequency-behavior was completely normalized after forskolin. Since depression of adenylate cyclase activity and intracellular cAMP levels may be even more pronounced in end-stage failing cardiomyopathy, we tested the influence of increasing concentrations of forskolin in ischemic and dilated cardiomyopathy. In the present study, force of contraction significantly declined at higher stimulation rates (negative force-frequency behavior) in end-stage failing myocardium from both ischemic and dilated cardiomyopathy. This negative force-frequency relation was beneficially affected by addition of 0.3 µM forskolin. At this low concentration of forskolin, the slope of the force-frequency relation was partially normalized and the optimum stimulation frequency did not differ from nonfailing myocardium (Fig. 7).

We could recently demonstrate that addition of forskolin results in Serine-16 and Threonin-17 phosphorylation of phospholamban in muscle strip preparations from failing human hearts (34). As a consequence, enhanced SR Ca^{2+} uptake capacity after forskolin may be the underlying mechanism for the partial normalization of the force-frequency-response in this study. These results are in agreement with the previous work of Mulieri et al. (26) and point to a similar defect in excitation-contraction coupling in moderately and severely failing myocardium which can be reversed by addition of low concentrations of forskolin. However, in contrast to moderately failing myocardium, in the present study forskolin normalized the force-frequency relation at low and intermediate stimulation rates, but did not prevent a decline in force at stimulation rates above 2.0 Hz in end-stage failing myocardium (Figs. 5 and 6). This might indicate exhaustion of the Ca^{2+} pump capacity at very high stimulation rates in end-stage failing myocardium despite relief of the inhibitory action of phospholamban, possibly related to reduced protein expression of the SR Ca^{2+} pump.

The observation that forskolin-mediated phosphorylation of phospholamban (and possibly of the SR Ca^{2+} pump itself (44)) has limited beneficial effects in failing human myocardium is underlined by the experiments at high concentrations of the drug. Higher concentrations of forskolin depressed frequency-response in nonfailing myocardium and had no effect on the negative force-frequency response in failing myocardium. Again, these findings are in agreement with previous work by Mulieri et al. (24) and may be attributable to excessive abbreviation of the twitch, which gets even more pronounced at higher stimulation rates (see Tables 1 and 2), a cAMP-mediated reduction in the Ca^{2+} sensitivity of the myofilaments (16), or Ca^{2+} overload of the myocytes. Furthermore, a high concentration of the β-adrenoceptor agonist isoproterenol reversed the positive force-frequency relation in nonfailing myocardium, while low concentrations of isoproterenol had beneficial effects on force-frequency response in failing human myocardium (39). In this context, it is interesting to note that phospholamban phosphorylation and lusitropy are achieved at lower intracellular cAMP levels than Ca^{2+} channel phosphorylation and positive inotropic effects (19).

Mulieri et al. (27) distinguished between altered expression and altered control of the SR Ca^{2+} pumps in failing human myocardium. In their study, they could normalize the blunted force-frequency relation in moderately failing myocardium due to mitral regurgitation with 0.5 μM forskolin. However, this normalization of the slope of the fore-frequency relation was associated with a significant abbreviation of the isometric twitch at each stimulation rate after forskolin as compared to nonfailing myocardium without forskolin. Because of these abnormally short relaxation times after forskolin, the authors concluded that restoration of the force-frequency in failing myocardium included a compensation for an additional defect in calcium pumping unrelated to protein kinase A control of SR Ca^{2+} pump activity. Accordingly, in our study, the partial normalization of the force-frequency relation at 0.3 μM forskolin was associated with a significant abbreviation of relaxation times of forskolin-treated failing myocardium as compared to untreated nonfailing myocardium at each stimulation rate (see Table 2). In other words, forskolin overcompensates reduced cAMP levels in failing myocardium, as can be seen from normalization of frequency-behavior associated with excess abbreviation of relaxation kinetics. This makes the combination of alterations in control of the activity (i.e., reduced cAMP, relative increase in phospholamban, or a defect in the phosphorylation sites of phospholamban) and a reduced expression of the SR Ca^{2+} pumps as underlying cause for altered frequency-behavior likely.

Clinical implications

The blunting and leftward shift of the force-frequency relation in failing hearts may be one underlying cause for the reduced exercise capacity of patients with heart failure. Furthermore, the presence of a negatively sloped force-frequency relation in the exercise range of heart rates may contribute to ventricular dilatation and the progression of heart failure. Under in-vivo conditions, adrenergic stimulation enhances frequency-potentiation of hemodynamic parameters of ventricular function (37). However, cAMP-dependent inotropic interventions have increased the risk for cardiovascular death in heart failure patients (29), and long-term β-blocker therapy may improve ventricular function and mortality, especially in patients with high heart rates (28, 42). Therefore, at this moment, long-term cAMP-dependent inotropic therapy is not recommended, but further clinical trials should try to identify a subgroup of patients who might benefit from interventions that stimulate cAMP production, possibly at very low dosages with only minimal inotropic effects.

Acknowledgment The excellent assistance of Ms. Mechthild Disch is gratefully acknowledged.

References

1. Böhm M, Beuckelmann D, Brown L, Feiler G, Lorenz B, Näbauer M, Kemkes B, Erdmann E (1988) Reduction of β-adrenoceptor density and evaluation of positive inotropic responses in isolated, diseased human myocardium. Eur Heart J 9: 844–852

2. Böhm M, Gierschik P, Jakobs KH, Pieske B, Schnabel P, Ungerer M, Erdmann E (1990) Increase of Giα in human hearts with dilated but not ischemic cardiomyopathy. Circulation 82: 1249–1265
3. Böhm M, Reiger B, Schwinger RH, Erdmann E (1994) cAMP concentrations, cAMP dependent protein kinase activity, and phospholamban in nonfailing and failing myocardium. Cardiovascr Res 28: 1713–1719
4. Bristow MR, Ginsburg R, Minobe W, Cubicciotti RS, Sageman WS, Lurie K, Billingham ME, Harrison DC, Stinson EB (1982) Decreased catecholamine sensitivity and beta-adrenergic-receptor density in failing human hearts. N Engl J Med 307: 205–211
5. Bristow MR, Ginsburg R, Strosberg A, Montgomery W, Minobe W (1984) Pharmacology and inotropic potential of forskolin in the human heart. J Clin Invest 74: 212–223
6. Bristow MR, Hershberger RE, Port JD, Minobe W, Rasmussen R (1988) β_1- and β_2-adrenergic receptor-mediated adenylate cyclase stimulation in nonfailing and failing human ventricular myocardium. Molec Pharmac 35: 295–303
7. Brodde OE (1991) β_1- and β_2-adrenoceptors in the human heart: Properties, function, and alterations in chronic heart failure. Pharmacol Rev 43: 203–242
8. Danielsen W, v. der Leyen H, Meyer W, Neumann J, Schmitz W, Scholz H, Starbatty J, Stein B, Doring V, Kalmar P (1989) Basal and isoprenaline-stimulated cAMP content in failing versus nonfailing human cardiac preparations. J Cardiovsc Pharmacol 14: 171–173
9. Eschenhagen T, Mende U, Nose M, Schmitz W, Scholz H, Haverich A, Hirt S, Döring V, Kalmar P, Höppner W, Seitz HJ (1992) Increased messenger RNA level of the inhibitory G-protein α-subunits Giα$_2$ in human end-stage heart failure. Circ Res 70: 688–696
10. Feldmann MD, Aldermann JD, Aroesti JM, Royal HD, Ferguson JJ, Owen RM, Grossmann W, McKay RG (1988) Depression of systolic and diastolic myocardial reserve during atrial pacing tachycardia in patients with dilated cardiomyopathy. J Clin Invest 82: 1661–1669
11. Feldmann AM, Cates AE, Veazey WB, Hershberger RE, Bristow MR, Baughman KL, Baumgartner WA, Van Dop C (1988) Increase in the 40,000-mol wt pertussis toxin sub-strate (G-protein) in the failing human heart. J Clin Invest 82: 189–197
12. Feldman MD, Copelas L, Gwathmey JK, Phillips P, Warren SE, Schoen FJ, Grossman W, Morgan JP (1987) Deficient production of cyclic AMP: pharmacologic evidence of an important cause of contractile dysfunction in patients with end-stage heart failure. Circulation 75: 331–339
13. Feldmann MD, Gwathmey JK, Phillips P, Schoen F, Morgan JP (1988) Reversal of the force-frequency relationship in working myocardium from patients with end-stage heart failure. J Appl Cardiol 3: 273–283
14. Flesch M, Schwinger RHG, Schiffer F, Frank K, Südkamp M, Kuhn-Regnier F, Arnold G, Böhm M (1996) Evidence for functional relevance of an enhanced expression of the Na^+/Ca^{2+} exchanger in failing human myocardium. Circulation 94: 922–1002
15. Gwathmey JK, Copelas L, MacKinnon R, Schoen FJ, Feldmann MD, Grossman W, Morgan JP (1987) Abnormal intracellular calcium handling in myocardium from patients with end-stage heart failure. Circ Res 61: 70–76
16. Hajjar RJ, Gao L, Solaro RJ, Gwathmey JK (1992) Differential effects of cAMP on Ca^{2+} activation and cross-bridge kinetics in control and myopathic myocardium. Circulation 86: I-282
17. Hasenfuss G, Holubarsch C, Hermann HP, Astheimer K, Pieske B, Just H (1994) Influence of the force-frequency relationship on hemodynamics and left ventricular function in patients with non-failing hearts and in patients with dilated cardiomyopathy. Europ Heart J 15: 164–170
18. Hasenfuss G, Reinecke H, Studer R, Meyer M, Pieske B, Holtz J, Holubarsch C, Posival H, Just H, Drexler H (1994) Relation between myocardial function and expression of sarcoplasmic reticulum Ca^{2+}-ATPase in failing and nonfailing human myocardium. Circ Res 75: 434–442
19. Kenakin TP, Amborse JR, Irving PE (1991) the relative efficiency of β-adrenoceptor coupling to myocardial inotropy and diastolic relaxation: organ selective treatment for diastolic dysfunction. J Pharmacol Exp Ther 257: 1189–1197
20. Limas CJ, Olivari MT, Goldenberg IF, Levine TB, Benditt DG, Simon A (1987) Calcium uptake by cardiac sarcoplasmic reticulum in human dilated cardiomyopathy. Cardiovasc Res 21: 601–605
21. Mercadier JJ, Lompre AM, Duc P, Boheler KR, Fraysse JB, Wisnewsky C, Allen PD, Komajda M, Schwartz K (1990) Altered sarcoplasmic reticulum Ca^{2+}-ATPase gene expression in the human ventricle during end-stage heart failure. J Clin Invest 85: 305–309
22. Meyer M, Schillinger W, Pieske B, Holubarsch C, Heilmann C, Posival H, Kuwajima G, Mikoshiba K, Just H, Hasenfuss G (1995) Alterations of sarcoplasmic reticulum proteins in failing human dilated cardiomyopathy. Circulation 92: 778–784
23. Mulieri LA, Hasenfuss G, Leavitt B, Allen PD, Alpert NR (1992) Altered myocardial force-frequency relation in human heart failure. Circulation 85: 1743–1750
24. Mulieri LA, Ittleman FP, Leavitt BJ, Martin BJ, Haeberle JR, Alpert NR (1992) Depressed myocardial force-frequency curve in mitral regurgitation heart failure is partially reversed by forskolin. Circulation 86: I-861
25. Mulieri LA, Leavitt B, Hasenfuss G, Allen PD, Alpert NR (1989) Protection of human left ventricular myocardium from cutting injury with 2,3-butanedione monoxime. Circ Res 65: 1441–1444

26. Mulieri LA, Leavitt BJ, Martin BJ, Haeberle JR, Alpert NR (1993) Myocardial force-frequency defect in mitral regurgitation heart failure is reversed by forskolin. Circulation 88: 2700–2704

27. Mulieri LA, Leavitt BJ, Wright RK, Alpert NR (1997) Role of cAMP in modulating relaxation kinetics and the force-frequency relation in mitral regurgitation heart failure. Basic Res Cardiol 92 (suppl I): 95–103

28. Packer M, Bristow MR, Cohn JN, Collucci WS, Fowler MB, Gilbert EM, Shusterman NH (1996) The effect of carvedilol on morbidity and mortality in patients with chronic heart failure. U.S. Carvedilol Heart Failure Study Group. New Engl J Med 334: 1349–1355

29. Packer M, Carver JR, Rodeheffer RJ, Ivanhoe RJ, DiBianco R, Zeldis SM, Hendrix GH, Bommer WJ, Elkayam U, Kukin ML, Mallis GI, Sollano JA, Shannon J, Tandon PK, DeMets DL (1991) Effect of oral milrinone on mortality in severe chronic heart failure. N Engl J Med 325: 1468–1475

30. Pieske B, Hasenfuss G, Holubarsch C, Schwinger R, Böhm M, Just H (1992) Alterations of the force-frequency relationship in the failing human heart depend on the underlying cardiac disease. Bas Res Card 87 (1): 213–221

31. Pieske B, Kretschmann B, Meyer M, Holubarsch C, Weirich J, Posival H, Minami K, Just H, Hasenfuss G (1995) Alterations in intracellular calcium handling associated with the inverse force-frequency relation in human dilated cardiomyopathy. Circulation 92: 1169–1178

32. Pieske B, Maier LS, Weber T, Bers DM, Hasenfuss G (1997) Alterations in sarcoplasmic reticulum Ca^{2+}-content in myocardium from patients with heart failure. Circulation 96 (suppl.): I-199

33. Pieske B, Sutterlin M, Schmidt-Schweda S, Minami K, Meyer M, Olschewski M, Holubarsch C, Just H, Hasenfuss G (1996) Diminished post-rest potentiation of contractile force in human dilated cardiomyopathy. Functional evidence for alterations in intracellular Ca^{2+} handling. J Clin Invest 98: 764–776

34. Pieske B, Zimber S, Bartel S, Karczewski P, Hasenfuss G, Just H, Scholz H, Stein B (1997) Frequency-induced inotropic and lusitropic effects in isolated human myocardium are cAMP independent. Europ Heart J 18 (suppl): P3544

35. Piot C, Lemaire S, Albat B, Seguin J, Nargeot J, Richard S (1996) High frequency-induced upregulation of human cardiac calcium currents. Circulation 93: 120–128

36. Reinecke H, Studer R, Vetter R, Holtz J, Drexler H (1996) Cardiac Na^+/Ca^{2+} exchange activity in patients with end-stage heart failure. Cardiovasc Res 31: 48–54

37. Ross J Jr, Miura T, Kambayashi M, Eising GP, Ryu KH (1995) Adrenergic control of the force-frequency relation. Circulation 92: 2327–2332

38. Schmidt U, Schwinger RH, Böhm M, Erdmann E (1994) Alterations of the force-frequency relation depending on stages of heart failure in humans. Am J Cardiol 74: 1066–1068

39. Schwinger RH, Böhm M, Müller-Ehmsen J, Uhlmann R, Schmidt U, Stäblein A, Überfuhr P, Kreuzer E, Reichart B, Eissner HJ, Erdmann E (1993) Effect of inotropic stimulation on the negative force-frequency relationship in the failing human heart. Circulation 88: 2267–2276

40. Schwinger RH, Böhm M, Schmidt U, Karczewski P, Bavendiek U, Flesch M, Krause EG, Erdmann E (1995) Unchanged protein levels of SERCA II and Phospholamban but reduced Ca^{2+} uptake and Ca^{2+}-ATPase activity of cardiac sarcoplasmic reticulum from dilated cardiomyopathy patients compared with patients with nonfailing hearts. Circulation 92: 3220–3228

41. Studer R, Reinecke H, Bilger J, Eschenhagen T, Böhm M, Hasenfuss G, Just H, Holtz J, Drexler H (1994) Gene expression of cardiac Na^+/Ca^{2+}-exchanger in end-stage human heart failure. Circ Res 75: 443–453

42. Waagstein F, Swedberg K, Hjalmarson A (1996) Improvement after metoprolol in idiopathic dilated cardiomyopathy is predicted by baseline systolic blood pressure and change in heart rate. JACC 27: 170A

43. Winegard S, Shanes AM (1962) Calcium flux and contractility in guinea pig atria. J Gen Physiol 45: 371–394

44. Xu A, Hawkins C, Narayanan N (1993) Phosphorylation and activation of the Ca^{2+}-pumping ATPase of cardiac sarcoplasmic reticulum by Ca^{2+}/calmodulin-dependent protein kinase. J Biol Chem 268: 8394– 8837

Author's address:
B. Pieske
Zentrum Innere Medizin
Abteilung Kardiologie und Pneumologie
Georg-August-Universität Göttingen
Robert-Koch-Str. 40
37075 Göttingen
Germany

Effect of inotropic interventions on the force-frequency relation in the human heart

U. Bavendiek, K. Brixius, G. Münch, C. Zobel, J. Müller-Ehmsen, R. H. G. Schwinger

Medizinische Klinik III, Labor für Herzmuskelphysiologie und molekulare Kardiologie, Universität zu Köln

Abstract

In severe human heart failure, an increase in frequency of stimulation is accompanied by a reduced force of contraction in vivo and in vitro. This contrasts the findings in nonfailing human hearts. To investigate influences of inotropic stimulation on the force-frequency relationship in human myocardium, the effects of the cAMP-independent positive inotropic agents ouabain (Na^+/K^+-ATPase inhibitor) and BDF 9148 (Na^+-channel modulator) as well as of the β-adrenoceptor agonist isoprenaline on the force-frequency relationship in electrically driven left ventricular papillary muscle strips from nonfailing and terminally failing human myocardium were studied. In nonfailing myocardium, force of contraction increased following an increase in stimulation frequency, whereas in failing human myocardium force of contraction gradually declined following an increase in stimulation frequency. Moderate stimulation of contractility by isoprenaline reversed the negative force-frequency relationship in failing myocardium and preserved the positive force-frequency relationship in nonfailing myocardium. In the presence of ouabain and BDF 9148 the positive force-frequency relationship was completely restored in failing myocardium. In contrast, in the presence of high concentrations of isoprenaline the former positive force-frequency relationship became negative even in nonfailing myocardium.

The negative force-frequency relationship in failing human myocardium is accompanied by alterations in the intracellular Ca^{2+}-homeostasis. The latter may be due to an impaired function of the sarcoplasmic reticulum (SR) in failing human myocardium. Therefore, the activity of the SR-Ca^{2+}-ATPase (SERCA2) of crude membrane preparations was investigated and was significantly reduced in failing compared to nonfailing human myocardium.

It is concluded that the negative force-frequency relationship may be due to alterations in the intracellular Ca^{2+}-handling caused by an impaired function of the SERCA2 in failing human myocardium. The beneficial effects of cAMP-increasing agents on the force-frequency relationship in failing human hearts could result from an enhanced phosphorylation status of phospholamban in the presence of β-adrenoceptor-stimulation. The effect of the $[Na^+]_i$-modulating agents BDF 9148 and ouabain demonstrates that the intracellular Na^+-homeostasis influences intracellular Ca^{2+}-handling as well. Differences observed in failing compared to nonfailing myocardium may be due to an altered expression or function of the Na^+/Ca^{2+}-exchanger, Na^+-channels or the Na^+/K^+-ATPase in addition to the blunted activity of the SERCA2 in failing myocardium.

Key words Heart failure – force-frequency relationship – inotropic stimulation – intracellular Ca^{2+}-homeostasis – SERCA2 – intracellular Na^+-homeostasis

Introduction

In nonfailing human myocardium, as in many other mammal species, frequency potentiation is a potent tool to increase inotropy (13). This phenomen first described about one hundred years ago by Bowditch (10) as "positive treppe" is used to increase blood flow during exercise. In terminaly heart failure, exercise is accompanied by a smaller decrease in endsystolic ventricular volume and a smaller increase in stroke volume compared to non-diseased hearts (18, 27). Additionally, peak rates of left ventricular pressure rise and fall are depressed and the frequency-dependent potentiation of these parameters is markedly reduced or even absent (18). Following these alterations the most obvious clinically consequences for patients with chronic heart failure is the complaint of dyspnoe and fatigue even at low exercise or even at rest, limiting them to perform activities of daily living.

Several investigators demonstrated an altered force-frequency relationship in failing human myocardium in vitro as well as in vivo studies (17, 38, 44). This failure to increase force of contraction following an increase in frequency of stimulation adds significantly to the already studied pathophysiological and pathobiochemical alterations in human heart failure, i.e., 1) altered β-adrenoceptor-effector-coupling due to downregulation of myocardial β-adrenoreceptors (11, 12), an increased level of inhibitory guanine nucleotid binding proteins (15), and reduced intracellular cAMP-levels (9, 14), 2) altered intracellular Ca^{2+} handling due to a reduced Ca^{2+} reuptake of the sarcoplasmic reticulum (31, 48) reported in isolated myocardial cells as well as in multicellular myocardial preparations (6, 7, 22, 41), 3) alterations at the level of the contractile apparatus as a reduced Mg^{2+}-ATPase activity (40), a slower cross-bridge cycling and an enhanced Ca^{2+} sensivity of the myofilaments (24, 25, 47, 53).

These alterations could have an influence on the negative force-frequency relationship in failing human hearts. To investigate mechanisms leading to a negative force-frequency relationship, inotropic interventions with different modes of action may help.

The present work mainly reviews previously performed investigations about cAMP-dependent and cAMP-independent inotropic interventions on the force-frequency relationship as well as data about an altered function of the SERCA2 in failing compared to nonfailing human myocardium.

Materials and methods

Myocardial tissue

Experiments were performed on isolated, electrically stimulated human left ventricular papillary muscle strips or trabecula. Tissue was obtained during cardiac transplantation. Patients suffered from heart failure clinically classified as NYHA IV on the basis of clinical symptoms and signs as judged by the attending cardiologist shortly before operation (DCM: n = 22, age 54.4 ± 3.5 y, ICM: n = 6, age 55.6 ± 2.5 y). Nonfailing human myocardium was obtained from donors who were brain dead as a result of traumatic injury and could not be transplanted for technical reasons (n = 8, age 51 ± 21 y). None of the patients had received Ca^{2+}-channel antagonists within 7 d of surgery. None of the patients received β-adrenoceptor agonists 48 h prior to operation. Drugs used for general anesthesia were flunitrazepam, fentanyl and pancuroniumbromide with isoflurane. Cardiac surgery was performed on cardiopulmonary bypass with cardioplegic arrest during hypothermia. Patients gave written informed consent before operation. The cardioplegic solution used was a modified Bretschneider solution containing (in mmol/l): NaCl 15; KCl 10; $MgCl_2$ 4; histidine HCl 180; tryptophan 2; mannitol 30; potassium dihydrogen oxoglutarate 1.

Contraction experiments

Immediately after excision, the myocardial tissue was placed in ice-cold preaerated Tyrode's solution (composition below) and delivered to the laboratory within 10 minutes. From each native myocardial tissue sample, left ventricular papillary muscle strips or trabeculae of 0.6–0.8 mm width and 8–10 mm length were carefully prepared under microscopic control (Axiovert 100, Carl Zeiss, Oberkochen, Germany) with muscle fibers running parallel to the length of the strips. Connective tissue if visible was carefully trimmed away. The muscles were suspended in an organ bath (20 ml) maintained at 37 °C and containing a modified Tyrode's solution of the following composition (in mmol/l): NaCl 119.8; KCl 5.4; $MgCl_2$ 1.05; $CaCl_2$ 1.8; Na HCO_3 22.6; NaH_2PO_4 0.42; glucose 5.05; ascorbic acid 0.28; Na_2EDTA 0.05. The bathing solution was continuously aerated with 95 % O_2 and 5 % CO_2. The muscles were stimulated by two platinum electrodes using field stimulation from a Grass S 88 stimulator (frequency 1 Hz; duration 5 ms; intensity 10 % to 20 % above threshold). Preparations were allowed to equilibrate for at least 90 min, with the bathing solution being changed once after 45 min. Isometric force of contraction was measured with an inductive force transducer (W. Fleck, Mainz, FRG) attached to a Hellige Helco scriptor (Hellige, Freiburg, FRG) or Gould recorder (Gould Inc., Cleveland, Ohio). Each muscle was streched to the length at which force of contraction was maximal. After complete mechanical stabilization, the force-frequency relationship was studied over a range of 0.5–3 Hz starting with a rate of 0.5 Hz before and after pharmacological intervention. Control strips show a decline of less then 10 % in baseline isometric tension during the period of time necessary to complete pharmacological testing. Frequency- or compound-dependent changes in force of contraction (FOC) were determined.

Preparation of the SR-vesicles and measurement of the activity of the SERCA2

The isolation of vesicles of the sarcoplasmic reticulum (SR) and the measurement of the activity of the SERCA2 were performed as described recently (48).

Materials

BDF 9148 (4-(3-(1-diphenylmethyl-azetidin-3-oxy)-2-hydroxy-propoxy)1 H-indol-2-carbonitrile) was kindly provided from Beiersdorf-Lilly AG (Hamburg, Germany). Ouabain, NADH, and Na_2ATP were obtained from Boehringer (Mannheim, Germany), phosphoenolpyruvat, PK/LDH-enzym-mixture, and isoprenaline from Sigma Chemical Co. (Deisenhofen, Germany). BDF 9148 was dissolved in DMSO. The final concentration of DMSO in the bathing solution never exceeded 0.05 %. All other chemicals were of analytical grade or the best grade commercially available. Only deionized and double-distilled water was used throughout.

Statistics

The data shown are means ± SEM. Statistical difference in the shape of the force-frequency relation in nonfailing human myocardium were analyzed as described previously (46). Statistical significance was analyzed using the Student's t-test for unpaired or paired observations (SPSS PC plus); $p < 0.05$ was considered to be significant.

Results

Force-frequency relationship in failing and nonfailing human myocardium

The rate-dependent change in force of contraction in nonfailing and failing myocardium is demonstrated in the original recordings given in Fig. 1. Only in the nonfailing heart was an increase in force of contraction linked with an enhanced stimulation frequency. Figure 2 shows the force-frequency relationship in failing and nonfailing human myocardium in a range from 0.5–3 Hz. Following an increase in stimulation frequency up to 3 Hz, the change in force of contraction gradually increased in nonfailing myocardium. In contrast, in failing myocardium an increase in the frequency of stimulation was accompanied by a decrease of change in force of contraction.

Force-frequency relationship and stimulation with isoprenaline

In order to investigate the influence of cAMP-dependent inotropic stimulation on the force-frequency relationship in failing and nonfailing myocardium, concentrations of 0.01 and

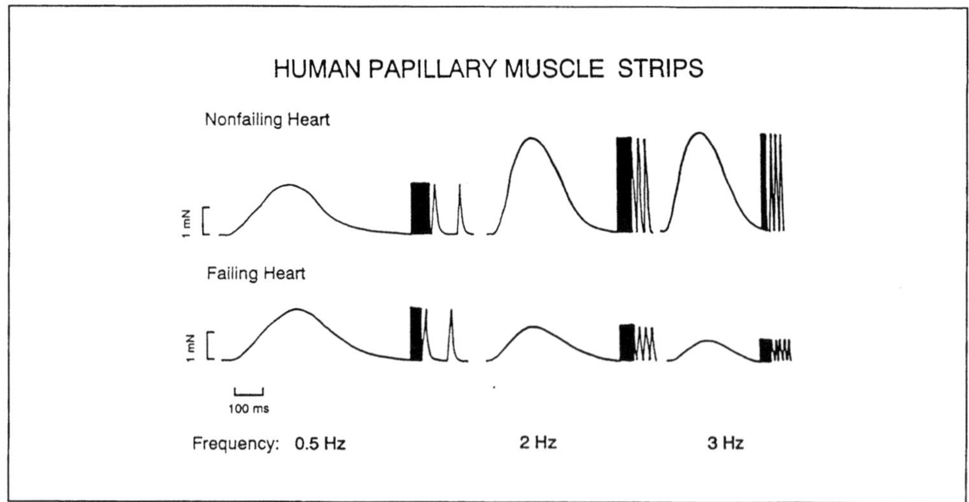

Fig. 1   Original recording of force of contraction in electrically driven papillary muscle strips from nonfailing and failing myocardium at various stimulation frequencies (adapted from Schwinger et al. 1993).

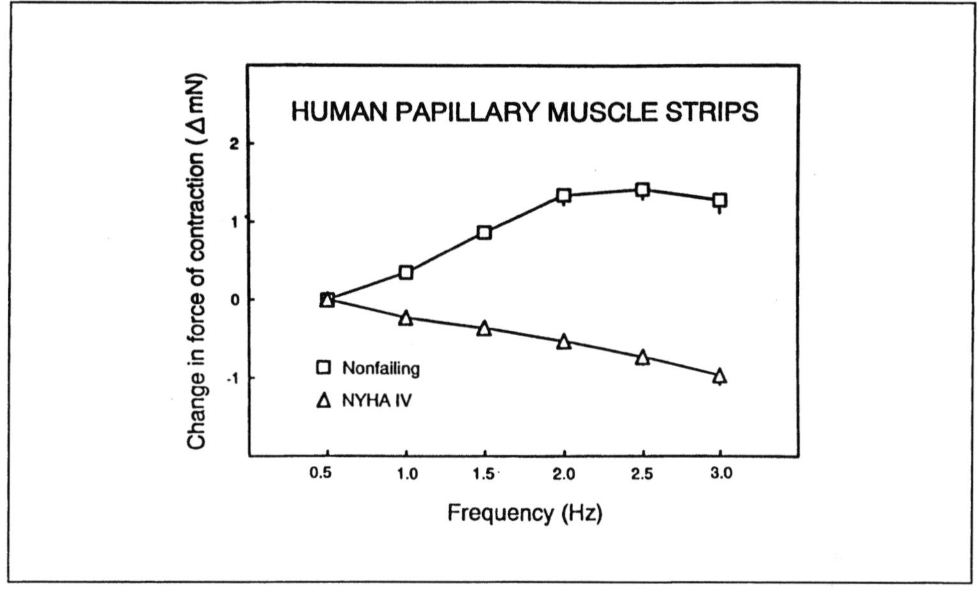

Fig. 2 Force-frequency relationship in electrically driven papillary muscle strips from nonfailing and terminally failing (NYHA IV) human myocardium. Increase in stimulation frequency is followed by an increase in force of contraction in nonfailing myocardium. In contrast in terminally failing myocardium, higher stimulation frequencies are followed by a decrease in force of contraction. Basal force of contraction at 0.5 Hz was 1.7 ± 0.2 mN in the nonfailing (13 muscle strips) and 2.4 ± 0.2 mN in the failing group (58 muscle strips). Force of contraction was significantly reduced in failing (1.8 ± 0.1 mN) compared to nonfailing hearts (3.1 ± 0.3 mN, $p < 0.05$) at a stimulation frequency of 2 Hz (adapted from Schwinger et al. 1993).

0.1 µmol/l isoprenaline in the organ bath were used. The application of a low concentration of isoprenaline (0.01 µmol/l) to the organ bath was not followed by a significant increase in force of contraction at basal conditions (0.5 Hz). In contrast application of a high concentration of isoprenaline (0.1 µmol/l) was followed by a significant increase in force of contraction as described previously (46). Stimulation with the low concentration of isoprenaline (0.01 µmol/l) did not influence the force-frequency relationship in nonfailing myocardium. In contrast in failing myocardium, the negative force-frequency relationship became even positive in the presence of 0.01 µmol/l isoprenaline (Fig. 3). Figure 4 shows the effect of a high concentration of isoprenaline (0.1 µmol/l) on the force-frequency relationship in nonfailing and failing human myocardium. In the presence of 0.1 µmol/l isoprenaline the previous positive force-frequency relationship in nonfailing myocardium became negative. In contrast to the improving influence of a low concentration of isoprenaline (0.01 µmol/l) on the negative force-frequency relationship in failing myocardium, the force-frequency relationship remained negative in the presence of a high concentration of isoprenaline (0.1 µmol/l) in failing myocardium.

Force-frequency relationship and stimulation with ouabain and BDF 9148

To examine the effect of various intracellular Na^+-concentrations the force-frequency relation was studied in the presence of the Na^+-channel-modulator BDF 9148 (0.1 µmol/l) and the cardiac glycoside ouabain (0.01 µmol/l). In the presence of ouabain plus BDF 9148

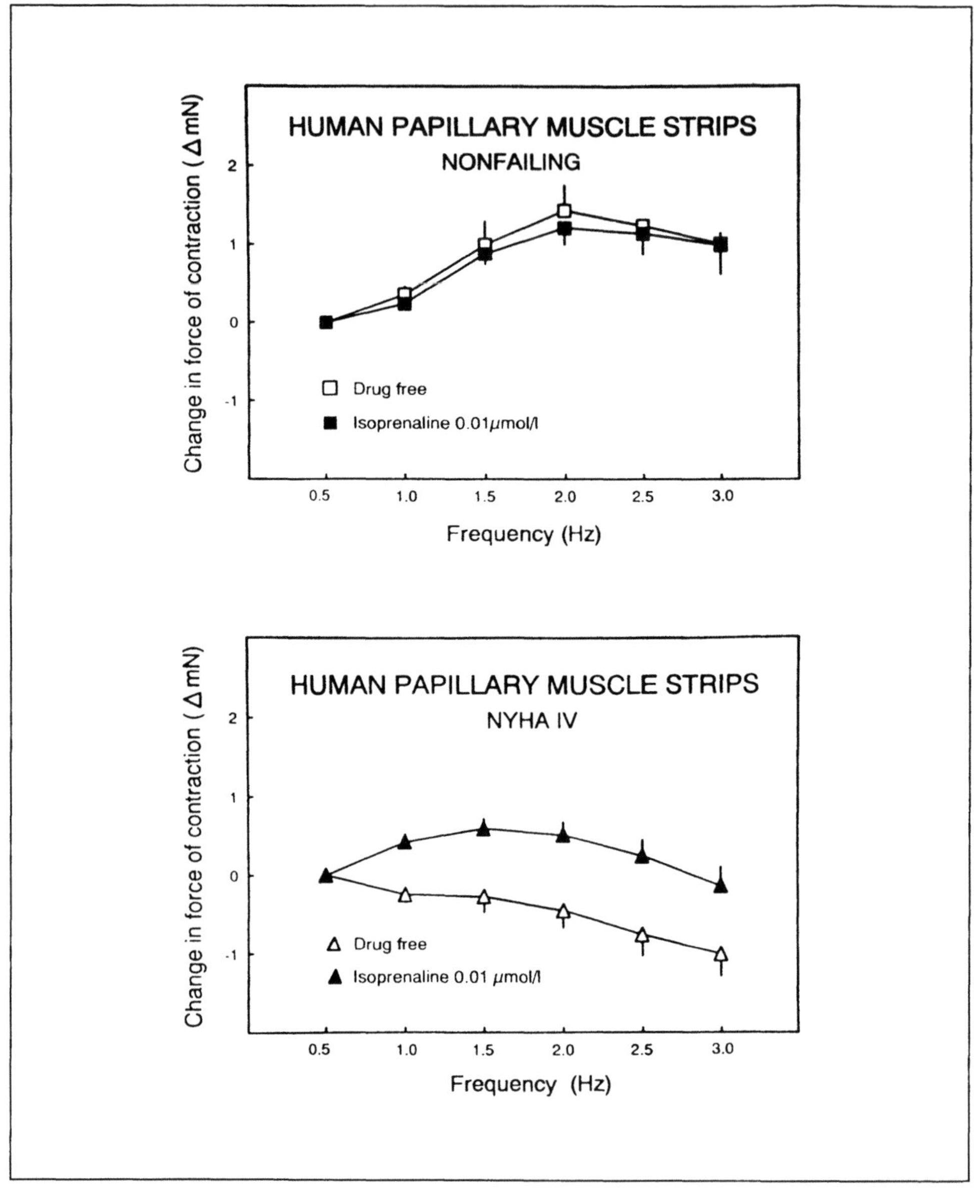

Fig. 3 Force-frequency relationship in failing and nonfailing myocardium under basal conditions and in the presence of a low concentration of isoprenaline (0.01 μmol/l) in isolated electrically driven papillary muscle strips from nonfailing (top) and failing (bottom) myocardium. The number of muscle strips studied was 7 in the failing and 4 in the nonfailing group. Whereas 0.01 μmol/l isoprenaline had no influence on the positive force-frequency relationship in nonfailing myocardium the former negative force-frequency relationship in failing myocardium became positive in the presence of 0.01 μmol/l isoprenaline. Basal force of contraction was 2.5 ± 0.4 mN and 2.7 ± 0.4 mN with as well as without pretreatment in failing tissue. The corresponding values in nonfailing myocardium were 1.9 ± 0.3 mN and 1.8 ± 0.4 mN (adapted from Schwinger et al. 1993).

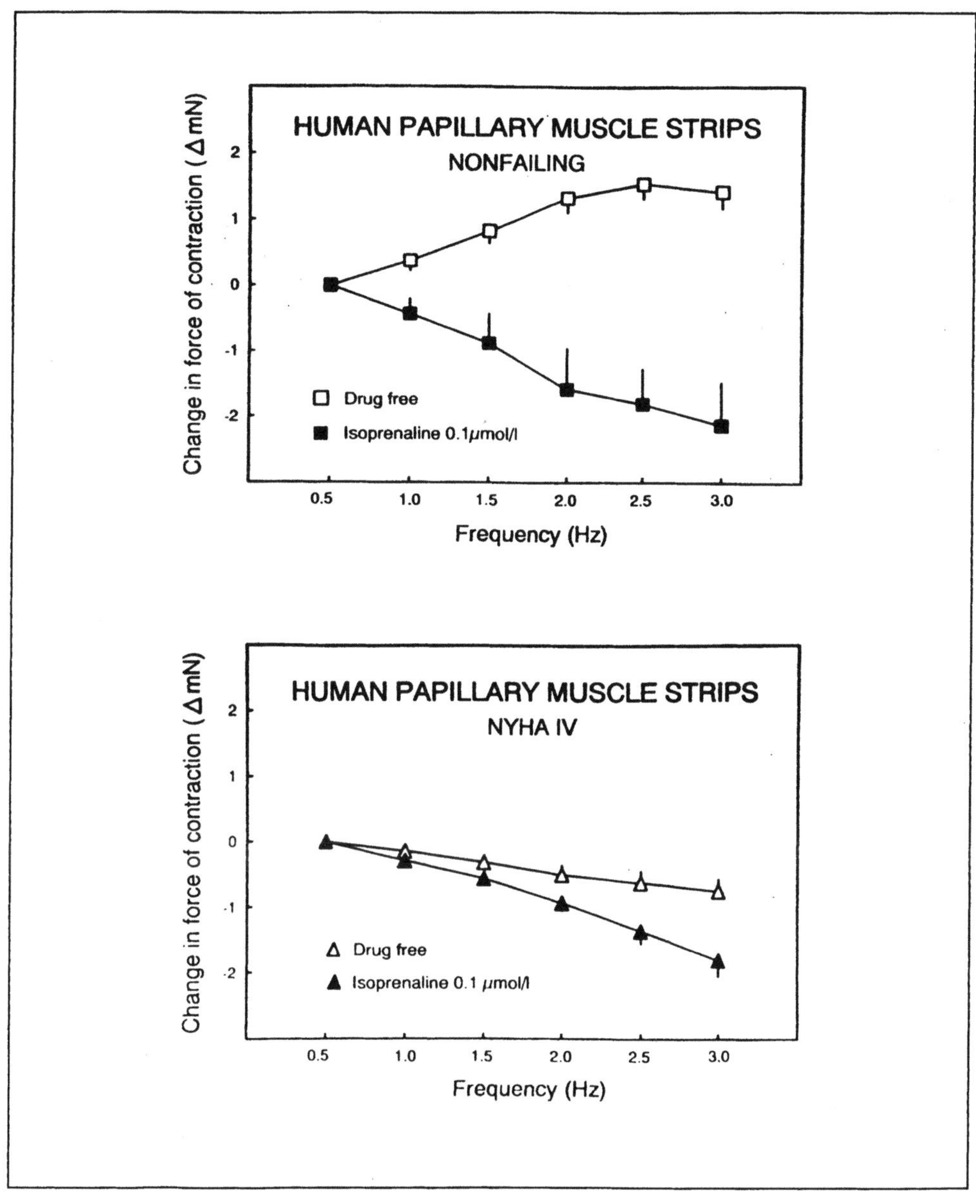

Fig. 4 Effect of inotropic stimulation with a high concentration of isoprenaline (0.1 μmol/l) on the force-frequency relationship in isolated electrically driven papillary muscle strips from nonfailing (top) and failing (bottom) myocardium. The number of muscle strips studied was 7 in the failing and 4 in the nonfailing group. In the presence of 0.1 μmol/l isoprenaline the former positive force-frequency relationship in nonfailing myocardium became negative and the force-frequency relationship remained still negative in failing myocardium. Basal force of contraction was 3.4 ± 0.4 mN and 1.7 ± 0.1 mN with as well as without pretreatment in failing tissue. The corresponding values in nonfailing myocardium were 7.5 ± 1.3 mN and 1.8 ± 0.2 mN (adapted from Schwinger et al. 1993).

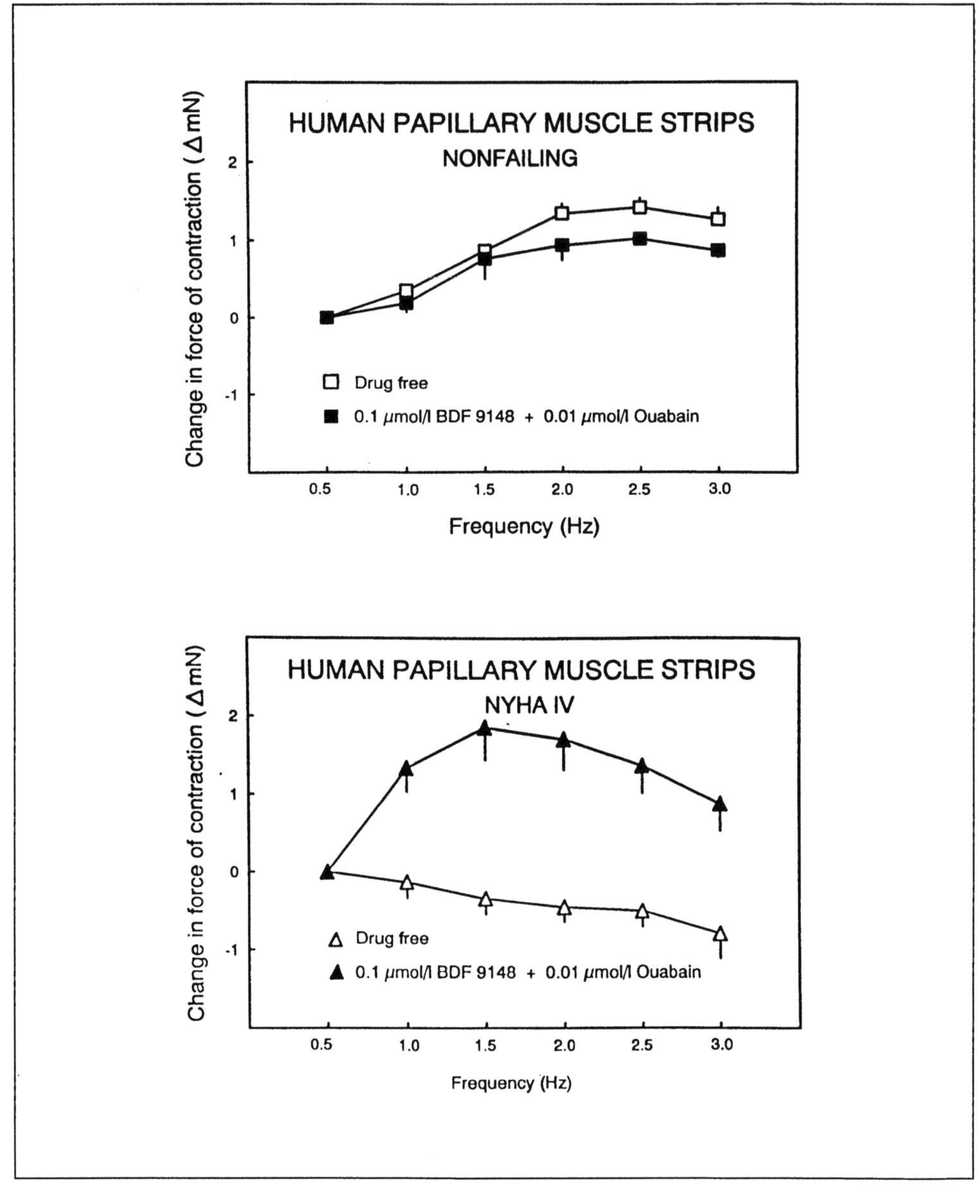

Fig. 5 Effect of BDF 9148 (0.1 µmol/l) plus ouabain (0.01 µmol/l) on the force-frequency relationship in isolated electrically driven papillary muscle strips from nonfailing (top) and failing (bottom) human myocardium. The number of muscle strips studied was 14 in the failing and 4 in the nonfailing group. Basal force of contraction with as well without pretreatment was 4.6 ± 0.2 mN and 2.4 ± 0.2 mN in the failing group and 1.9 ± 0.2 mN and 1.7 ± 0.2 mN in the nonfailing group, respectively. Prestimulation with BDF 9148 (0.1 µmol/l) plus ouabain (0.01 µmol/l) was able to restore the former negative force-frequency relationship in failing human myocardium (adapted from Schwinger et al. 1993).

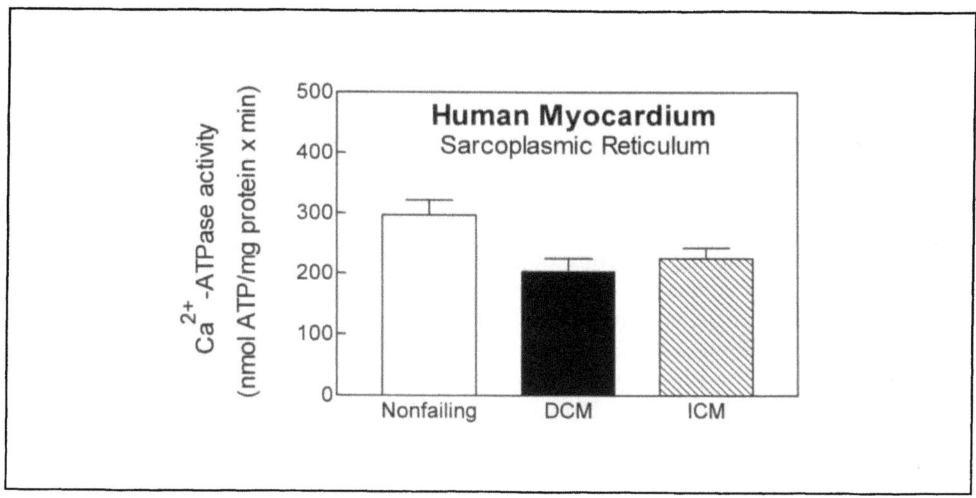

Fig. 6 Activity of the SERCA2 in crude membrane preparations from nonfailing and failing myocardium from patients with idiopathic dilated cardiomyopathy (DCM) and ischemic dilated cardiomyopathy (ICM). Activity of the SERCA2 in DCM as well as in ICM was significantly reduced compared to nonfailing human myocardium (p < 0.05). The activity of the SERCA2 in nmol ATPx mg protein^{-1} x min^{-1} was 279 ± 23 in nonfailing myocardium (n = 7), 195 ± 21 in DCM (n = 10), and 213 ± 18 in ICM (n = 6).

the change in force of contraction increased following an increase in stimulation frequency even in terminally failing myocardium (Fig. 5). BDF 9148 (0.1 µmol/l) plus ouabain (0.01 µmol/l) did not affect the force-frequency relation in nonfailing tissue. As previously published, also under the influence of BDF 9148 as well as ouabain alone the negative force-frequency relationship in failing myocardium became positive and the positive force-frequency relationship in nonfailing myocardium remained positive (8, 19). Thus, differences in the protein expression and function of regulatory proteins of the Na$^+$-homeostasis may occur in failing human myocardium to result in different modifications on the force-frequency relationship in failing compared to nonfailing myocardium.

Activity of the SERCA2 in human failing and nonfailing myocardium

The activity of the SERCA2 was measured by an optical assay in sarcoplasmic reticulum membrane preparations as described previously (48). The activity of the SERCA2 was measured at a free Ca^{2+}-concentration of 10 µmol/l in the presence of the calcium ionophore A 23187 (3 µmol/l) in failing and nonfailing human myocardium, respectively. As illustrated in Fig. 6 in crude membrane preparations of the sarcoplasmic reticulum the activity of the SERCA2 was significantly reduced in failing (DCM, ICM) compared to nonfailing (NF) human myocardium. This holds true for both, ischemic and dilated cardiomyopathic hearts (activity of the SERCA2 in nmol ATP x mg protein^{-1} x min^{-1}: NF 279 ± 23, DCM 195 ± 21, ICM 213 ± 18).

Discussion

Force-frequency relationship and intracellular Ca^{2+}-handling

Several studies have demonstrated a blunted force-frequency relationship in terminally human heart failure (17, 38, 44). The latter has been suggested to be due to alterations in intracellular Ca^{2+}-handling in failing human myocardium. Gwathmey et al. (22, 23) and Pieske et al. (41) have measured frequency dependent changes in developed tension and intracellular Ca^{2+}-transients using the bioluminescent bioprotein aequorin in multicellular preparations in failing and nonfailing human myocardium. Both groups found a negative force-frequency relationship as well as alterations in the intracellular Ca^{2+}-homeostasis in failing compared to nonfailing human myocardium. However, at higher stimulation frequencies Gwathmey et al. (22, 23) found no alterations in the systolic peak $[Ca^{2+}]_i$ but a significant increase in diastolic $[Ca^{2+}]_i$ and diastolic tension in failing compared to nonfailing myocardium. In contrast, Pieske et al. (41) did not detect alterations in diastolic tension or diastolic Ca^{2+} but a significant decrease in peak Ca^{2+}-transients and a close correlation between peak intracellular Ca^{2+} signals and isometric tension at a given frequency of stimulation. Additionally, Beuckelmann et al. (6) have reported a decreased peak $[Ca^{2+}]_i$ concentration and an increased diastolic $[Ca^{2+}]_i$ concentration in failing compared to nonfailing human hearts in measurements of electrically stimulated isolated myocardial cells using the Ca^{2+} indicator fura-2; however, these studies refer only to the basal condition as frequency of stimulation was not changed. Although this is an increasing evidence for an altered Ca^{2+}-handling in failing human myocardium, it remains still a matter of debate whether alterations of tension development and Ca^{2+}-handling at increasing frequencies are due to systolic and/or diastolic changes. The use of different intracellular Ca^{2+}-indicating dyes (aequorin vs. fura) with different sensivities to measure diastolic or systolic $[Ca^{2+}]_i$, the lack of quantification of intracellular Ca^{2+} concentrations (22, 41), and the use of unphysiological low experimental temperatures (30 °C) or low stimulation rates (22, 23) probably explain some of the observed differences in intracellular Ca^{2+}-handling. However, additional measurements comparing failing and nonfailing human myocardium are necessary to solve these controversal results described above. It remains an unresolved issue whether the systolic Ca^{2+} level, the diastolic Ca^{2+} level or both affect the force-frequency relationship and hence may be responsible for the negative force-frequency relationship found in failing myocardial tissue.

Activity of the SERCA2 influences the force-frequency relationship

The impaired Ca^{2+} sequestration by the sarcoplasmic reticulum may be one candidate for the altered Ca^{2+}-handling and the altered force-frequency relationship in failing myocardium. Although a reduced mRNA-expression of the SERCA2 and of phospholamban has been found in failing compared to nonfailing myocardium (2, 3, 16, 32, 48, 52) studies investigating the protein levels or function of the SERCA2 reveal contradictory results. Movsesian et al. (37), Schwinger et. al. (48), and Linck et al. (32) found no difference in the protein expression of SERCA2 and phospholamban between nonfailing and failing myocardium. In contrast, one group (26, 34, 52) found a reduced SERCA2 protein expression in failing human myocardium compared to nonfailing tissue. However, whereas Movsesian et al. (35) found no difference in Ca^{2+}-uptake between failing and nonfailing human myocardium, Ca^{2+}-uptake and activity of the SERCA2 in diseased hearts have been shown to be reduced compared to nonfailing hearts by several investigators (31, 48, this study). Consistently, Beuckelmann et al. (7) measured a significant slower decline of a caffeine induced intracellular Ca^{2+}-transient after maximal preloading of the sarcoplasmic reticulum with Ca^{2+} in isolated myocardial cells in failing compared to nonfailing myocardium. Beuckelmann and coworkers (7) interpreted this alteration to be due to a diminished activity of the SERCA2 in failing myocardium, as other important mechanisms of Ca^{2+} extrusion out of the cytosol, e.g., Na^+/Ca^{2+}-exchange were not present at the given experimental conditions.

Furthermore the Ca^{2+} sensivity of the SERCA2 may be altered (49). This altered function of the SERCA2 could be the result of an altered phosphorylation of phospholamban via the cAMP-dependent or Ca^{2+}/calmodulin-dependent proteinkinase (33, 49), an altered phosphorylation of the SERCA2 via the Ca^{2+}/calmodulin-dependent proteinkinase (54) or changes of intracellular regulatory proteins, e.g., calmodulin (28).

Consistenly, recently published data highlight the need of an unimpaired function of the sarcoplasmic reticulum for the positive force-frequency relationship in human myocardium. As the inhibition of the SERCA2 by the high selective inhibitor cyclopiazonic acid led to a negative force-frequency relationship even in nondiseased human myocardium (5, 50) a close correlation between force-frequency behaviour and SR-Ca^{2+}-uptake measured in identical nonfailing and failing human hearts has also been shown (41).

cAMP and the force-frequency relationship

The positive force-frequency relationship has been suggested to be due to changes in the Ca^{2+} content of the sarcoplasmic reticulum, possibly as a result of changes in net Ca^{2+} influx into the cell secondary to an increase in $[Na]_i$ (20). If a reduced Ca^{2+}-loading of the sarcoplasmic reticulum is the cause, then agents that facilitate Ca^{2+}-reuptake would be beneficial. Stimulation with a low concentration of isoprenaline caused an increase in the force of contraction following an increase in stimulation rate in failing human myocardium with a former negative force-frequency relationship and was able to preserve the "positive treppe" phenomenon observed in nonfailing human myocardium. In contrast, prestimulation with a high concentration of isoprenaline resulted in a pronounced negative force-frequency relationship in both failing and nonfailing human myocardium. This has been demonstrated also after increasing the extracellular Ca^{2+} concentration and may result from "Ca^{2+}-overload" after significant inotropic stimulation (46). In failing human myocardium basal and isoprenaline stimulated cAMP levels were reported to be reduced (9, 14). This seems not to be caused by an increased phosphodiesterase activity (36, 51) but rather because of a downregulation of β-adrenoceptors (11, 12) or increased levels of inhibitory G-proteins (15) in failing human hearts. One major target of phosphorylation through the cAMP-dependent proteinkinase is the regulatory protein of the SERCA2 phospholamban (33). Phospholamban decreased the Ca^{2+} sensivity of the SERCA2 in its unphosphorylated form. Phospholamban looses its inhibitory effect on the SERCA2 after phosphorylation through the cAMP-dependent or Ca^{2+}/Calmodulin-dependent proteinkinase leading to an increased Ca^{2+} sensivity of the SERCA2. As recently described, there is a decreased Ca^{2+} sensivity of the SERCA2 and cAMP-dependent phosphorylation level of phospholamban in failing compared to nonfailing myocardium possibly as a result of reduced cAMP levels in failing human myocardium (49). Altered regulatory processes through cAMP-dependent phosphorylation may be an important reason for the impaired force-frequency relationship and Ca^{2+}-handling in failing human myocardium. As low concentrations of isoprenaline (46) or forskolin (39), which enhance intracellular cAMP levels and thereby increase Ca^{2+}-reuptake of the sarcoplasmic reticulum, were able to restore the positive force-frequency relationship in failing hearts, there seems to be no cAMP-dependent post-receptor defect in failing human myocardium. In addition as described in guinea pig atria, lusitropy and phospholamban phosphorylation occurred at lower cAMP levels than positive inotropic responses and Ca^{2+} channel phosphorylation (29). In the presence of low concentrations of isoprenaline, maximal rate of tension decay increased more in relation to developed force of contraction at higher frequencies of stimulation (46). As in myopathic cells diastolic intracellular Ca^{2+} is already augmented (6), a further increase by cAMP-dependent or cAMP-independent positive inotropic agents may be detremential. Only moderate stimulation of cAMP will be effective to improve myocardial function by facilitating diastolic Ca^{2+} sequestration by cAMP-dependent phosphorylation of phosholamban. In human heart failure the excessively enhanced endogenous catecholamine levels could impair myocardial function due to an enhanced diastolic Ca^{2+} load. In this situation, application of β-adrenoceptor antagonists may improve myocardial function not only by lowering heart rate but also by reducing stimulatory effects on intracellular Ca^{2+}-homeostasis. This could hold true especially for the newer class of β-adrenoceptor antagonists, which may not increase the number of stimulatory β-adrenoceptors during treatment, e.g., carvedilol.

Intracellular Na$^+$ and the force-frequency relationship

The combination of ouabain plus BDF 9148 was effective in restoring the positive force-frequency relationship in failing human myocardium. Cardiac glycosides enhance intracellular Na^+ possibly via blockade of the Na^+/K^+-ATPase (1). The Na^+ channel activator BDF 9148 increases intracellular Na^+ that activates the Na^+/Ca^{2+}-exchanger to increase intracellular Ca^{2+}. In contrast to β-adrenergic stimulation, both compounds remain effective in increasing force of contraction in failing human myocardium (45). Prestimulation with BDF 9148 has been reported to enhance sensivity to ouabain in human myocardium (45). Both compounds activate membrane-bound Na^+/Ca^{2+}-exchange mechanisms and thereby influence the sarcolemmal Ca^{2+}-transient and intracellular Ca^{2+}-homeostasis. As only in failing human myocardium the force-frequency relationship became positive in the presence of low concentrations of ouabain plus BDF 9148, the protein expression and function of regulatory proteins of the Na^+-homeostasis, e.g., the Na^+/Ca^{2+}-exchanger, the Na^+/K^+-ATPase and Na^+ channels, may be different in failing compared to nonfailing human myocardium. Pretreatment with low concentrations of ouabain plus BDF 9148 or isoprenaline influenced the force-frequency relationship similarily, indicating that the underlying mechanisms responsible for improvement of the force-frequency relationship may represent not only cAMP-dependent mechanisms rather than other effects influencing directly or indirectly intracellular Ca^{2+}-handling. Recent studies have shown that there may be no difference in the number of binding sites for cardiac glycosides, i.e., the Na^+/K^+-ATPase between nonfailing and failing human myocardium (43). However, as recently reported the Na^+/K^+-ATPase-isoform expression may be changed in failing compared to nonfailing tissue, thus, leading to a decreased Na^+/K^+-ATPase activity in failing human myocardium (21). Studer et al. reported an increased mRNA- and protein-expression as well as an increased activity of the Na^+/Ca^{2+}-exchanger in the failing human heart compared to nonfailing tissue (42, 52). As a consequence, an increased Ca^{2+}-influx via activation of the Na^+/Ca^{2+}-exchanger (4) followed by an enhanced Ca^{2+}-induced Ca^{2+}-release (30) in failing compared to nonfailing myocardium may be caused by one or both of the above mentioned alterations: an increased expression and function of the Na^+/Ca^{2+}-exchanger or an increased intracellular $[Na^+]$ due to a reduced Na^+/K^+-ATPase activity in failing compared to non-failing tissue. These studies might be an indicative for an altered Na^+-homeostasis in addition to the altered Ca^{2+}-homeostasis in failing human myocardium as well.

Conclusions

The present study demonstrates that increasing intracellular Ca^{2+}-concentrations may have a detrimental effect on the force-frequency relationship in man. The negative force-frequency relationship may result from an altered intracellular Ca^{2+}-handling. The lack of systolic Ca^{2+} augmentation and/or the presence of an enhanced diastolic Ca^{2+} level may lead to a failure of the heart to increase force after enhancing the frequency of stimulation. In addition, the intracellular Na^+-homeostasis seems to be altered in failing myocardium as well. Functional alterations of the Ca^{2+}- and Na^+-regulatory systems – SERCA2, Na^+/K^+-ATPase, Na^+/Ca^{2+}-exchanger – rather than alterations of the protein expression seem to be responsible for the inversed force-frequency relationship in heart failure. New therapeutical approaches in treatment of heart failure should adress these pathophysiological alterations. Pharmacological stimulation of the SERCA2, phospholamban-inhibitors, or genetic modification leading to an enhanced activity of the SERCA2 may be therapeutical interventions in the future.

Acknowledgment Our special thanks are due to Professor Dr. B. Reichart (Dept. of Cardiac Surgery, University of Munich) and Professor Dr. de Vivie (Dept. of Cardiac Surgery, University of Cologne) and their colleagues for providing the myocardial tissue. We thank Heidrun Villena, Tatjana Schewior, and Andrea Herber for their excellent technical assistance. Experimental work was supported by the Deutsche Forschungsgemeinschaft (DFG: R.H.G.S.) and the Zentrum für Molekulare Medizin Köln (ZMMK: R.H.G.S.: Projekt 26). We are although thankful for the support of the "Sandoz Stiftung für therapeutische Forschung". This work contains data of the Doctoral Thesis of U.B. (University of Cologne, in preparation).

References

1. Akera T, Brody TM (1978) The role of the Na^+-K^+-ATPase in the inotropic action of digitalis. Pharmacol Rev 29: 187–220
2. Arai M, Alpert NR, MacLennan DH, Barton P, Periasamy M (1993) Alterations in sarcoplasmic reticulum gene expression in human heart failure: a possible mechanism for alterations in systolic and diastolic properties of the failing myocardium. Circ Res 72: 463–469
3. Arai M, Matsui H, Periasamy M (1994) Sarcoplasmic reticulum gene expression in cardiac hypertrophy and heart failure. Circ Res 74: 555–564
4. Barcenas-Ruiz L, Beuckelmann DJ, Wier WG (1987) Sodium-channel exchange in heart: membrane currents and changes in $[Ca^{2+}]_i$. Science 238: 1720–1722
5. Bavendiek U, Brixius K, Frank K, Reuter H, Pietsch M, Groß A, Müller-Ehmsen J, Erdmann E, Schwinger RHG (1996) Altered inotropism in the failing human myocardium. Basic Res Cardiol 91 (Suppl 2): 9–16
6. Beuckelmann DJ, Näbauer M, Erdmann E (1992) Intracellular calcium handling in isolated ventricular myocytes from patients with terminal heart failure. Circulation 85: 1046–1055
7. Beuckelmann DJ, Näbauer M, Krüger C, Erdmann E (1995) Altered diastolic $[Ca^{2+}]_i$ in human ventricular myocytes from patients with terminal heart failure. Am Heart J 129: 684–689
8. Böhm M, La Rosee K, Schmidt U, Schulz C, Schwinger RHG, Erdmann E (1992) Force-frequency relationship and inotropic stimulation in the nonfailing and failing human myocardium: implications for the medical treatment of heart failure. Clin Invest 70: 421–425

9. Böhm M, Reiger B, Schwinger RHG, Erdmann E (1994) cAMP concentrations, cAMP dependent protein-kinase activity, and phospholamban in non-failing and failing myocardium. Cardiovasc Res 28: 1713–1719

10. Bowditch HP (1871) Über die Eigentümlichkeiten der Reizbarkeit, welche die Muskelfasern des Herzens zeigen. Berl Sächs Ges (Akad) Wiss: 652–689

11. Bristow MR, Ginsburg R, Minobe W, Cubicciotti RS, Sageman WS, Lurie K, Billingham ME, Harrison DC, Stinson EB (1982) Decreased catecholamine sensitivity and β-adrenergic-receptor density in failing human hearts. N Engl J Med 307: 205–211

12. Brodde O-E (1991) β_1- and β_2-adrenoceptors in the human heart: properties, function, and alterations in chronic heart failure. Pharmacol Rev 43: 203–242

13. Buckley NM, Penefsky ZJ, Litwak RS (1972) Comparative force-frequency relationship in human and other mammalian ventricular myocardium. Pflugers Arch 332: 259–270

14. Danielsen W, von der Leyen H, Meyer W, Neumann J, Schmitz W, Scholz H, Starbatty J, Stein B, Döring V, Kalmar P (1989) Basal and isoprenaline-stimulated cAMP content in failing versus nonfailing human cardiac preparation. J Cardiovasc Pharmacol 14: 171–173

15. Feldman AM, Cates AE, Veazey WB, Hershberger RE, Bristow MR, Raughman KL, Baumgartner WA, Van Dop C (1988) Increase of the 40000-mol wt pertussis toxin substrate (G protein) in the failing human heart. J Clin Invest 82: 189–197

16. Feldman AM, Ray PE, Silan CM, Mercer JA, Minobe W, Bristow MR (1991) Selective gene expression in failing human heart: quantification of steady-state levels of messanger RNA in endomyocardial biopsies using the polymerase chain reaction. Circulation 83: 1866–1872

17. Feldman MD, Gwathmey JK, Phillips P, Schoen F, Morgan JP (1988) Reversal of the force-frequency-relationship in working myocardium from patients with endstage heart failure. J Appl Cardiol 3: 273–283

18. Feldman MD, Alderman JD, Aroesty JM, Royal HD, Ferguson JJ, Owen RM, Grossman W, McKay RG (1988) Depression of systolic and diastolic myocardial reserve during atrial pacing tachycardia in patients with dilated cardiomyopathy. J Clin Invest 82: 1661–1669

19. Flesch M, Schwinger RHG, Schiffer F, Frank K, Südkamp M, Kuhn-Regnier F, Arnold G, Böhm M (1996) Evidence for a functional relevance of an enhanced expression of the Na^+-Ca^{2+}-exchanger in the failing human myocardium. Circulation 94: 992–1002

20. Framton JE, Harrison SM, Boyett MR, Orchard CH (1991) Ca^{2+} and Na^+ in rat myocytes showing different force-frequency relationships. Am J Physiol 261: C739– C750

21. Frank K, Schwinger RHG, Wang J, Müller-Ehmsen J, McDonough A, Erdmann E (1996) Die α_1-, α_3-, β_1-Isoform-Expression sowie die Gesamtaktivität der Na^+, K^+-ATPase ist am insuffizienten menschlichen Myokard vermindert. Z Kardiol 85 (Suppl 2): 644

22. Gwathmey JK, Copelas L, Mackkinnon R, Schoen FJ, Feldman MD, Grossman W, Morgan JP (1987) Abnormal intracellular calcium handling in myocardium from patients with end-stage heart failure. Circ Res 61: 70–76

23. Gwathmey JK, Slawsky MT, Hajjar RJ, Briggs GM, Morgan JP (1990) Role of the intracellular calcium handling in force-interval relationships of human ventricular myocardium. J Clin Invest 85: 1599–1613

24. Hajjar RJ, Gwathmey JK (1992) Cross-bridge dynamics in human ventricular myocardium: regulation of contractility in the failing myocardium. Circulation 86: 1819–1826

25. Hasenfuss G, Mulieri LA, Leavitt BJ, Allen PD, Haeberle JR, Alpert NR (1992) Alteration of contractile function and excitation-contraction coupling in dilated cardiomyopathy. Circ Res 70: 1225–1232

26. Hasenfuss G, Reinecke H, Studer R, Markus M, Pieske B, Holtz J, Holubarsch C, Posival H, Just H, Drexler H (1994) Relation between myocardial function and expression of sarcoplasmic reticulum Ca^{2+}-ATPase in failing and nonfailing myocardium. Circ Res 75: 434–442

27. Higginbotham MB, Morris KG, Williams RS, McHale PA, Coleman RE, Cobb FR (1986) Regulation of stroke volume during submaximal and maximal upright exercise in normal man. Circ Res 58: 281–291

28. Jeck CD, Zimmermann R, Schaper J, Schaper W (1994) Decreased expression of calmodulin mRNA in human end-stage heart failure. J Mol Cell Cardiol 26: 99–107

29. Kenakin TP, Ambrose JR, Irving PE (1991) The relative efficiency of beta adrenoreceptor coupling in myocardial inotropy and diastolic relaxation: organ selective treatment for diastolic dysfunction. J Pharmacol Exp Ther 257: 1189–1197

30. Leblanc N, Hume JR (1990) Sodium current-induced release of calcium from cardiac sarcoplasmic reticulum. Science 248: 372–376

31. Limas CJ, Olivari MT, Goldenberg IF, Levine TB, Benditt DG, Simon A (1987) Calcium uptake by sarcoplasmic reticulum in human dilated cardiomyopathy. Cardiovasc Res 21: 601–605

32. Linck B, Boknik P, Eschenhagen T, Müller FU, Neumann J, Nose M, Jones LR, Schmitz W, Scholz H (1996) Messanger RNA expression and immunological quantification of phospholamban and SR-Ca^{2+}-ATPase in failing and nonfailing human hearts. Cardiovasc Res 31: 625–632

33. Lompre AM, Anger M, Levitsky D (1994) Sarco(endo)plasmic reticulum calcium pumps in the cardiovascular system: function and gene expression. J Mol Cell Cardiol 26: 1109–1121

34. Meyer M, Schillinger W, Pieske B, Holubarsch C, Heilmann C, Posival H, Kuwajima G, Mikoshiba K, Just H, Hasenfuss G (1995) Alterations of sarcoplasmic reticulum proteins in failing human dilated cardiomyopathy. Circulation 92: 778–784
35. Movsesian MA, Bristow RB, Krall J (1989) Ca^{2+}-uptake by sarcoplasmic reticulum from patients with idiopathic dilated cardiomyopathy. Circ Res 65: 1141–1144
36. Movsesian MA, Smith CJ, Krall J, Bristow MR, Manganiello VC (1991) Sarcoplasmic reticulum-associated cyclic adenosine 5'-monophoshate phosphodiesterase activity in normal and failing human hearts. J Clin Invest 88: 15–19
37. Movsesian MA, Karimi M, Green K, Jones LR (1994) Ca^{2+}-transporting ATPase, phospholamban, and calsequestrin levels in nonfailing and failing myocardium. Circulation 90: 653–657
38. Mulieri LA, Hasenfuss G, Leavitt B, Allen PD, Alpert NR (1992) Altered myocardial force-frequency relation in human heart failure. Circulation 85:1743–1750
39. Mulieri LA, Leavitt BJ, Martin BJ, Haeberle JR, Alpert NR (1993) Myocardial force-frequency defect in mitral regurgitation heart failure is reversed by forskolin. Circulation 88: 2700–2704
40. Pagani ED, Alousi AA, Grant AM, Older TM, Dziuban SW Jr, Allen PD (1988) Changes in myofibrillar content and Mg-ATPase activity in ventricular tissues from patients with heart failure caused by coronary artery disease, cardiomyopathy, or mitral valve insufficiency. Circ Res 63: 380–385
41. Pieske B, Kretschmann B, Meyer M, Holubarsch C, Weirich J, Posival H, Minami K, Just H, Hasenfuss G (1995) Alterations in intracellular calcium handling associated with the inverse force-frequency relation in human dilated cardiomyopathy. Circulation 92: 1169–1178
42. Reinecke H, Studer R, Vetter R, Holtz J, Drexler H (1996) Cardiac Na^+/Ca^{2+} exchange activity in patients with end-stage heart failure. Cardiovasc Res 31: 48–54
43. Schwinger RHG, Böhm M, Erdmann E (1990) Effectiveness of cardiac glycosides in human myocardium with and without downregulation of β-adrenoceptors. J Cardiovasc Pharmacol 15: 692–697
44. Schwinger RHG, Böhm M, Erdmann E (1992) Inotropic and lusitropic dysfunction in myocardium from patients with dilated cardiomyopathy. Am Heart J 123: 116–128
45. Schwinger RHG, Böhm M, La Rosee K, Schmidt U, Schultz C, Erdmann E (1992) Na^+-channel activators increase cardiac glycoside sensivity in failing human myocardium. J Cardiovasc Pharmacol 19: 554–561
46. Schwinger RHG, Böhm M, Müller-Ehmsen J, Uhlmann R, Schmidt U, Stäblein A, Überfuhr P, Kreuzer E, Reichart B, Eissner HJ, Erdmann E (1993) Effect of inotropic stimulation on the negative force-frequency-relationship in the failing human heart. Circulation 88: 2267–2276
47. Schwinger RHG, Böhm M, Koch A, Schmidt U, Morano I, Eissner HJ, Überfuhr P, Reichart B, Erdmann E (1994) The failing human heart is unable to use the Frank-Starling mechanism. Circ Res 74: 959–969
48. Schwinger RHG, Böhm M, Schmidt U, Karczewski P, Bavendiek U, Flesch M, Krause EG, Erdmann E (1995) Unchanged protein levels of SERCA II and phospholamban but reduced Ca^{2+}-uptake and Ca^{2+} ATPase-activity of cardiac sarcoplasmic reticulum from patients with dilated cardiomyopathy compared to nonfailing patients. Circulation 92: 3220–3228
49. Schwinger RHG, Bavendiek U, Hörter S, Karczewski P, Schmidt U, Bölck S, Hoischen S, Krause E-G, Erdmann E (1996) Verminderte Ca^{2+}-Sensivität der SERCA II bei DCM aufgrund einer verminderter PKA-abhängigen Phosphorylierung von Phospholamban. Z Kardiol 85 (Suppl 2): 970
50. Schwinger RHG, Brixius K, Bavendiek U, Hoischen S, Müller-Ehmsen J, Bölck B, Erdmann E (1997) Effect of cyclopiazonic acid on the force-frequency-relationship in human nonfailing myocardium. J Pharmacol Exp Ther 283: 286–292
51. Steinfarth M, Danielsen W, von der Leyen H, Mende U, Meyer W, Neumann J, Nose M, Rech T, Schmitz W, Scholz H, Starbatty J, Stein B, Döring V, Kalmar P, Haverich A (1992) Reduced α_1 and β_2-adrenoceptor-mediated positive inotropic effects in human end-stage heart failure. Br J Pharmacol 105: 463–469
52. Studer R, Reinecke H, Bilger J, Eschenhagen T, Böhm M, Hasenfuss G, Just H, Holtz J, Drexler H (1994) Gene expression of the cardiac Na^+-Ca^{2+} exchanger in end-stage human heart failure. Circ Res 75: 443–453
53. Wolff MR, Love RB, Canver CC, Mentzer RM (1995) Myofibrillar calcium sensivity of tension is increased in human heart failure: role of reduced β-adrenergically-mediated myofibrillar protein phosphorylation. Circulation 92 (Suppl I 8): 2802
54. Xu A, Hawkins C, Narayanan N (1993) Phosphorylation and activation of the Ca^{2+}-pumping ATPase of cardiac sarcoplasmic reticulum by Ca^{2+}/calmodulin-dependent-proteinkinase. J Biol Chem 268: 8394–8397

Author's address:
R. H. G. Schwinger
Universität zu Köln
Medizinische Klinik III
Labor für Herzmuskelphysiologie und
molekulare Kardiologie
Joseph-Stelzmann-Str. 9
50924 Köln, Germany

Effects of cytokines and nitric oxide on myocardial E-C coupling

R. Haque, H. Kan, M. S. Finkel

Departments of Medicine (Cardiology), Pharmacology, and Toxicology
West Virginia University School of Medicine, Robert C. Byrd Health Sciences Center
Louis A. Johnson V.A. Medical Center, Morgantown, USA

Abstract

Compelling evidence now exists that pro-inflammatory cytokines and nitric oxide (NO) are newly identified endogenous regulators of myocardial contractility. The mechanism(s) responsible for the inotropic and chronotropic effects of these novel mediators can be explained on the basis of recently established principles of myocardial excitation contraction coupling (E-C). A novel hypothesis is proposed that cytokines and NO-mediated alterations in E-C coupling contribute to the reversible myocardial depression and β-adrenergic desensitization observed in a diverse group of clinical conditions that activate host inflammatory responses, including congestive heart failure. The results of in vitro studies indicate that cytokines and NO have both immediate, short-term, as well as long-term effects on cardiac performance. Basic studies into these cytokine signaling pathways in cardiac myocytes have the potential to provide important new insights relevant to the design of new management strategies for the treatment of congestive heart failure patients.

Key words Cytokines – nitric oxide – myocardium – congestive heart failure

Introduction

Myocardial ischemia followed by reperfusion was first shown to be associated with a transient period of depressed contractility in the opened chest dog model (16, 21, 43, 82). The clinical implications of these experimental observations were not fully appreciated until sophisticated imaging techniques enabled clinicians to assess myocardial contractility and viability non-invasively in patients (12, 19). It has become increasingly apparent that a number of clinical conditions result in reversible depression of myocardial contractility. Reversible myocardial depression following reperfusion of ischemic myocardium has been documented in patients following myocardial infarction, cardiopulmonary bypass, thrombolytic therapy, and coronary angioplasty (12, 19). This condition has been referred to as "stunned" myocardium.

A number of non-ischemic conditions have also been shown to be associated with reversible myocardial depression in animal models and humans (8, 22, 27, 46, 64, 74, 75,

78, 84, 94). The systemic inflammatory response syndrome (SIRS) is one such condition that may serve as a paradigm for reversible myocardial depression associated with both ischemic and non-ischemic etiologies (89). The myocardial effects of sepsis-induced SIRS have three characteristics shared by trauma, myocardial ischemia, cardiac transplant rejection, and congestive heart failure (4, 8, 12, 16, 18, 19, 21, 22, 27, 33, 43, 46, 57, 58, 63, 64, 74, 75, 78, 82, 84, 88, 94):
(1) activation of inflammatory mediators, (2) reversible component of myocardial depression, (3) β-adrenergic desensitization.

Compelling evidence now exists that pro-inflammatory cytokines and nitric oxide (NO) are newly identified endogenous regulators of myocardial function (5–7, 10, 11, 28, 29, 31, 35, 37, 40–42, 52, 55, 59, 64, 67, 68, 71, 80, 81, 90, 97). The mechanism(s) responsible for the inotropic and chronotropic effects of these novel mediators can be explained on the basis of recently established principles of myocardial excitation – contraction coupling (E-C coupling). A novel hypothesis is proposed that cytokine and NO-mediated alterations in E-C coupling contribute to the reversible myocardial depression and β-adrenergic desensitization observed in a diverse group of clinical conditions that activate host inflammatory responses including, sepsis, ischemia, and congestive heart failure.

Myocardial excitation-contraction (E-C) coupling

The major regulators of the transsarcolemmal entry of calcium include L-type calcium channels and autonomic receptors (9, 14, 15, 38, 45, 51, 54, 76, 79, 83) (Fig. 1). These membrane bound proteins all contribute to the influx of only a minute quantity of calcium from outside the cell into the myocyte. The small quantity of calcium that traverses the L-type calcium channel during membrane depolarization causes the release of the large reservoir of calcium stored in the sarcoplasmic reticulum (SR) through the SR calcium release channel (ryanodine receptor) (9, 23). This large reservoir of calcium then interacts with tropomyosin to allow the actin and myosin filaments to overlap. This results in systolic myocardial contraction. Diastolic relaxation results with the resequestration of this large reservoir of calcium back into the sarcoplasmic reticulum through the SR calcium/ATPase (9, 39, 49). Calcium exits the cell through the Na^+/Ca^{++} exchanger and sarcolemmal $Ca^{++}ATPase$ (9, 89).

Autonomic receptors further regulate calcium influx through the sarcolemma (Fig. 1) (9, 14, 15, 38, 45, 51, 54, 76, 83). β-Adrenergic stimulation results in the association of a catalytic subunit of a G-protein coupled to the β receptor. This stimulates the enzyme, adenylate cyclase, to convert ATP to cAMP. Increasing cAMP production results in cAMP dependent phosphorylation of the L-type calcium channel. Phosphorylation results in an increase in the probability for the open state of the channel. This translates into an increase in transsarcolemmal calcium influx during phase 2 (i.e., the plateau phase) of the action potential. Alpha adrenergic receptor stimulation results in the phospholipase C-mediated breakdown of phosphatidylcholine to inositol triphosphate (IP_3) and diacyl glycerol (DAG). These second messengers further enhance mobilization of both transsarcolemmal calcium influx and SR calcium efflux.

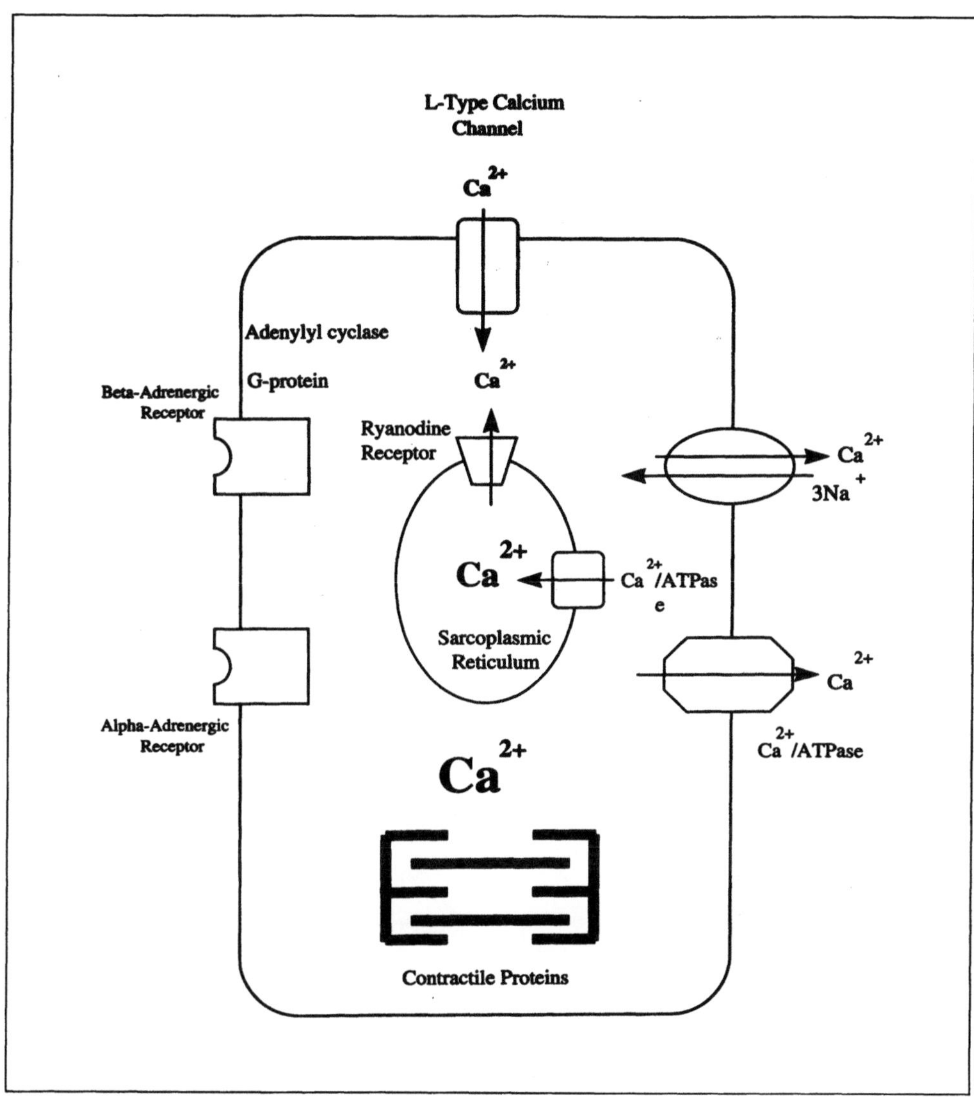

Fig. 1 Schematic diagram illustrating the movement of calcium from the extracellular space to trigger intracellular release of calcium followed by extrusion of calcium back into the extracellular space. Calcium enters the myocyte through L-type calcium channels that are modulated by adrenergic receptors. This small quantity of calcium triggers the release of the large reservoir of intracellular calcium stored in the SR (sarcoplasmic reticulum) by activation of the SR calcium release channel (ryanodine receptor). Calcium is resequestered into the SR by the SR calcium/ATPase. Calcium is extruded from the cell largely through the Na^+/Ca^{++} exchanger and the sarcolemmal calcium ATPase.

The mechanism by which transsarcolemmal calcium activates the release of SR calcium is not completely understood. It does appear to involve an allosteric conformational change in the SR release channel caused by the binding of calcium to a specific site (23). It has been shown that sulfhydryl reagents regulate calcium release from skeletal and cardiac SR vesicles. The physiologic gating of the ryanodine-sensitive SR release channel was proposed to be dependent on the redox state of critical sulfhydryl groups residing on the SR membrane. We have shown that the oxidation or reduction of free sulfhydryls on the SR calcium release channel plays an important role in the reversible component of myocardial depression in the hamster cardiomyopathy model (30).

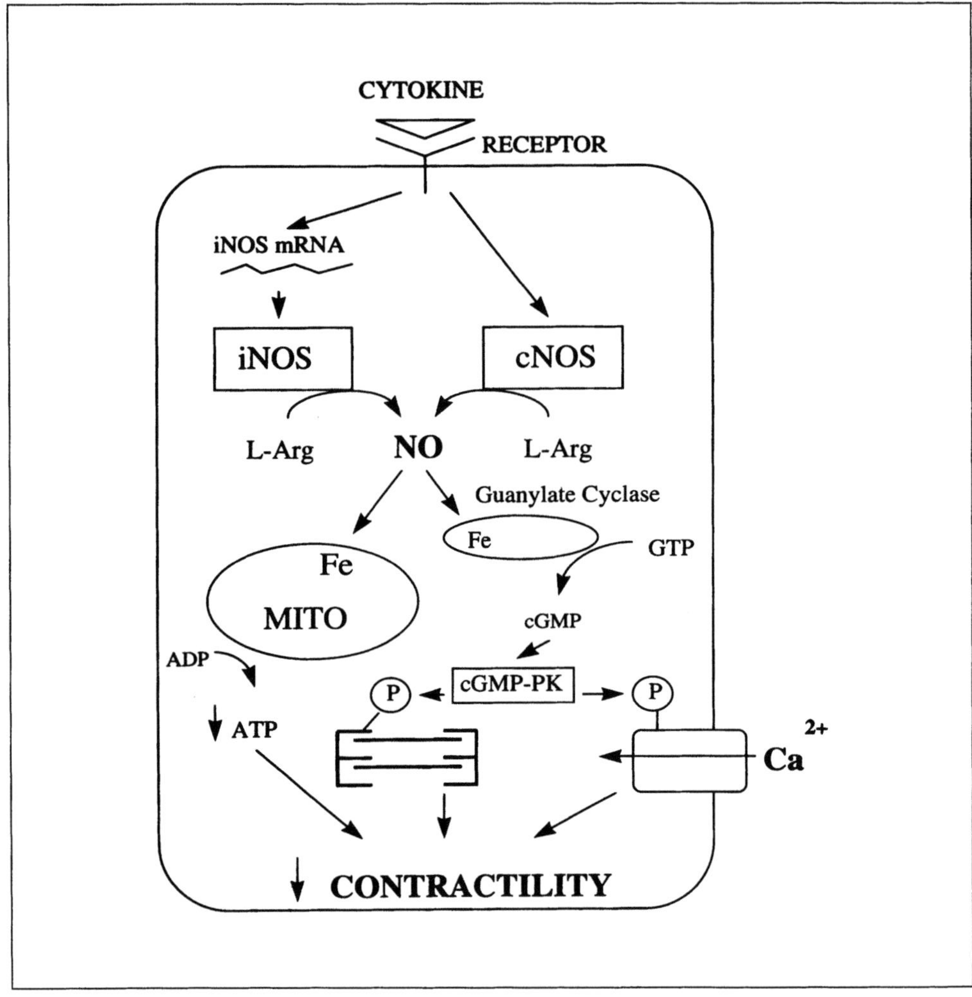

Fig 2 Schematic diagram illustrating the effects of the binding of a pro-inflammatory cytokine to a receptor on the surface of a cardiac myocyte. This stimulates iNOS mRNA and protein production over several hours. Additionally, immediate inotropic effects are apparent within minutes that are dependent on the presence of myocardial cNOS. NO production from either of these enzymes activates guanylate cyclase by binding to iron which converts GTP to cGMP. cGMP can depress myocardial contractility by phosphorylating sarcolemmal L-type calcium channels and/or contractile proteins. Phosphorylation of calcium channels diminishes the influx of extracellular calcium while phosphorylation of contractile proteins impairs their affinity for calcium. In addition, the large quantities of NO that result from iNOS activation depress mitochondrial activity by binding to iron in succinate dehydrogenase. Depression of L-type calcium channel activity, lowering the affinity of contractile proteins for calcium, and the suppression of mitochondrial activity all can contribute to depression in myocardial contractility.

Nitric oxide and cytokines

Nitric oxide (NO) has been reported to play a role in a wide range of cellular processes including cellular proliferation, apoptosis, and mitochondrial electron transport (20, 60). Nitric oxide is formed from the oxidation of one of the two chemically equivalent guanidino nitrogens of the amino acid, L-arginine, by a distinct family of NO synthases (13, 20, 47, 50, 60, 61, 73, 74, 96). Two different constitutive (present all the time) (cNOS) and a single inducible (requires gene expression) (iNOS) enzymes have been cloned and sequenced (13, 50, 61, 96). cNOS have been described in neural tissue (type I) and endothelium (type II). Cytokines induce a third type of NOS (type III). Arginine analogues such as L-NMMA block the production of NO by competitively inhibiting NO synthase enzyme activity (20, 60). The addition of L-arginine can overcome this inhibition (20, 60). NO has been shown to have a variety of effects on cells, including raising cGMP levels by activating soluble guanylate cyclase (30, 47) (Fig. 2).

Proinflammatory cytokines are a class of secretory polypeptides that are synthesized and released locally by macrophages, leukocytes, and endothelial cells in response to injury (1).

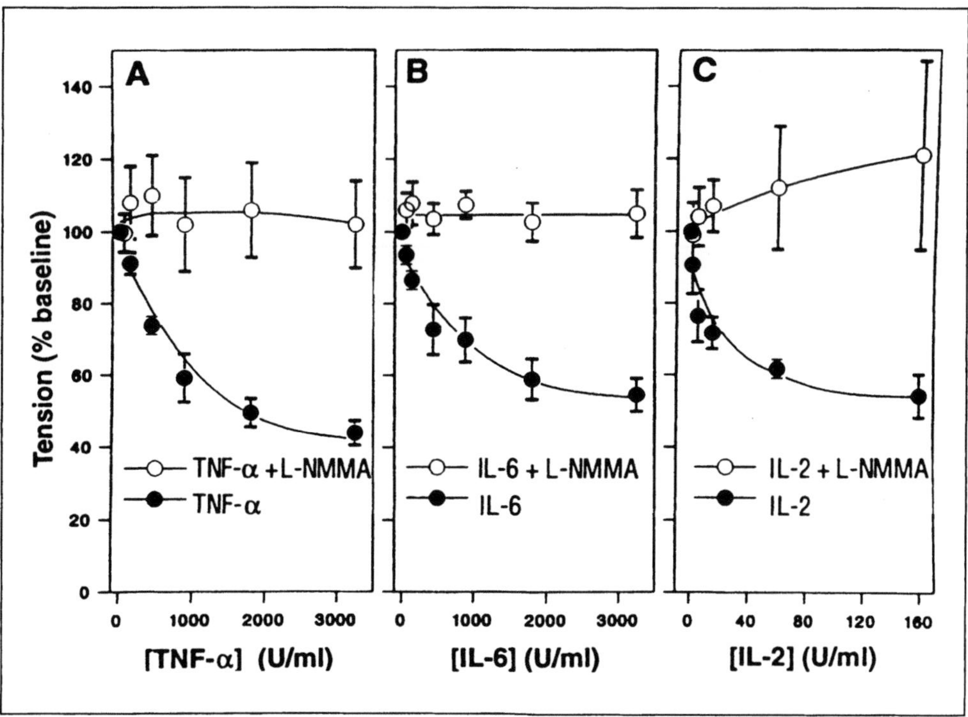

Fig. 3 Graphs depicting the negative inotropic effects of increasing concentrations of TNF-a (A), IL-6 (B), and IL-2 (C) alone (closed circles) or in the presence of L- NMMA (10 μM) (open circles). L-NMMA alone (10^{-7} to 10^{-3} M) had no significant inotropic effect (n = 6). Values represent the means ± SEM of six different determinations in six different papillary muscle preparations. (Reproduced with permission from Science 257: 367–389, 1992.)

Interleukins 1,2,6 and TNF (Tumor Necrosis Factor) are cytokines that are produced by immune cells in response to challenge or injury (1). Interleukin (IL)-2 administration to animal models and cancer patients elicited reversible hemodynamic changes similar to those seen in shock due to gram-negative bacterial sepsis (69, 85, 93, 98). Patients

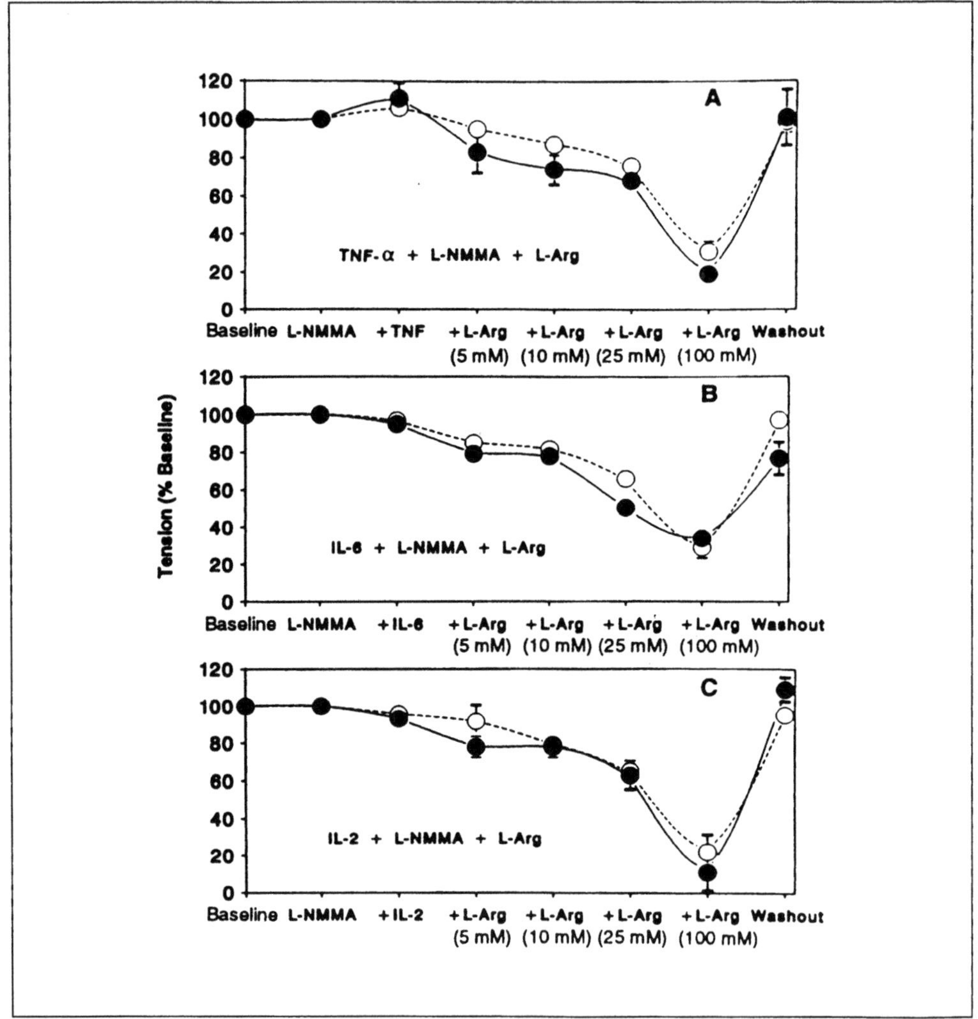

Fig. 4 Inhibition of inotropic effects of cytokines by treatment of muscle with l-NMMA (10 μM) and reversal of that inhibition by L-Arg. Intact papillary muscles (closed circles) or muscles lacking endothelium (open circles) were treated with L-NMMA (10 μM) for 10 min. TNF-α (100 U/ml) (A), IL-6 (1000 U/ml) (B), or IL-2 (160 U/ml) (C) was added for 10 min. Subsequently, L-Arg was added in increasing concentrations for 10 min. Tension returned to baseline within 30 min after the medium containing inotropic agents was removed and replaced with unsupplemented medium. L-Arg alone (100 mM) reduced tension to 31 ± 6 % of baseline (n = 6). No inotropic effect of L-Arg was observed at concentrations from 10^{-7} to 10^{-3} M (n = 6). Values represent the means ± SEM of six different determinations in six different papillary muscles. Chemically denuding the endothelium did not alter the inotropic responses of the papillary muscles to the cytokines. (Reproduced with permission from Science 257: 387–389, 1992.)

developed sinus tachycardia, decreased mean arterial pressure, increased cardiac index, decreased systemic vascular resistance, and a fall in left ventricular ejection fraction.

These hemodynamic effects of gram-negative bacteria have been attributed to endotoxin (lipopolysaccharide-LPS) in the bacterial membrane (26, 87). LPS has been shown to mediate effects through stimulation of mononuclear phagocytes (26, 87). Of the variety of mediators released by these cells, TNF, IL-1, and IL-6 appear to play a pivotal role in mediating the hemodynamic effects of gram-negative sepsis and shock. IL-1, TNF, and LPS have been demonstrated to cause hypotension (95). Plasma IL-6 levels have been found to be significantly increased in septic patients (36).

Reperfusion of ischemic myocardium is associated with infiltration of leukocytes and macrophages that may be responsible for a transient depression of myocardial contractility ("stunned myocardium"). We investigated possible immediate (within minutes), direct inotropic effects of these cytokines on the heart (27). TNF, IL-6, and IL-2 all reversibly depressed contractility of isolated left ventricular papillary muscles (27) (Fig. 3). The NO synthase inhibitor, L-NMMA, blocked these negative inotropic effects (Fig. 3). L-Arginine reversed the inhibition by L- NMMA by providing additional substrate for NO production (Fig. 4). These results suggested that the direct negative inotropic effects of cytokines on the heart were dependent on the enhanced activity of a myocardial cNOS enzyme. This was the first report of a myocardial depressant effect of endogenous NO. Subsequent molecular and cellular studies definitively demonstrated the presence of a functional cNOS in cardiac myocytes (7, 52).

Inflammatory cytokines have also been shown to reduce the positive inotropic response of isolated cardiac myocytes to the β-adrenergic agonist, isoproterenol, through a mechanism possibly involving NO (6, 35, 44, 81). TNF and IL-1 have been shown to uncouple agonist-occupied receptors from adenylate cyclase in isolated cardiac myocytes (35). These findings implicated guanine nucleotide binding protein (G-protein) function in the direct or indirect action of cytokines on the heart. G-protein mediated depression of cardiac myocyte L-type calcium channels by IL-1 has recently been reported (59). This is consistent with a cGMP-mediated effect of NO on cardiac L-type calcium channels. Thus, b-adrenergic desensitization (hyporesposiveness) could result from a cytokine-mediated, NO dependent suppression of cardiac L-type calcium channels.

Cytokines have also been demonstrated to regulate each other's effects on the heart. Transforming growth factor (TGF)-α has been shown to antagonize the chronotropic effects of IL-1 on isolated neonatal cardiac myocytes (80). The spontaneous beating rates of neonatal cardiac myocytes are also dependent on sarcolemmal L-type calcium channel activity (9, 54). Thus, the regulation of the sarcolemmal L-type calcium channel could explain both the inotropic and chronotropic effects of cytokines on the heart.

Stunned myocardium

The observed inotropic effects of proinflammatory cytokines raised the possibility that they participate in reversible post-ischemic myocardial depression ("stunning"). In another study conducted in our laboratory, elevated levels of IL-6 were detected in patients immediately following aortocoronary bypass grafting (29). These same concentrations of IL-6 were also shown by us to reversibly depress contractility in human cardiac tissue (29) (Fig. 5). Other laboratories have independently confirmed the presence of elevated IL-6 levels

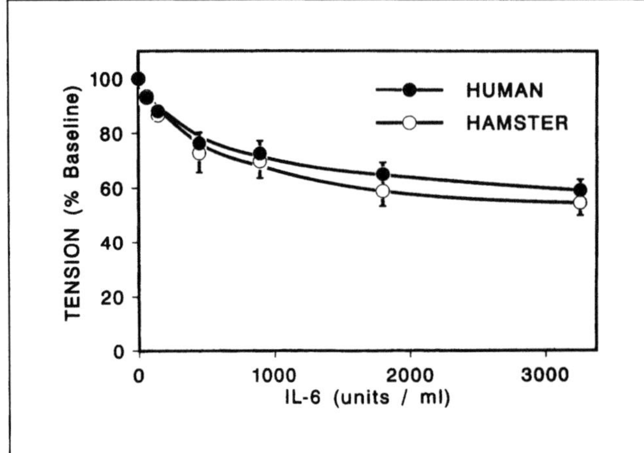

Fig. 5 Graph depicting the inotropic effects of adding increasing concentrations of IL-6 on tension generated by isolated human pectinate muscles (closed circles) and hamster papillary muscles (open circles). Values represent means ± SEM of 6 different experiments conducted using 6 different preparations from 6 different patients and hamsters. (Reprinted with permission from the Am. J. Cardiol 71: 1231–1232, 1993.)

in cardiac surgical patients (32, 86). Serum IL-6 levels have also been reported to be elevated in patients and animal models following myocardial infarction (34, 48). From these observations, it is intriguing to speculate that IL-6 could contribute to the transient myocardial depression, "stunning", that is known to occur following cardiopulmonary bypass and myocardial infarction. We further explored the potential role for NO in post-CABG myocardial stunning by assaying for its stable end-products, NO_2^- (nitrite) and NO_3^- (nitrate) (40, 41). Coronary sinus nitrite and nitrate levels were increased 10-fold in patients following coronary artery bypass surgery. In addition, NO synthase enzyme activity was increased 3-fold in pectinate muscles from these patients following the same surgery. These elevated levels of NO products were temporally associated with post-operative myocardial stunning. Taken together, our findings support a cytokine-stimulated, NO-mediated mechanism for myocardial stunning following cardiopulmonary bypass. The potential therapeutic implications of these studies justify future efforts to elucidate the molecular mechanisms involved in the effects of cytokines and NO on the heart.

Congestive heart failure

Focusing exclusively on the immediate effects of cytokines on the heart provides only a uni-dimensional appreciation of the complex relationship between the heart and the immune system (Fig. 2). We and others have shown that cytokines also induce the expression of iNOS in cardiac myocytes (5, 6, 10, 11, 65, 67, 68, 80). This revelation has now provided a novel approach to understanding the role of cytokines and iNOS in congestive heart failure patients (CHF). We have recently reported that cytokine-stimulated NO production reversibly inhibited mitochondrial enzyme activity in cardiac myocytes (67) (Fig. 6). We have also shown that norepinephrine, TNF, and cAMP increase NO production in cardiac myocytes through different molecular mechanisms (52, 66, 68). These observations in cardiac myocytes may provide important insights into the molecular mechanisms

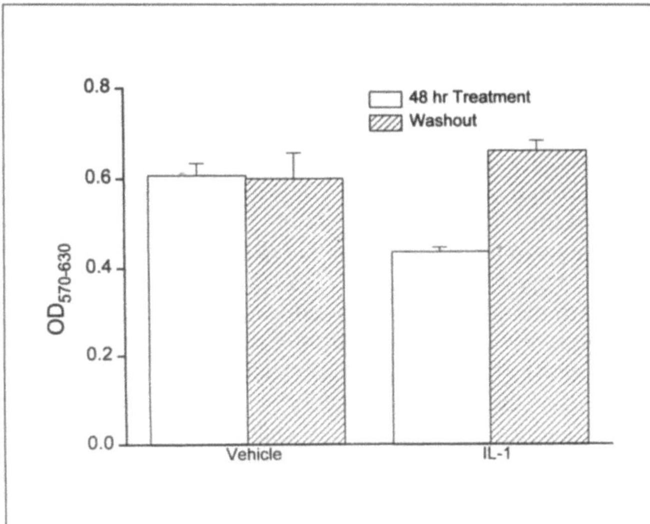

Fig. 6 Bar graph depicting the effect of cytokine treatment and washout on mitochondrial activity measured as $OD_{570-630}$. Cells were treated with vehicle (0.608 ± 0.026) or 500 U/ml IL-1 (0.436 ± 0.010) for 48 h. Cells were also treated with vehicle or 500 U/ml IL-1 for 48 h, washed, and allowed to incubate for another 48 h in serum-free media with no additives at which time the $OD_{570-360}$ was measured for the cells treated with vehicle (0.601 ± 0.056) or 500 U/ml IL-1 (0.0622 ± 0.022). Values represent the means ± SEM of 12 replicate wells from 3 separate experiments. (Reprinted with permission from Biochem and Biophys Res Comm, 213: 1002–1009, 1995.)

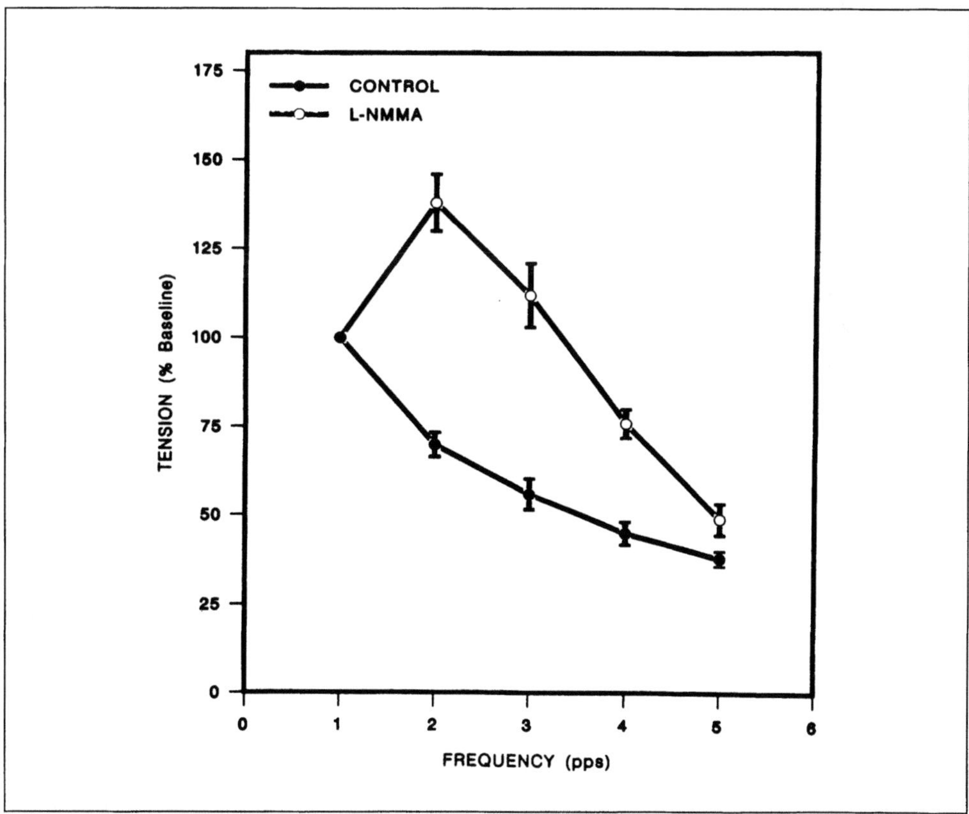

Fig. 7 Graph of the immediate effects (within 1 to 2 beats) of increasing stimulation rate from 1 to 5 Hz on tension generated by isolated hamster papillary muscles alone (closed circles) or in the presence of 10 µM L-NMMA (open circles). The values represent the means ± S.E.M. of 6 determinations from 6 different preparations (P < 0.01; ANOVA). (Reprinted with permission from J. Pharm Exp Ther 272: 945–952, 1995.)

responsible for the deleterious effects of cAMP elevating agents and the poor prognosis associated with elevated circulating levels of norepinephrine and TNF in CHF (17, 53, 56, 91). The recently reported improvements in both ventricular function and survival with the combined alpha and beta adrenergic blocker, carvedilol, in CHF supports the clinical relevance of our molecular studies (70). A similar improvement in both ventricular function and survival in CHF was also reported with the use of a novel inotrope with cytokine inhibitory properties, vesnarinone (24, 63).

We have previously reported that the NO synthase inhibitor, L-NMMA, reversed the negative inotropic effect of increasing stimulation frequency in isolated hamster papillary muscles (negative force-frequency; negative "staircase") (28) (Fig. 7). L-NMMA also blunted the negative inotropic effect of the sarcoplasmic reticulum calcium release channel regulator, ryanodine (Fig. 8). Papillary muscles isolated from CHF patients also demonstrate a negative force-frequency response (25). The inotropic response of cardiac myocytes to stimulation frequency is dependent on the relationship between the sarcolemmal L-type calcium channel, sarcoplasmic reticulum calcium release channel and the Na^+/Ca^{++} exchanger (E-C coupling; Fig. 1) (9, 54, 92). Cytokine-mediated, NO dependent alterations in E-C coupling could result in changes in the force-frequency relationship. Taken together, these basic and clinical observations support a pathophysiologically relevant role for cytokines and NO in CHF, as well.

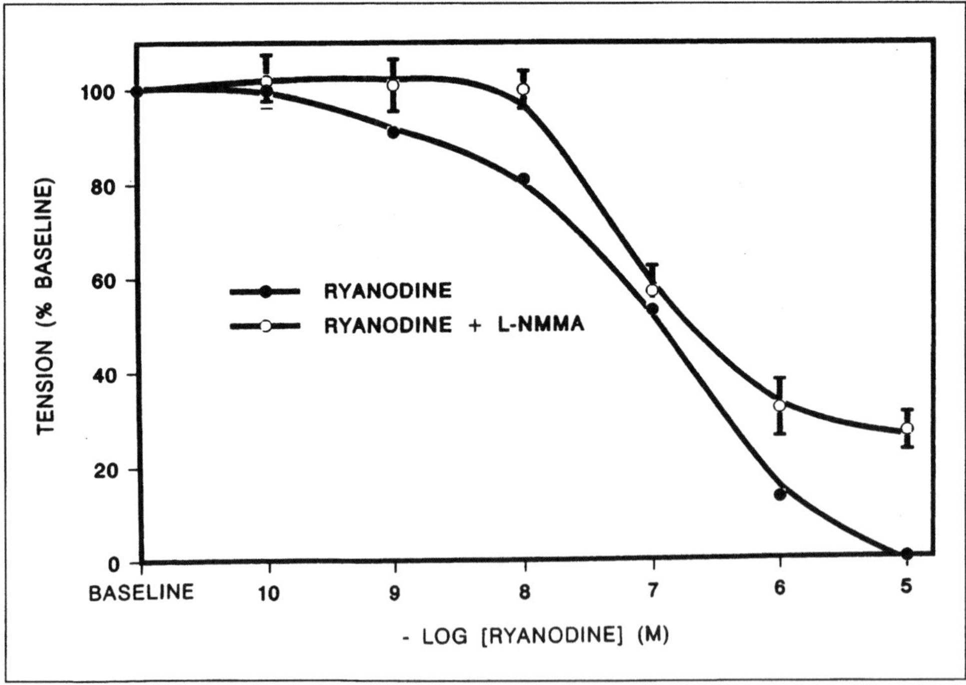

Fig. 8 Graph of the inotropic effects of increasing concentrations of ryanodine alone (closed circles) and in the presence of 10 μM L-NMMA (open circles). Values represent the means ± S.E.M. of 6 determinations from 6 different preparations (P < 0.01; ANOVA). (Reprinted with permission from J. Pharm Exp Ther 272: 945–952, 1995.)

Conclusions

Pro-inflammatory cytokines and NO are newly identified endogenous regulators of myocardial E-C coupling. The in vitro inotropic effects of these immunomodulators suggest that they may contribute to the pathogenesis of the reversible myocardial depression and β-adrenergic desensitization observed clinically in patients with sepsis, trauma, ischemia, cardiac transplant rejection, myocarditis, and congestive heart failure. Basic studies of cytokine signaling pathways in cardiac myocytes have the potential to provide important new insights relevant to the design of new management strategies for the treatment of cardiac patients.

Acknowledgments   This research was supported by the National Institutes of Health, Grant #HL-53372, and the Ohio-West Virginia Affiliate of the American Heart Association.

References

1. Abbas AK, Lichtman AH, Pober JS (1991) Cellular and Molecular Immunology. Philadelphia: W. B. Saunders Company, pp 226–242
2. Abramson JJ (1987) Regulation of the sarcoplasmic reticulum calcium permeability by sulfhydryl oxidation and reduction. J Memb Sci 33: 241–248
3. Abramson JJ, Trimm JL, Weden L and Salama G (1983) Heavy metals induce rapid calcium release from sarcoplasmic reticulum vesicles isolated from skeletal muscle. Proc Natl Acad Sci USA 80: 1526–1530
4. Baan CC, Van Emmerik NEM, Balk AHMM, Quint WGV, Mochtar B, Jutte NHPM, Niesters HGM, Weimar W (1994) Cytokine mRNA expression in endomyocardial biopsies during acute rejection from human heart transplants. Clin and Exp Immunol 97 (2): 293–298
5. Balligand JL, Ungureanu-Longrois D, Simmons WW, Pimental D, Malinski TA, Kapturczak M, Taha Z, Lowenstein CJ, Davidoff AJ, Kelly RA, Smith TW, Michel T (1994) Cytokine-inducible nitric oxide synthase (iNOS) expression in cardiac myocytes. J Biol Chem 269: 27580–27588
6. Balligand JL, Ungureann D, Kelly RA, Kobzik L, Pimental D, Michael T, Smith TW (1993) Abnormal contractile function due to induction of nitric oxide synthesis in rat cardiac myocytes follow exposure to activated macrophage-conditioned medium. J Clin Invest 91: 2314–2319
7. Balligand JL, Kobzik L, Han X, Kaye DM, Belhassen L, O'Hara DS, Kelly RA, Smith TW and Michel T (1995) Nitric oxide-dependent parasympathetic signaling is due to activation of constitutive endothelial (Type III) nitric oxide synthase in cardiac myocytes. J Biol Chem 270 (4): 14582– 14586
8. Barry WH (1994) Mechanisms of Immune-mediated myocyte injury. Circ 89: 2421– 2432
9. Bers DM (1991) Excitation-Contraction Coupling and Cardiac Contractile Force. Norwell: Kluwer Academic Publishers, pp 119–145
10. Brady AJB, Poole-Wilson PA, Harding SE, Warren JB (1992) Nitric oxide production within cardiac myocytes reduces their contractility in endotoxemia. Am J Physiol (Heart Circ Physiol 32) 263: H1963–H1966
11. Brady AJB, Warren JB, Poole-Wilson PA, Williams TJ, Harding SE (1993) Nitric oxide attenuates cardiac myocyte contraction. Am J Physiol 265: H176–H182
12. Braunwald E and Kloner RA (1982) The stunned myocardium: Prolonged, postischemic ventricular dysfunction. Circulation 66: 1146–1149
13. Bredt DS, Hwang PM, Glatt CE, Lowenstein C, Reed RR, Snyder SH (1991) Cloned and expressed nitric oxide synthase structurally resembles cytochrome P-450 reductase. Nature 351: 714–718
14. Brown AM and Birnbaumer L (1988) Direct G protein gating of ion channels. Am J Physiol 254: H401–H410
15. Brown JH and Jones LG (1986) Phosphoinositide metabolism in the heart. In: Putney JW Jr. (ed) Phospho-inositides and Receptor Mechanisms. Alan R. Liss, pp 245–270
16. Charlat ML, O'Neill PG, Hartley CJ, et al. (1989) Prolonged abnormalities of left ventricular diastolic wall thinning in the "stunned" myocardium in conscious dogs: Time course and relation to systolic function. J Am Coll Cardiol 13: 185–194
17. Cohn JN, Levine TB, Olivari MT, et al. (1984) Plasma norepinephrine as a guide to prognosis in patients with chronic congestive heart failure. N Eng J Med 311: 819

18. Cristmas JW, Holden EP, Blackwell TS (1995) Strategies for blocking the systemic effects of cytokines in the sepsis syndrome. Crit Care Med 23: 955–963
19. Dilsizian V, Bonow RO (1993) Current diagnostic techniques of assessing myocardial viability in patients with hibernating and stunned myocardium. Circulation 87 (1): 1–20
20. Dinerman JL, Lowenstein CJ, Snyder SH (1993) Molecular mechanisms of nitric oxide regulation: Potential relevance to cardiovascular disease. Circ Res 73 (No 2): 217–222
21. Ellis SG, Henschke CI, Sandor T, et al. (1983) Time course of functional and biochemical recovery of myocardium salvaged by reperfusion. J Am Coll Cardiol 1: 1047–1055
22. Ellrodt AG, Riedinger MS, Kimchi A, Berman DS, Maddahi J, Swan HJC, Murata GH (1985) Left ventricular performance in septic shock: Reversible segmental and global abnormalities. Am Heart J 110: 402–409
23. Fabiato A, Fabiato F (1978b) Calcium induced release of calcium from the sarcoplasmic reticulum and skinned fibers from adult human, dog, cat, rabbit, rat, and frog hearts and fetal and newborn rat ventricles. Ann NY Acad Sci 307: 491–522
24. Feldman AM, Bristow MR, Parmley WW, Carson PE, Pepine CJ, Gilbert EM, Strobeck, JE, Hendrix GH, Power ER, Bain RP (1993) Effects of vesnarinone on morbidity and mortality in patients with heart failure. Vesnarinone Study Group. New Eng J Med 329 (3): 149–155
25. Feldman MC, Gwarthmey JC, Phillips P, Schoen F, Morgan JP (1988) Reversal of the force-frequency relationship in working myocardium from patients with end-stage heart failure. J Appl Cardiol 3: 273–283
26. Filkins JP (1985) Monokines and the metabolic pathophysiology of septic shock. Federation Proceedings 44: 300–304
27. Finkel MS, Oddis CV, Jacobs TD, Watkins SC, Hattler BG, Simmons RL (1992) Inotropic effects of cytokines on the heart mediated by nitric oxide. Science 257: 387–389
28. Finkel MS, Oddis CV, Mayer OH, Hattler BG, Simmons RL (1995) Nitric oxide synthase inhibitor alters papillary muscle force-frequency relationship. J Pharm Exp Ther 272: (No 2): 945–952
29. Finkel MS, Shen L, Oddis CV, Hoffman RA, Romeo RC, Simmons RL, Hattler BG (1993) IL-6 as a mediator of stunned myocardium. Am J of Cardiol 71: 1231– 1232
30. Finkel MS, Oddis CV, Romeo RC, Salama G (1993) Positive inotropic effect of acetylcysteine in the cardiomyopathic Syrian hamster. J Card Pharm 21: 29–34
31. Freeswick PD, DiSilvio M, Nussler AK, Shah NS, Nguyen D, Billiar TR, Finkel MS, Hattler BG (1993) Evidence for inducible nitric oxide synthase expression in the heart. Surgical Forum 44: 267–269
32. Frering B, Philip I, Dehoux M, Rolland C, Langlois JM, Desmonts JM (1994) Circulating cytokines in patients undergoing normothermic cardiopulmonary bypass. J Thorac Cardiovasc Sur 108: 636–641
33. Giroir BP, Horton JW, White DJ, McIntyre KL, Lin CQ (1994) Inhibition of tumor necrosis factor prevents myocardial dysfunction during burn shock. Am J Physiol 267 (Heart Circ Physiol 36): H118–H124
34. Guillen I, Blanes M, Gomez-Lechon MJ, Castell JV (1995) Cytokine signaling during myocardial infarction: Sequential appearance of IL-1 and IL-6. Am J Physiol 269 (Regulatory Integrative Comp Physiol 38): R229–R235
35. Gulick T, Chung MK, Peiper SJ, Lange LG, Schreiner GF (1989) Interleukin-1 and tumor necrosis factor inhibit cardiac myocytes β-adrenergic responsiveness. Proc Natl Acad Sci USA 86: 6753–6757
36. Hack CE, DeGroot ER, Felt-Bersma RJF, Nujens JH, Strack Van Schijndel RJM, Erenberg-Belmer AJM, Thys LG, Aarden LA (1989) Increased plasma levels of interleukin-6 in sepsis. Blood 74: 1704–1710
37. Harding P, Carretero OA, LaPointe MC (1995) Effects of interleukin-1 beta and nitric oxide on cardiac myocytes. Hypertension 25 (3): 421–430
38. Hartzell HC (1988) Regulation of cardiac ion channels by catecholamines, acetylcholine and second messenger systems. Prog Biophys Molec Biol 52: 165–247
39. Hasselbach W and Oetliker H (1983) Energetics and electrogenicity of the sarcoplasmic reticulum calcium pump. Annu Rev Physiol 45: 325–339
40. Hattler BG, Gorcsan JIII, Shah N, Oddis CV, Billiar TR, Simmons RL, Finkel MS (1994) A potential role for nitric oxide (NO) in myocardial stunning. J Card Surg 9: 425–429
41. Hattler BG, Oddis CV, Zeevi A, Luss H, Shah N, Geller DA, Billiar TR, Simmons RL, Finkel MS (1995) Regulation of constitutive nitric oxide synthase activity by the human heart. Am J Cardiol 76: 957– 959
42. Hattler BG, Zeevi A, Oddis CV, Finkel MS (1995) Cytokine Induction during cardiac surgery: analysis of TNF-α expression pre- and post-cardiopulmonary bypass. J Card Surg 10: 418–422
43. Heyndrickx GR, Millard RW, McRitchie RJ, et al. (1975) Regional myocardial functional and electrophysiological alterations after brief coronary occlusion in conscious dog. J Clin Invest 56: 978–985
44. Hoffman BB, Lefkowitz RJ (1996) Goodman and Gilman's the Pharmacologic Basis of Therapeutics 8th Edition: Gilman AG, Rall TW, Nies AS, Taylor P. Pergamon Press, Inc., pp 187–243
45. Hosey MM, Lazdunski M (1988) Calcium channels: Molecular pharmacology, structure and regulation. J Membr Biol 104: 81–105
46. Hung JW, Lew YW (1993) Cellular mechanisms of endotoxin-induced myocardial depression in rabbits. Circulation Research 73: 125–134

47. Ignarro LJ, Buga GM, Wood KS, Byrns RE, Chaudhuri G (1987) Endothelium-derived relaxing factor produced and released from artery and vein is nitric oxide. Proc Natl Acad Sci USA 84: 9265–9269

48. Ikeda U, Ohkawa F, Seino Y, Yamamotor K, Hidaka Y, Kasahara T, Kawai T, Shimada K (1992) Serum interleukin 6 levels become elevated in acute myocardial infarction. J Mol Cell Cardiol 24: 579–584

49. Ikemoto N (1982) Structure and function of the calcium pump protein of sarcoplasmic reticulum. Ann Rev Physiol 44: 297–315

50. Janssens SP, Shimouchi A, Quertermous T, Bloch DB, Bloch KD (1992) Cloning and expression of cDNA encoding human endothelium-derived relaxing factor/nitric oxide synthase. J Biol Chem 267: 14519– 14522

51. Jones LG, Goldstein D and Brown JH (1988) Guanine nucleotide-dependent inositol triphosphate formation in chick heart cells. Circ Res 62: 299–305

52. Kanai AJ, Mesaros S, Finkel MS, Oddis CV, Strauss HC, Malinski T (1997) Nitric oxide release measured directly with a porphyrinic microsensor reveals adrenergic control of constitutive nitric oxide synthase in cardiac myocytes. Am J Physiol 273 (42): C1371–C1377

53. Katz SD, Rao R, Berman JW, Schwarz M, Demopoulos L, Bijoi R, LeJemtel TH (1994) Pathophysiological correlates of increased serum tumor necrosis factor in patients with congestive heart failure. Circulation 90: 12–16

54. Katz AM (1992) Physiology of the Heart, 2nd ed. New York: Raven Press

55. Kawamura T, Wakusawa R, Okada K, Inada S (1993) Elevation of cytokines during open heart surgery with cardiopulmonary bypass: Participation of interleukin 8 and 6 in reperfusion injury. Can J Anaesth 40: 11; 1016–1021

56. Levine B, Kalman J, Mayer L, Filit HM, Packer M (1990) Elevated circulating levels of tumor necrosis factor in severe chronic heart failure. N Eng J of Med 323 (4): 236–241

57. Liu MS, Xuan YT (1986) Mechanisms of endotoxin-induced impairment in Na⁺-Ca⁺⁺ exchange in canine myocardium. Am J Physiol 251 (Regulatory Integrative Comp Physiol 20): R1078–R1085

58. Liu MS, Wu LL (1991) Reduction in the Ca^{2+}-induced Ca^{2+} release from canine cardiac sarcoplasmic reticulum following endotoxin administration. Biochem and Biophys Res Comm 174 (No. 3): 1248– 1254

59. Liu S, Schreur KD (1995) G protein-mediated suppression of L-type Ca^{2+} current by interleukin-1 beta in cultured rat ventricular myocytes. Am J Physiol 268 (2Pt1): C339–349

60. Lowenstein CJ, Snyder SH (1992) Nitric oxide, a novel biologic messenger. Cell 70: 705–707

61. Lyons C, Orloff B, Cunningham J (1992) Molecular cloning and functional expression of an inducible nitric oxide synthase from a murine macrophage cell line. J Biol Chem 267: 6370–6374

62. Mann DL, Young JB (1994) Basic mechanisms in congestive heart failure. Recognizing the role of proinflammatory cytokines. Chest 105: 897–904

63. Matsumori A, Shioi T, Yamada T, Matsui S, Sasayama S (1994) Vesnarinone, a new inotropic agent, inhibits cytokine production by stimulated human blood from patients with heart failure. Circ 89: 955– 958

64. Neumann DA, Lane R, Allen GS, Herskowitz A, Rose, NR (1993) Viral myocarditis leading to cardio-myopathy: Do cytokines contribute to pathogenesis? Clin Immunology and Immunopathology 68 (No 2): 181–190

65. Oddis CV, Simmons RL, Hattler BG, Finkel MS (1994) Chronotropic effects of cytokines and the nitric oxide synthase inhibitor, L-NMMA, on cardiac myocytes. Biochem and Biophys Res Comm 205 (No 2): 992–997

66. Oddis CV and Finkel MS (1995) Norepinephrine enhances expression of inducible nitric oxide synthase by cardiac myocytes. Circulation 92 (8): I567

67. Oddis CV and Finkel MS (1995) Cytokine-stimulated nitric oxide production inhibits mitochondrial activity in cardiac myocytes. Biochem and Biophys Res Comm 213: (No 3): 1002–1009

68. Oddis CV, Simmons RL, Hattler BG, Finkel MS (1995) cAMP enhances inducible nitric oxide synthase mRNA stability in cardiac myocytes. Am J Physiol H38 (6): 2044–2050

69. Ognibene FP, Rosenberg SA, Lotze MT, Skibber J, Parker MM, Shelhamer JH, Parillo JE (1988) Interleukin-2 administration causes reversible hemodynamic changes and left ventricular dysfunction similar to those seen in septic shock. Chest 94: 750-754

70. Packer M, Bristow MR, Cohn JN, Colucci WS, Fowler MB, Gilbert EM (1995) Effect of carvedilol on the survival of patients with chronic heart failure. Supplement 1 Circ 92 (8): I-142

71. Pagani FD, Baker LS, Hsi C, Knox M, Fink MP, Visner MS (1992) Left ventricular systolic and diastolic dys-function after infusion of tumor necrosis factor-α in conscious dogs. J Clin Invest 90: 389–398

72. Palmer RMJ, Ashton DS, Moncada S (1988) Vascular endothelial cells synthesize nitric oxide from L-arginine. Nature 333: 664–666

73. Palmer RMJ, Ferrige AG, Moncada S (1987) Nitric oxide release accounts for the biological activity of endothelium-derived relaxing factor. Nature 327: 524–526

74. Parillo JE (1993) Mechanisms of disease: Pathogenic mechanisms of septic shock. N Eng J Med 328: 1471–1477

75. Parker MM, Shelhamer JH, Bacharach SL, Green MV, Natanson C, Frederick TM, Damske BA, Parrillo JE (1985) Profound but reversible myocardial depression in patients with septic shock. Annals of Internal Medicine 100: 483–490

76. Poggioli J, Sulpice JC and Vassort G (1986) Inositol phosphate production following α_1-adrenergic, muscarinic, or electrical stimulation in isolated rat heart. FEBS Lett 206: 292–298
77. Prabhu SD and Salama G (1990) The heavy metal ions Ag^+ and Hg^+ trigger calcium release from cardiac sarcoplasmic reticulum. Arch Biochem Biophys 277: 47–55
78. Reilly JM, Cunnion RE, Burch-Whitman C, Parker MM, Shelhamer JH, Parrillo JE (1989) A circulating myocardial depressant substance is associated with cardiac dysfunction and peripheral hypoperfusion (lactic acidemia) in patients with septic shock. Chest 95: 1072–1080
79. Reuter H and Scholtz H (1977) The regulation of the Ca^{++} conductance of cardiac muscle by adrenaline. J Physiol 264: 49–62
80. Roberts AB, Roche NS, Winokur TS, Burmester JK, Sporn MB (1992) Role of transforming growth factor-B in maintenance of function of cultured neonatal cardiac myocytes. J Clin Invest 90: 2056–2062
81. Rozanski GJ, Witt RC (1994) IL-1 inhibits beta-adrenergic control of cardiac calcium current: Role of L-arginine/nitric oxide pathway. Am J Phys 267 (5Pt2): H1753– 1758
82. Saven JJ, Peirce G, Katcher AH, Sheldon WF (1961) Correlation of intramyocardial electrocardiograms with polarographic oxygen and contractility in the nonischemic and regional ischemic left ventricle. Circ Res 9: 1268–1275
83. Scholtz JB, Schaeffer W, Schmitz H, Scholtz M, Steinfath M, Lohse U, Schwabe, Puurunen J (1988) Alpha-1 adrenoreceptor-mediated positive inotropic effect and inositol triphosphate increase in mammalian heart. J Pharmacol Exp Ther 245: 335–337
84. Smith LW, McDonough KH (1988) Inotropic sensitivity to β-adrenergic stimulation in early sepsis. Am J Physiol 255 (Heart Circ Physiol 24): H699–H703
85. Sobotka PA, McMannis J, Fisher RI, Stein DG, Thomas JX Jr (1990) Effects of interleukin-2 on cardiac function in the isolated rat heart. J Clin Invest 86: 845–850
86. Steinberg JB, Kapelanski DP, Olson JD, Weiler JM (1993) Cytokine and complement levels in patients undergoing cardiopulmonary bypass. J Thorac Cardiovasc Surg 106: 1008–1016
87. Sultzer BM (1968) Genetic control of leukocyte responses to endotoxin. Nature 219: 1253–1254
88. Suter PM, Suter S, Girardin E, Roux-Lombard P, Grau GE, Dayer JM (1992 High brochoalveolar levels of tumor necrosis factor and its inhibitors, interleukin-1, interferon and elastase, in patients with adult respiratory distress syndrome after trauma, shock or sepsis. Am Rev Respir Dis 145: 1016–1022
89. Tanford C (1983) Mechanism of free energy coupling in active transport. Ann Rev Biochem 52: 379–409
90. Thaik CM, Calderone A, Takahashi N, Colucci WS (1995) Interleukin-1 beta modulates the growth and phenotype of neonatal rat cardiac myocytes. J Clin Inv 96 (2): 1093–1099
91. Thomas JA, Marks BH (1978) Plasma norepinephrine in congestive heart failure. Am J Cardiol 41: 233
92. Tiaho F, Piot C, Nargeot J, Richard S (1994) Regulation of the frequency-dependent facilitation of L-type Ca^{2+} currents in rat ventricular myocytes. J Physiol 477.2: MS2249: 237–252
93. Vaitkus PT, Grossman D, Fox KR, McEvoy MD, Doherty JV (1990) Complete heart block due to interleukin-2 therapy. Am Heart J, pp 978–980
94. Vincent JL, Bakker J, Marecaux G, Schandene L, Kahn RJ, Dupont E (1992) Administration of anti-TNF antibody improves left ventricular function in septic shock patients. Chest 101: 810–815
95. Weinberg JR, Wright DJM, Guz A (1988) Interleukin-1 and tumor necrosis factor cause hypotension in the conscious rabbit. Clinical Science 75: 251–255
96. Xie QW, Cho HJ, Calaycay J, Mumford RA, Swiderek KM , Lee TD, Ding A, Troso T, Nathan C (1992) Cloning and characterization of inducible nitric oxide synthase from mouse macrophages. Science 256: 225–228
97. Yoshida T, Okumura H, Kaya H, Okabe Y, Matano S, Ohtake S, Nakamura S, Matsuda T (1993) Prevention of doxuribicin-induced cardiotoxicity by recombinant interleukin-1 in hamsters. Doxorubicin cardiotoxicity and interleukin-1. Biotherapy 6 (2): 125–132
98. Zeilender S, Davis D, Fairman RP, Glauser FL (1989) Inotropic and vasoactive drug treatment of interleukin-2 induced hypotension in sheep. Cancer Research 49: 4423– 4426

Author's address:
M. S. Finkel
Departments of Medicine (Cardiology),
Pharmacology, and Toxicology
West Virginia University School of Medicine
Robert C. Byrd Health Sciences Center
Louis A. Johnson V.A. Medical Center
Morgantown, WV 26506-9157
USA

Adrenergic regulation of the force-frequency effect

J. Ross Jr.

University of California San Diego, Department of Medicine, La Jolla, USA

Abstract

An important interaction between β-adrenergic receptor (AR) stimulation and the myocardial contractile response to increased heart rate has only recently been identified. The effect of β-AR stimulation to amplify the force-frequency effect is responsible for a large component of the positive inotropic effect of exercise in conscious dogs and also can be demonstrated at rest with dobutamine infusions over a range of paced heart rates. The interaction is apparent across species (dog, pig, mouse, rabbit, man). Amplification of the heart rate effect on myocardial contractility by dobutamine is lost in heart failure, which may play an important role in impaired exercise tolerance in that setting. In syndromes of chronotropic incompetence when adrenergic control is intact, it may be expected that a normal response of myocardial contractility to exercise will be achieved only when the interaction with heart rate is optimized by use of a rate-responsive cardiac pacemaker.

Key words Heart rate – myocardial contractility – cardiac frequency – exercise

Introduction

A number of features of the force-frequency relation in isolated cardiac muscle are described elsewhere in this symposium. This brief review will focus primarily on recent studies concerned with force-frequency responses of the intact left ventricle, largely in the conscious state, in several mammalian species. Past research has significantly underestimated the importance of the force-frequency relation in the normal regulation of cardiac contractility, in part due to limitations in methodology for assessing myocardial contractility but in particular because of the lack of studies during exercise or stress (10, 14). More recent experiments have emphasized the importance of the interaction between neurohumoral activation of the heart by sympathetic stimulation and the heart rate, an interaction which carries significant implications not only for normal physiological control but for several disease states. Recently, we have proposed (25) that the three intrinsic factors generally considered to modulate myocardial contractility in the whole heart (length-dependent myofilament activation which participates in the Frank Starling effect, direct β-adrenergic receptor activation of myocardial contractility, and the basal force-frequency effect) should be supplemented by a fourth factor: β-adrenergic regulation of the force-frequency effect, which operates during exercise and other forms of stress (Fig. 1).

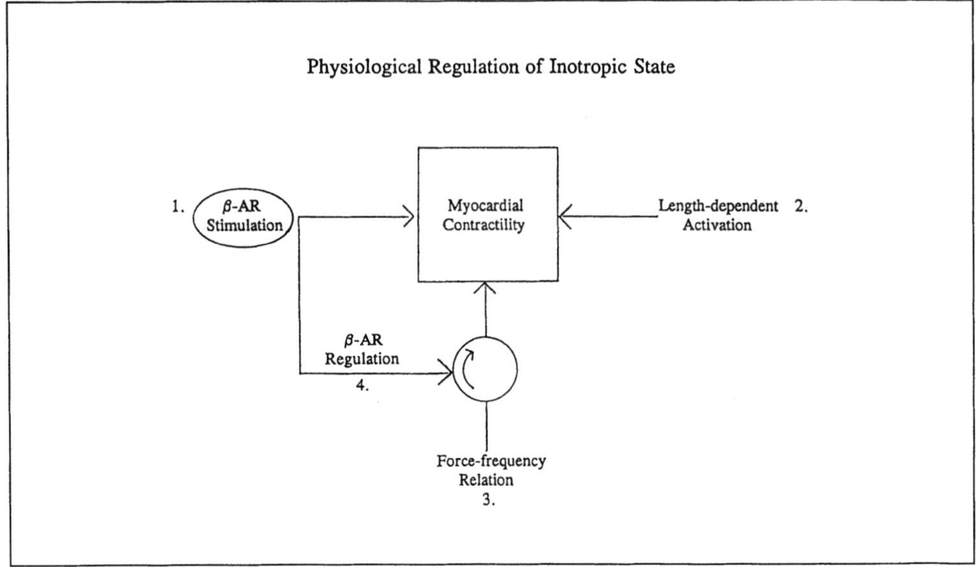

Fig. 1 Expanded scheme of the intrinsic factors regulating myocardial contractility in vivo showing the direct myocardial effect of β-adrenergic receptor (β-AR) stimulation (1), length-dependent activation (2), the basal force-frequency relation (3), and the regulatory effect of enhanced β-AR stimulation on the force-frequency relation (4). (Reproduced with permission from Ross et al. (25))

Exercise and the force-frequency response in dogs

Our attention was first drawn to the pronounced effect of neurohumoral activation of the heart on the response to changes in cardiac frequency during studies in the conscious, exercising dog (16). In these experiments, dogs were preinstrumented with sets of implanted ultrasonic crystals, which allowed calculation of left ventricular volumes, a high-fidelity micromanometer in the left ventricular (LV) cavity, and pacing electrodes on the left atrium. A selective sinus node inhibitor, UL-FS 49 or zatebradine, an I_f channel blocker (8), which is known to have no direct effect on myocardial contractility (4, 11) including the conditions used in these experiments (16), was used to slow the intrinsic sinus node rate. The dogs performed sustained, strenuous steady-state exercise on a treadmill at an average heart rate of about 240 beats per minute (bpm) and atrial pacing was then commenced at a level slightly faster rate, following which UL-FS 49 was administered. While steady-state exercise continued, we were then able to pace down to lower heart rates for 30–45 seconds to reach a steady-state while continuously recording the maximum first derivative of left ventricular pressure (LV dP/dt_{max}), LV end-diastolic pressure (LVEDP) and left ventricular dimensions, returning to 240 bpm between each rate change. As heart rate was reduced stepwise from 240 to 160 bpm a striking reduction in LV dP/dt_{max} was observed which was proportional to the reduction of heart rate (Fig. 2). While it is recognized that LV dP/dt_{max} is directly proportional to the preload (13), the left ventricular EDP rose substantially at the

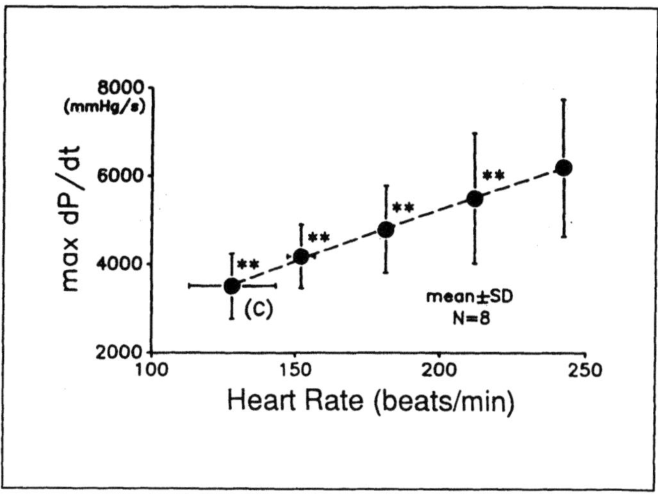

Fig. 2 Plot showing the relation between heart rate and max dP/dt (left ventricular maximum dP/dt) in conscious dogs standing at rest and during sustained exercise at several heart rates. The lowest heart rate represents the resting condition (C) and the highest heart rate that during exercise with atrial pacing at 240 beats per minute. The intermediate heart rates show the effects of pacing to slower rates during continued exercise, with the sinus node rate controlled at a low level by zatebradine. ** = p < 0.001 vs. 240 beats/min. Values are mean ± SD. (Reproduced with permission from Miura et al. (16))

lower heart rates, as might be expected, which by itself should increase rather than decrease LV dP/dt$_{max}$. The effect on contractility of slowing heart rate during exercise, despite continued adrenergic neurohumoral activation, was quite marked; in fact well over 50 % of the positive inotropic effect of exercise appeared to depend on a normal increase in heart rate. In a few experiments we were able to measure end-systolic LV pressure-volume relations at two levels of heart rate, during exercise using transient inferior vena caval occlusion, and could show that the slope of the end-systolic pressure-volume relationship was reduced at the lower heart rate (16).

Effects of direct β-adrenergic receptor activation at rest

In other experiments, conscious resting dogs were pretreated with UL-FS 49 to allow study of a wide range of heart rates induced by atrial pacing before and after infusion of the β-adrenergic agonist dobutamine at 3 dosage levels (12). When heart rate was progressively increased stepwise during each condition from approximately 100 bpm to 200 bpm, there was little increase in dP/dt$_{max}$ under control resting conditions (Fig. 3A); we consider this response to result primarily from the progressive fall in left ventricular end-diastolic pressure as heart rate is increased, counteracting any effect on dP/dt$_{max}$ (Fig. 3B). However, with low, medium, and high dose dobutamine the force-frequency responses were shifted upward and steepened, indicating dose-dependent amplification of the force-frequency effect by β-adrenergic stimulation (Fig. 3A). During β-adrenergic stimulation, the higher the paced heart rate the larger the increase in LV dP/dt$_{max}$, and amplification occurred despite similar reductions in left ventricular EDP over the range of heart rates studied, reflected by increasing slopes of the relation between left ventricular EDP and LV dP/dt$_{max}$ as the dose of dobutamine was augmented Fig. 3B).

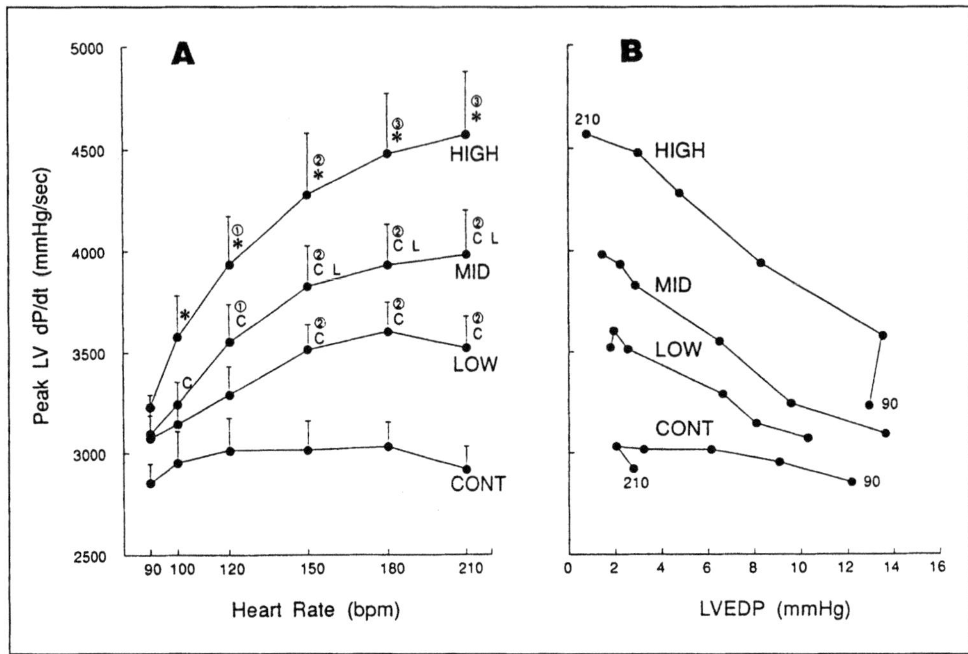

Fig. 3 Panel A: Plot of average relations between peak left ventricular (LV) dP/dt and heart rate during control (CONT) and during dobutamine infusion at three doses (LOW, MID, and HIGH) in conscious dogs. Data are shown as mean ± SEM. * $p = 0.05$ vs. CONT, LOW and MID; (1) < 0.05 vs. pacing rate of 90 beats per minute (bpm); (2) < 0.05 vs. pacing rates of 100 bpm; (3) $p < 0.05$ vs. pacing rates of 100, 120, and 150 bpm; C, $p,0.05$ vs. CONT; L, $p < 0.05$ vs. LOW. Panel B: LV dP/dt$_{max}$ is plotted against LV end-diastolic pressure (LVEDP). Numbers indicate heart rates. Note that ranges of LVEDP are almost identical for control and the three dobutamine doses. (Reproduced with permission from Kambayashi et al. (12))

Under these resting conditions there was shortening of the time constant of left ventricular relaxation (tau) under control conditions as heart rate was increased, and tau was further progressively reduced at increasing doses of dobutamine (12). In other experiments, it also was shown that slowing of the heart rate response during exercise using UL-FS 49 resulted in prolongation of tau along with upward displacement of the left ventricular diastolic pressure-volume relationship during early LV filling (17).

Force-frequency responses in the mouse

Rodent isolated cardiac muscle generally shows a negative force-frequency response (3). In studies in the intact mouse, initial experiments were performed in anesthetized openchest conditions, with pacing wires attached to the right atrium and a 1.8 French Millar cathetertip micromanometer inserted retrograde into the LV via the carotid artery (21).

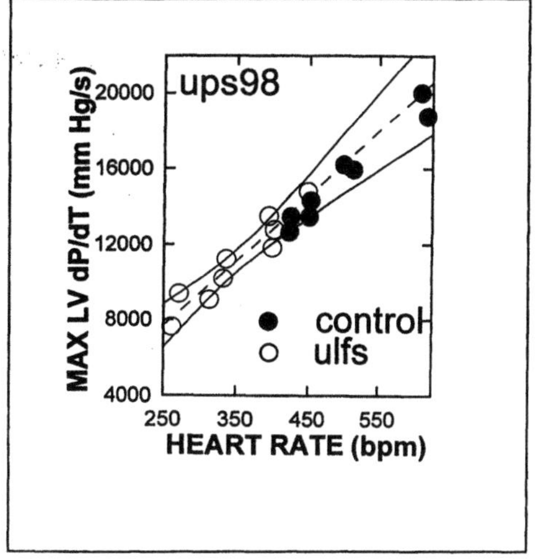

Fig. 4 Example of the relation between heart rate and maximum LV dP/dt in a mouse, following recovery from anesthesia. Data points were recorded with and without spontaneous body movements. Solid circles: data prior to administration of the sinus node inhibitor zatebradine (UL-FS 49). Open circles: data obtained after administration of zatebradine.

UL-FS 49 was administered to reduce the heart rate to about 200 bpm. As heart rate was increased by electrical stimulation of the atrium, LV end-diastolic pressure fell, and LV dP/dt$_{max}$ increased up to a heart rate averaging approximately 300 bpm; above that level, dP/dt began to fall as heart rate was further increased (descending limb of the force-frequency relation). Dobutamine was then administered and the experiment repeated; with β-adrenergic stimulation, the force-frequency relation was displaced upward and a descending limb was apparent only at an average heart rate in excess of 400 bpm (21).

In the conscious mouse, the resting heart rate averages 450 to 500 bpm, and therefore studies were performed in unanesthetized mice. Prior to study, the animals are chronically instrumented with pacing wires on the left atrium, and after recovery for several days they were anesthetized (ketamine-xylazine) and a 1.8 French Millar catheter is inserted retrograde via the carotid artery into the LV. The mice were then allowed to recover from anesthesia over the course of one to two hours until they intermittently moved spontaneously. The intrinsic heart rate, LV pressure and LV dP/dt$_{max}$ were then recorded for about 10–15 minutes at rest and during spontaneous movements when the heart rate reaches frequencies of up to 600 bpm. Incremental doses of UL-FS 49 were then administered, and pressure recordings made at rest and during spontaneous movements for an additional 10–15 minutes as the sinus rate as heart rate slowed due to the drug effect. The results of a representative experiment are shown in Fig. 4 (21). A linear relationship was observed between heart rate and LV dP/dt$_{max}$, before and after UL-FS 49 administration, with similar conditions of rest and intermittent spontaneous activity before and after heart rate slowing, implying a similar degree of neurohumoral stimulation. This observation indicates that the heart rate is a primary, powerful determinant of myocardial contractility in the mouse. A descending limb of the force-frequency relation was seen only with pacing under open-chest conditions, and interaction between the heart rate and the β-adrenergic stimulation appeared to prevent a descending limb at high cardiac frequencies under intact conditions (21). Other studies in mice using atrial pacing at the same heart rates before and after UL-FS 49 administration indicate lack of any direct negative inotropic effect of UL-FS 49, as shown in other species (4, 11, 21, 27).

Force-frequency relations in heart failure

Studies in the pig

Initial studies on the effects of β-adrenergic stimulation on the force-frequency effect in heart failure were carried out in the swine model of pacing-induced cardiac failure. Pigs were chronically instrumented with pacing wires and a high-fidelity micromanometer (Konigsburg) and studied before and after rapid ventricular pacing for 3 weeks to produce marked depression of LV function, documented by echocardiography (6). Animals were studied in the conscious state following administration of UL-FS 49 to lower the initial heart rate, and atrial pacing was performed over a range of 100 to approximately 225 bpm. Before heart failure (as noted in the normal dog) the force-frequency relation was flat with no increase in LV dP/dt$_{max}$ as LV end-diastolic pressure fell during increases in heart rate; administration of dobutamine caused upward displacement and increased slope of the heart rate-LV dP/dt$_{max}$ relation as the heart rate was increased, indicating amplification of the force-frequency relation in the normal pig (Fig. 5, left panel) (6).

Following induction of heart failure, the administration of UL-FS was repeated and the control force-frequency relation was shown to be displaced downward with a small positive effect of increasing heart rate. With dobutamine administration, there was only a small upward displacement of the force-frequency relation, but the amplification was entirely lost (Fig. 5, right hand panel) (6).

These findings indicate loss of an important reserve mechanism in severe heart failure, and the absence of adrenergic amplification of contractility with increasing heart rate is likely to play a significant role in the impaired exercise performance observed in this setting.

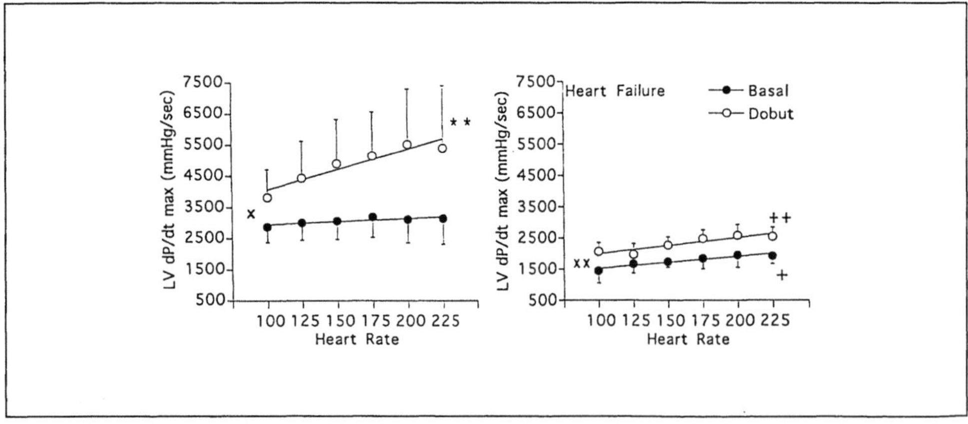

Fig. 5 (A) Heart rates (beats/min) and the mean first derivative of maximum left ventricular (LV) pressure (LV dP/dt$_{max}$) before (left panel) and after (B) heart failure (right panel). Data are shown without (Basal, solid circles) and during (open ciroles) dobutamine (dobut) infusion. Data are mean ± SD, n = 6 animals. Before heart failure: slope of force-frequency relation (FFR) basal, not significant; after dobutamine, P < 0.003; FFR basal vs. dobutamine (x), P < 0.006). After heart failure, FFR basal slope, P < 0.001; slope FFR basal vs. dobutamine, NS. FFR basal shifted downward vs. before HF (xx), P < 0.006. (Reproduced with permission from Eising et al. (6))

Studies in the rabbit

Heart failure is being produced in rabbits by rapid atrial pacing (26). Rabbits are chronically instrumented with pacing wires and an implanted carotid sheath and then after 3 weeks of rapid pacing they are studied by echocardiography to document severe depression of LV function, followed by studies under conscious conditions using retrograde catheterization of the left ventricle with a 2 French Millar catheter-tip micromanometer (26). Before heart failure a slightly positive forcefrequency effect was observed with atrial pacing following UL-FS 49 over a range of 200 to 350 bpm, which showed amplification with dobutamine administration. Above 375 bpm up to 425 bpm a descending limb of the force-frequency relation was observed, characterized by a falling LV dP/dt_{max} with constant LVEDP. Dobutamine attenuated this descending limb.

After heart failure, similar studies showed a depressed and flat force-frequency relation at rest, with loss of amplification of the force-frequency relation by dobutamine up to a heart rate of about 350 bpm, despite slight upward displacement of the entire relationship. In heart failure, there was a pronounced descending limb of the force-frequency relation between heart rates of 350 to 425 bpm. As in control studies, the LV end-diastolic pressure fell on the ascending limb, but it remained constant on the descending limb of the force-frequency relation, suggesting depression of myocardial contractility at high heart rates. Dobutamine infusion in high dose prevented the descending limb of the force-frequency relation in heart failure (26).

Preliminary studies in human subjects

Ongoing studies in human subjects suggest that responses to β-adrenergic stimulation in the normal and failing heart are similar to those observed experimentally. Thus, in relatively normal hearts (patients undergoing cardiac catheterization who have no severe coronary stenosis or inducible ischemia) studied by retrograde high-fidelity catheter-tip micromanometry, right atrial pacing over a range of approximately 65 to 160 bpm produced a progressive fall in LVEDP at rest with little change or slight rise in LV dP/dt_{max}, and administration of dobutamine with repetition of the pacing sequence shows amplification of the force-frequency effect characterized by progressively increasing LV dP/dt_{max} as heart rate is increased over the same range of heart rates. Lack of amplification of a depressed force-frequency relation by β-adrenergic stimulation with dobutamine has now been found in several patients with chronic heart failure (see appendix).

Discussion

The force-frequency effect in the intact heart differs in some respects from that observed in cardiac muscle contracting isometrically, but in both the mechanisms underlying the increase in contractility are related to the increased number of action potentials per minute resulting in increased transsarcolemmal Ca^{2+} influx into the myocardial cell, decreased diastolic time for Ca^{2+} efflux via the Na/Ca^{2+} exchanger, and a possible lag in the Na pump; all of which lead to enhanced Ca^{2+} storage in the sarcoplasmic reticulum associated with enhanced Ca^{2+} release accompanying each cardiac contraction (2, 19). In the studies described herein in the intact heart, this basal force-frequency effect is enhanced by β-adrenergic receptor stimulation, which is undoubtedly related to increased phosphorylation of the calcium channel, allowing enhanced Ca^{2+} influx, together with phosphorylation of phospholamban which disinhibits sarcoplasmic reticulum (SR) Ca^{2+} ATPase, leading to further enhancement of Ca^{2+} storage and release (28, 30). The mechanism of the progressive enhancement of LV dP/dt_{max} at higher heart rates, which we have termed amplification, during β-adrenergic stimulation is less clear. We have considered the possibility that catecholamines might induce additional phosphorylation of phospholamban by activation of Ca^{2+} calmodulin-dependent protein kinase (1), although there is no direct evidence on this possibility. A potentially important mechanism is frequency-dependent facilitation of the transmembrane Ca^{2+} current, recently described by Piot et al. (23).

In normal mouse and rabbit hearts we found a descending limb of the force-frequency effect at high cardiac frequencies, which was also evident in the failing rabbit heart. Several explanations are possible for these observations. The observed descending limb may represent decreasing myocardial contractility, as shown in control and failing human muscle strips contracting isometrically (20). Recent observations by Pieske and coworkers in such muscle strips have nicely proven a close correlation between intracellular Ca^{2+} transients and peak muscle twitch tension, both on the ascending and descending limbs of the force-frequency relation (22). Our observation that LV end-diastolic pressure remained constant as LV dP/dt fell on the ascending limb is consistent with, but does not prove, a negative inotropic effect since diastolic cardiac dimensions were not measured. Dysfunction of the SR Ca^{2+} ATPase pump seems likely to play an important role in the failing heart (9, 29), although impairment of intrasarcoplasmic reticulum Ca^{2+} transport to release sites may be involved (32), and there is also evidence that delayed mechanical restitution may occur in heart failure (24) possibly due to impaired function of the calcium release channel (31). Finally, impaired ventricular filling might also be an important mechanism in the descending limb of the whole heart, which could be compounded by delayed relaxation consequent to reduced filling; also, at high heart rates atrial stimulation may occur during late ventricular systole and contribute to impaired cardiac filling (21). Thus, the mechanism of the descending limb in the whole heart remains uncertain at present, although its occurrence could impair ventricular function and cardiac output at high heart rates during exercise or tachyarrhythmias in heart failure.

Our finding that dobutamine administration ameliorated the descending limb in the normal heart and prevented it in the failing heart is consistent with any of the above mechanisms, since β-adrenergic stimulation appears to favorably affect mechanical restitution (5), improve AV conduction, and also enhance cardiac filling by increasing LV relaxation rate (18).

The finding that expression of the positive inotropic effect of β-adrenergic stimulation during exercise is highly dependent upon the heart rate response carries important implications not only for physiologic control, but also for disease settings. For example, in the sick sinus syndrome or atrio-ventricular block, the β-adrenergic receptor system is usually intact and rate-responsive cardiac pacemaking therefore can be expected to benefit the cardiac output during exercise not only by increasing the number of heart beats per minute but also by markedly enhancing myocardial contractility through amplification of the force-frequency effect. In heart failure, the situation is more complex since both β-adrenergic system dysfunction and chronotropic incompetence occur. Clearly, it would be desirable to restore both β-adrenergic receptor function and the heart rate response during exercise, but probably not at rest; thus, the effects of chronic β-adrenergic system activation in transgenic mouse models which overexpress either the β-adrenergic receptor (15) or GSα (7) have proven toxic to the heart, and unfavorable effects of sympathomimetic agents in patients with heart failure are well-known. β-blockade may upregulate the β-adrenergic receptor system but cause impairment of the heart rate response to exercise which might then be corrected by rate-responsive pacing. Thus, additional research is needed on the cellular mechanisms of the interaction between heart rate and β-adrenergic receptor interaction, as well as on ways to improve it in heart failure.

Conclusion

These findings demonstrate the importance of integrated stimulation of the sinus node and the myocardium by β-adrenergic activation in regulating normal myocardial contractility during exercise or stress. Thus, the expression of the effect of β-adrenergic stimulation on myocardial contractility depends upon the heart rate response. Amplification of the force-frequency relation by β-adrenergic stimulation appears to be operative under conscious conditions across mammalian species including the mouse, rabbit, dog, pig, and human. Impairment of the β-adrenergic receptor system, as well as abnormalities of sinus node function or electrical conduction leading to chronotropic incompetence, can lead to loss of this important physiologic mechanism for regulating myocardial contractility during exercise or stress.

Acknowledgment   Supported by an endowed chair awarded to Dr. Ross by the San Diego County Affiliate of the American Heart Association and by the Richard D. Winter Fund.

References

1. Bers DM (1991) Excitation-contraction coupling and cardiac contractile force. Kluwer Academic Publishers, Dordrecht Boston London, pp 95
2. Bers DM (1991) Excitation-contraction coupling and cardiac contractile force. Kluwer Academic Publisher, Dordrecht Boston London, pp 155–158, 167–170
3. Buckley NM, Penefsky ZJ, Litwak RS (1972) Comparative force-frequency relationships in human and other mammalian ventricular myocardium. Pflügers Arch 332: 259–270
4. Chen Z, Slinker BK (1992) The sinus node inhibitor UL-FS 49 lacks significant inotropic effect. J Clin Pharmacol 19: 264–271
5. Drake-Holland AJ, Sitsapesan R, Herbacznska-Cedro K, Seed WA, Noble MIM (1992) Effect of adrenaline on cardiac force-interval relationship. Cardiovasc Res 26: 496–501
6. Eising GP, Hammond HK, Helmer GA, Gilpin E, Ross J Jr (1994) Force-frequency relations during heart failure in the pig. Am J Physiol 267: H2516–H2522
7. Gaudin C, Ishikawa Y, Wight DC, Mahdavi V, Nadal-Ginard B, Wagner TE, Vatner DE, Homcy CJ (1995) Overexpression of Gs alpha protein in the hearts of transgenic mice. J Clin Invest 95: 1676–1683
8. Goethals M, Raes A, Van Bogaert PP (1993) Use-dependent block of the pacemaker current I_f in rabbit sino-atrial node cells by zatebradine (UL-FS 49). On the mode of action of sinus node inhibitors. Circulation 88 (part 1): 2389–2401
9. Gwathmey JK, Slawsky MT, Hajjar RJ, Briggs GM, Morgan JP (1990) Role of intracellular calcium handling in force-interval relationships of human ventricular myocardium. J Clin Invest 85: 1599–1613
10. Higgins CB, Vatner SF, Franklin D, Braunwald E (1973) Extent of regulation of the heart's contractile state in the conscious dog by alteration in the frequency of contraction. J Clin Invest 52: 1189–1194
11. Indolfi C, Guth BD, Miura T, Miyazaki S, Schultz R, Ross J Jr (1989) Mechanism of improved ischemic regional dysfunction by bradycardia. Circulation 80: 983–993

12. Kambayashi M, Miura T, Oh B-H, Rockman HA, Murata K, Ross J Jr (1992) Enhancement of the force-frequency effect on myocardial contractility by adrenergic stimulation in conscious dogs. Circulation 86: 572–580
13. Little WC (1985) The left ventricular dP/dt_{max}-end-diastolic volume relation in closed-chest dogs. Circ Res 56: 808–815
14. Mahler F, Yoran C, Ross J Jr (1974) Inotropic effects of tachycardia and poststimulation potentiation in the conscious dog. Am J Physiol 227: 569–575
15. Milano CA, Dolber PC, Rockman HA, Bond RA, Venable ME, Allen LF, Lefkowitz RJ (1994) Myocardial expression of a constitutively active α_{1B}-adrenergic receptor in transgenic mice induces cardiac hypertrophy. Proc Natl Acad Sci, USA 91: 10109–10113
16. Miura T, Miyazaki S, Guth BD, Kambayashi M, Ross J Jr (1992) Influence of the force-frequency relation on left ventricular function during exercise in conscious dogs. Circulation 86: 563–571
17. Miura T, Miyazaki S, Guth BD, Indolfi C, Ross J Jr (1994) Heart rate and force-frequency effects on diastolic function of the left ventricle in exercising dogs. Circulation 89: 2361–2368
18. Miyazaki S, Guth BD, Miura T, Indolfi C, Schulz R, Ross J Jr (1990) Changes of left ventricular diastolic function in exercising dogs without and with ischemia. Circulation 81: 1058–1070
19. Morgan JP (1991) Abnormal intracellular modulation of calcium as a major cause of cardiac contractile dysfunction. N Engl J Med 325: 625–632
20. Mulieri LA, Hasenfuss G, Leavitt B, Allen PD, Alpert NR (1992) Altered myocardial force-frequency relation in human heart failure. Circulation 85: 1743–1750
21. Palakodeti V, Oh S, Oh B-H, Mao L, Hongo M, Peterson KL, Ross J Jr (1997) The force-frequency effect is a powerful determinant of myocardial contractility in the mouse. Am J Physiol 273: H1283–H1290
22. Pieske B, Kretschmann B, Meyer M, Holubarsch C, Weirich J, Posival H, Minami K, Just H, Hasenfuss G (1995) Alterations in intracellular calcium handling associated with the inverse force-frequency relation in human dilated cardiomyopathy. Circulation 92: 1169–1178
23. Piot C, Lemaire S, Albat B, Seguin J, Nargeot J, Richard S (1996) High Frequency-induced upregulation of human cardiac calcium currents. Circulation 93: 120–128
24. Prabhu SD, Freeman GL (1995) Effect of tachycardia heart failure on the restitution of left ventricular function in closed-chest dogs. Circulation 91: 176–185
25. Ross J Jr, Miura T, Kambayashi M, Eising GP, Ryu K-H (1995) Adrenergic control of the force-frequency relation. Circulation 92: 2327–2332
26. Ryu K-H, Tanaka N, Dalton N, Ross J Jr (1995) Adrenergic responses and the descending limb of force-frequency relations in the failing rabbit heart. FASEB J 9: A558 (Abstract)
27. Ryu K-H, Tanaka N, Ross J Jr (1996) Effects of a sinus node inhibitor on the normal and failing rabbit heart. Basic Res Cardiol 90: 131–139
28. Sasaki T, Inui M, Kimura Y, Kuzuya T, Tada M (1992) Molecular mechanism of regulation of Ca^{2+} pump ATPase by phospholamban in cardiac sarcoplasmic reticulum. J Biol Chem 267: 1675–1679
29. Schwinger RHG, Schmidt U, Bavendiek U, Erdmann E (1995) Ca^{2+}-uptake of sarcoplasmic reticulum plays a functional role for the force-frequency relationship in man. J Am Coll Cardiol February: 371A (Abstract)
30. Trautwein W, Heschler J (1990) Regulation of cardiac L-type calcium current by phosphorylation and G proteins. Annu Rev Physiol 52: 257–274
31. Vatner DE, Naoki S, Kiuchi K, Shannon RP, Vatner SF (1994) Decrease in myocardial ryanodine receptors and altered excitation-contraction coupling early in the development of heart failure. Circulation 90: 1423–1430
32. Wier WG, Yue DT (1986) Intracellular calcium transients underlying the short-term force-interval relationship in ferret ventricular myocardium. J Physiol 376: 507–530

Author's address:
John Ross, Jr., M.D.
University of California San Diego
Department of Medicine 0613B
9500 Gilman Drive
La Jolla, CA 92093-0613
USA

Appendix

In studies completed after the submission of this paper, patients without significant cardiac disease (controls) and patients with cardiac failure secondary to severe dilated cardiomyopathy were studied using high fidelity LV micromanometry and graded right atrial pacing from the resting rate up to 150–160 beats/min before and after dobutamine infusion. The relation between heart rate and $LVdP/dt_{max}$ showed a positive slope during dobutamine infusion in controls, whereas in patients with heart failure this relation was depressed and showed no amplification with β-adrenergic stimulation; however, in the patients with heart failure the relation between heart rate and relaxation time was improved by dobutamine (Bhargava V, Shabetai R, Mathiäsen RA, Dalton N, Hunter JJ, Ross J Jr. Loss of adrenergic control of the force-frequency relation in heart failure secondary to idiopathic or ischemic cardiomyopathy. American Journal of Cardiology 81: 1130–1137, 1998).

Influence of left ventricular pressures and heart rate on myocardial high-energy phosphate metabolism

S. Neubauer

Medizinische Universitätsklinik Würzburg

Abstract

This review describes the effects of changes in left ventricular pressures and heart rate on myocardial high-energy phosphate metabolism. When cardiac workload is substantially increased, creatine kinase flux will increase markedly, phosphocreatine will show a small but detectable decrease, and ATP will not change. In this context, heart rate is a much weaker acute metabolic stimulus than left ventricular developed pressure. However, in heart failure, chronic reduction of heart rate has beneficial effects on alterations of high-energy phosphate metabolism.

Key words   Heart rate – left ventricular developed pressure – ATP – phosphocreatine – creatine kinase reaction velocity

For an understanding of the interrelations between myocardial workload and high-energy phosphates, one should be aware of the emerging role of high-energy phsphate metabolism in cardiac and skeletal muscle (Fig. 1). Incidentially, creatine phosphate (or phosphocreatine, which is a synonymous term) was discovered in 1927 four years before ATP (6) and was first thought to be the molecule providing the energy for contraction, which was replenished by ATP (Model 1). This reaction is catalyzed by creatine kinase. In 1962, Cain and Davies (4) inhibited creatine kinase with fluorodinitrobenzene and found that contractions continued at least for a short time, during which ATP decreased and phosphocreatine remained constant. Thus, ATP was indentified as the primary fuel for contraction, and phosphocreatine was assigned a diminished role to act purely as an energy reservoire (Model 2). In the 1970s, however, experiments showed that in ischemia, muscle contraction stopped after about one minute. At this time, phosphocreatine was almost completely exhausted, but ATP was still at 80 % of control levels (8). Thus, a number of groups including Gudbjarnason et al. (8, 21) postulated Model 3 implementing functional compartimentation. In this model, the high-energy phosphate bond is transferred from ATP to creatine at the site of ATP production (mitochondria), yielding phosphocreatine and ADP. This reaction is catalyzed by the mitochondrial isoenzyme of creatine kinase. Phosphocreatine

Supported by DFG grant SFB 355 „Pathophysiologie der Herzinsuffizienz“, Teilprojekt A3, and by grant BMBF „Klinisches Forschungszentrum, Teilprojekt F2“

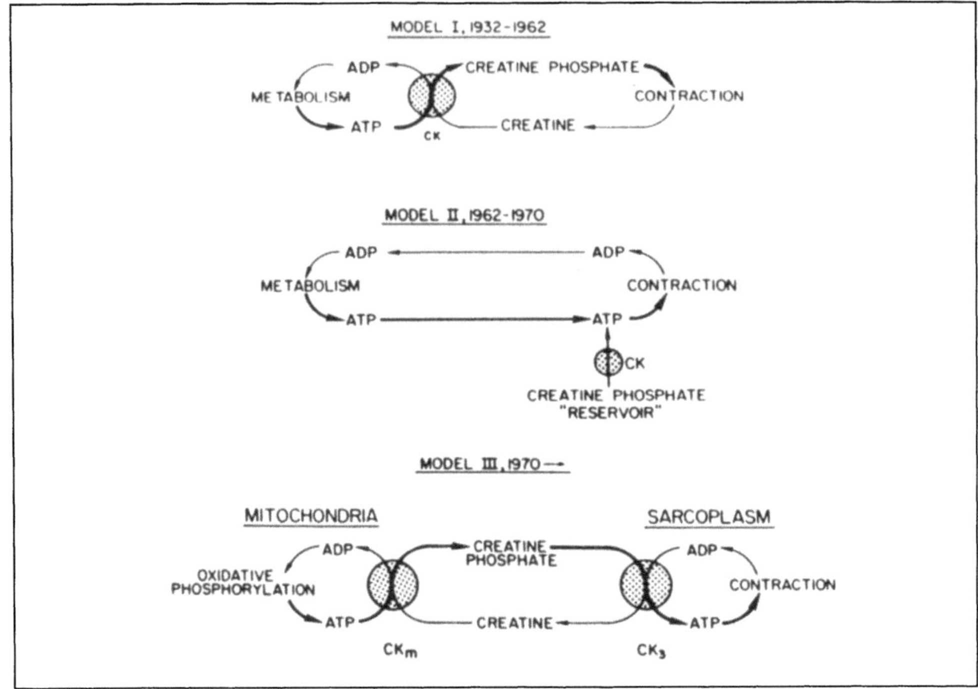

Fig. 1 History of the emerging role of myocardial high-energy phosphates. For further details, see manuscript text. Adapted from: Ingwall JS, Bittl JA (1987) Regulation of heart creatine kinase. Basic Res Cardiol 82 (2): 93–101. Reproduced with permission.

then diffuses to the site of ATP utilization, the myofibrils, where the back reaction occurs, ATP is reformed and is used for contraction. This reaction is catalyzed by the myofibrillar-bound MM-creatine kinase isoenzyme. Free creatine then diffuses back to the mitochondria. It was shown that a major limitation of Model 2 is that the very low free cytosolic ADP concentration (40–80 µM) does not provide sufficient capacity for the back diffusion to the mitochondria (21). This function is therefore assigned to free creatine, which is present at concentrations that are at least two orders of magnitude higher than ADP.

The various components of high-energy phosphate metabolism are analyzed using a wide range of methods: ATP and phosphocreatine can be determined noninvasively and repetitively using 31P magnetic resonance (MR) spectroscopy. A high resolution 31P MR spectrum from a perfused rat heart can be obtained with a high-field MR spectrometer within two to five minutes. ATP and phosphocreatine can also be determined analytically after rapid freezing and perchloric acid extraction using high-pressure liquid chromatography or spectrophotometric methods (17, 20). Free creatine does not have a phosphorus atom and can, therefore, not be determined with 31P MR spectroscopy. It can, however, be measured with HPLC (20) or with a fluorometric assay developed by Kammermeier (11). Total creatine kinase activity is measured spectrophotometrically, creatine kinase iso-enzymes by agarose gel electrophoresis. Inorganic phosphate is best determined with 31P MR spectroscopy; analytical methods will determine erroneously high values due to degradation of ATP and phosphocreatine during freezing and extraction. Fig. 2 shows a typical 31P MR spectrum from an isolated rat heart. A major advantage of the MR spectroscopy

Fig. 2 31P MR spectrum of an isolated rat heart acquired at 7 tesla. Pulse angle 45 degrees, pulse repetition time 1.93 s, number of acquisitions 152. MPE = monophosphate esters.

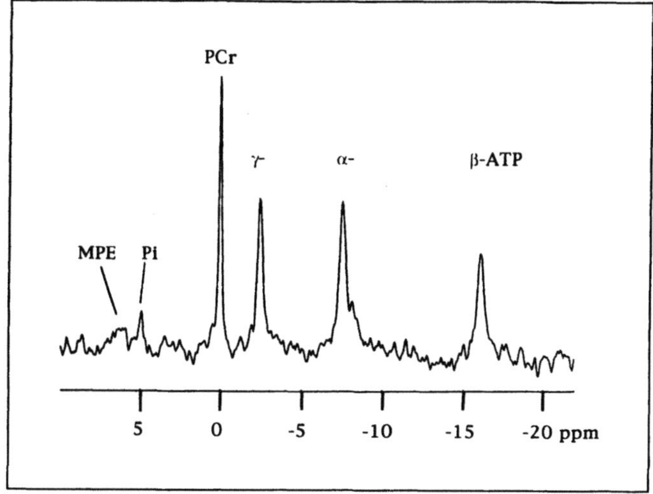

method is that it not only allows to determine steady state concentrations but also true chemical flux. Using 31P MR saturation transfer (7), creatine kinase reaction velocity („creatine kinase flux") can be determined, which represents ATP transfer from the mitochondria to the myofibrils (9). The saturation transfer method is described in detail elsewhere (2); this methods yields the T1 (spin lattice relaxation time) of phosphocreatine, the rate constant (k_{for}), and the reaction velocity (flux), which is in the order of 8–15 mM/sec.

Free cytosolic ADP cannot be measured directly with any method. The values found by HPLC mostly represent myofibrillar-bound ADP, which is biochemically irrelevant. Free ADP has to be calculated from the creatine kinase equilibrium according to:

$$ADP = (ATP \times creatine) : (phosphocreatine \times H^+ \times K_{eq})$$

where H^+ is the intracellular hydrogen ion concentration, measured from 31P MR spectra by the chemical shift difference of inorganic phosphate and phosphocreatine; K_{eq} is the equilibrium constant of the creatine kinase reaction determined as 1.66×10^{-9} M^{-1} (15).

ADP is, thus, calculated to be in the order of 40–80 µM, i.e., two orders of magnitude lower than all the other metabolites of the creatine kinase reaction. The free energy change of ATP hydrolysis (ΔG) is a measure of the efficiency of ATP utilization and is given in KJ/mol ATP that is hydrolyzed according to Kammermeier et al. (12).

$$\Delta G = \Delta G_o + RT \ln (ADP \times inorganic\ phosphate) : ATP$$

where
ΔG_o is the standard free energy change at 37 °C, $Mg^{2+} = 1$ mM
R = gas constant
T = temperature [K]

In normal cardiomyocytes, ΔG is in the order of –59 KJ/mol. Below a threshold value for ΔG, many intracellular enzymes such as $SR\text{-}Ca^{++}\text{-}ATPase$ (–52 KJ/mol) or $Na^+/K^+\text{-}ATPase$ (–46 KJ/mol) will not function properly (12).

The interrelations between high-energy phosphate metabolism and cardiac workload have been studied at various levels of complexity: In vitro perfused rodent hearts, in vivo

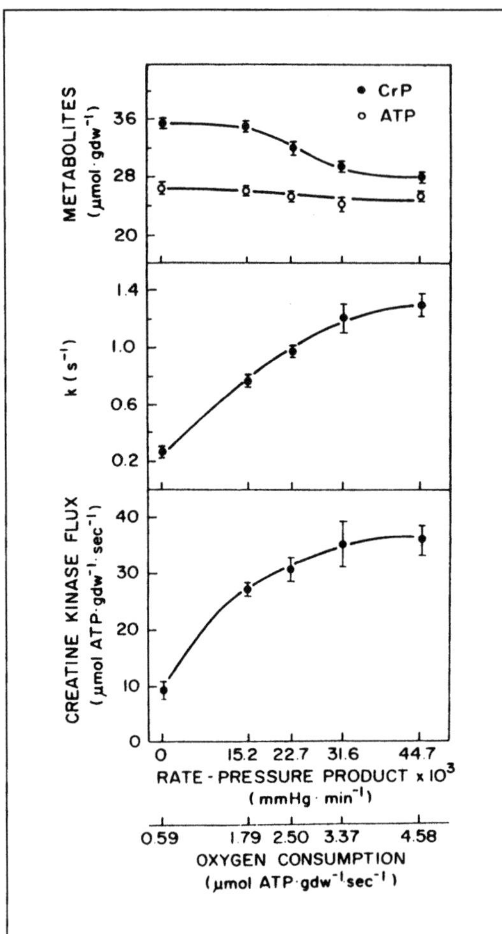

Fig. 3   Tissue contents of ATP and PCr, rate constant k, and creatine kinase flux for rat hearts working at five levels of performance. Adapted from: Ingwall JS, Bittl JA (1987) Regulation of heart creatine kinase. Basic Res Cardiol 82 (2): 90–101. Reproduced with permission.

rodent hearts, in vivo dog hearts and the human heart. Fig. 3 shows results from the „classic" isolated heart experiment by Bittl and Ingwall (2). In this glucose-perfused rat heart model, high-energy phosphates, the creatine kinase rate constant, and creatine kinase flux were measured noninvasively by 31P MR spectroscopy. Hearts were studied during cardioplegia and under four different workload conditions achieved by increasing left ventricular balloon volume and, thus, end-diastolic pressure, in a stepwise manner. This increased the rate-pressure product from about 15 000 to about 45 000 (mmHg/min) only by increasing left ventricular developed pressure, while heart rate remained unchanged. With increased left ventricular pressure development and oxygen consumption, there was a small but significant decrease of phosphocreatine, no change in ATP, a dramatic increase of both the creatine kinase rate constant and creatine kinase flux. While Bittl et al. (2) changed left ventricular developed pressure, Field et al. (5) altered heart rate by pacing perfused rat hearts at 120, 240, and 360/min. Although developed pressure decreased with increasing heart rate, rate-pressure products incrased by up to 60 %. 31P MR spectra obtained under these conditions demonstrated that myocardial high-energy phosphate concentrations remained completely unchanged during this protocol.

Using an in vivo rat model, where a surface coil was placed over the heart after thoracotomy, Bittl and Ingwall (3) studied the effects of workload changes on high-energy phosphates. When the in vivo rat heart was paced at frequencies ranging from 300 to 600/min, rate-pressure products increased by up to 30 %. Under these conditions, ATP, phosphocreatine, rate constant, and creatine kinase flux all remained constant. However, when both heart rate and developed pressure were altered, results were different. When rats were studied under 2 % halothane, 1 % halothane, and isoproterenol infusion, rate-pressure products increased by 64 and 149 %. Under these conditions, ATP remained constant, phosphocreatine decreased, and the rate constant as well as creatine kinase flux showed marked increases.

The correlation between workload and creatine kinase flux also holds in postischemic myocardium. We have subjected perfused ferret hearts to 20, 40 or 60 min of total ischemia followed by reperfusion. Rate-pressure products during reperfusion recovered to about 70, 40, and 10 % of control levels. Creatine kinase flux very closely followed the changes of workload in postischemic myocardium as well (18).

For many years a controversy has raged as to whether changes in high-energy phosphates can be induced in the in vivo dog heart with increasing workload. Balaban's group has demonstrated no changes with work (1 for review). Similarly, Chance's group has reported that when the in vivo dog heart is paced with 120 or 240/min, high-energy phosphate levels measured with 31P MR spectroscopy do not change (16). The most sophisticated large-animal MR methodology has been developed by Zhang et al. (23). Using the 31P MR localization technique FLAX-ISIS (Fourier series window longitudinally modulated adiabatic excitation – image-selected in vivo spectroscopy), these authors were able to resolve high-energy phosphate metabolism in 5 voxels spanning the left ventricular wall, localizing spectra to the subendocardium, midmyocardium and subepicardium. Under control conditions, there were no transmural differences of high-energy phosphates, and inorganic phosphate was not visible. During stimulation with high-dose dopamine and dobutamine, leading to about a 170 % increase of rate-pressure products due to increases of both left ventricular developed pressure and heart rate, inorganic phosphate became visible, phosphocreatine decreased, but again, there was no transmural difference. When this experiment was repeated in flow-limited myocardium due to LAD-stenosis, transmural differences became visible. Fig. 4 taken from the work by Zhang et al. (23) clearly demon-

Fig. 4 Change in whole wall ΔPi/Cr as a function of whole wall oxygen consumption. Adapted from Zhang J et al. (1995) Am J Physiol 268: H1891–H1905. Reproduced with permission.

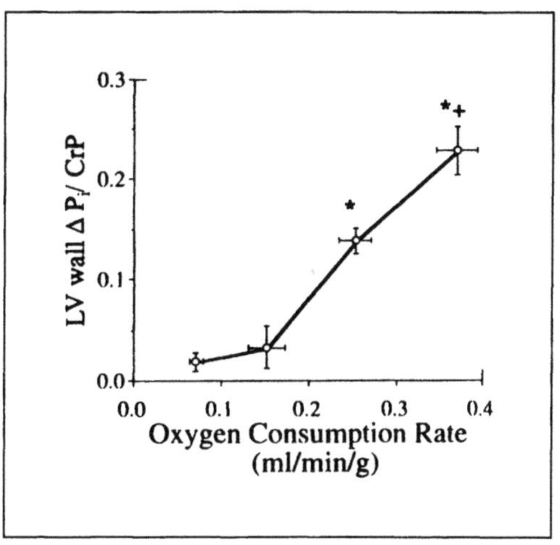

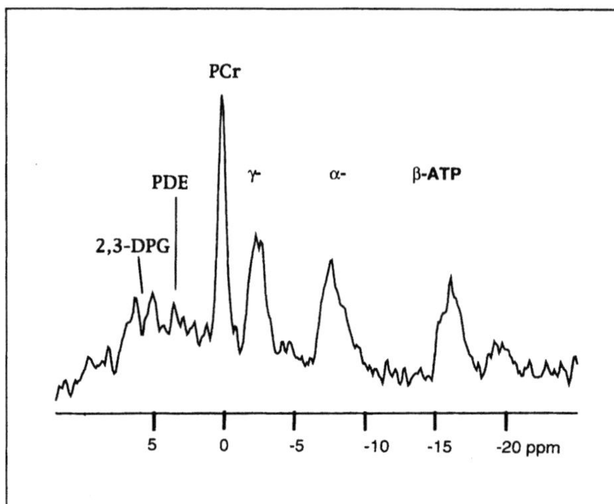

Fig. 5 ^{31}P MR spectrum of the anterior myocardium from a healthy volunteer acquired at 1.5 tesla. Adiabatic pulses, repetition time 15 s, number of acquisitions 128. ISIS localization. PDE = phosphodiesters; 2-3-DPG = 2,3-diphosphoglycerate.

strates that with moderate increases of workload and oxygen consumption, there is no change of inorganic phosphate and phosphocreatine; but at higher workload states, there is a clear correlation between work and high-enery phosphates. In dog hearts, high-energy phosphate levels therefore will change only with more striking increases of workload but remain constant in the low workload range.

In the human heart, the only technique that allows the study of workload-dependent changes of high-energy phosphates is 31P MR spectroscopy. In conjunction with localization methods, myocardial volumes of 30–80 cm^3 can be interrogated. Fig. 5 shows a human cardiac 31P MR spectrum obtained with the localization technique ISIS (image-selected in vivo spectroscopy). Weiss et al. (22) have studied volunteers and patients with LAD-stenosis > 70 % during handgrip exercise leading to a 20–30 % increase of heart rate. Under these conditions, myocardial high-energy phosphates remained constant in volunteers. However, in patients with LAD-stenosis, i.e., in flow-limited myocardium, even this very moderate increase of workload significantly reduced phosphocreatine/ATP ratios. This effect was partially reversible upon recovery. However, Lamb et al. (14) recently showed that workload-dependent changes of high-energy phosphates occur even in normal human myocardium. This group subjected volunteers to high-dose dobutamine infusion (40 µg/kg x min) combined with atropine. This increased rate-pressure products about 3-fold. Under these conditions, phosphocreatine/ATP ratios decreased significantly from about 1.4 to less than 1.2. Thus, similar to the findings in dog myocardium, in human heart small workload changes do not but major workload changes do change myocardial high-energy phosphate levels, i.e., decrease phosphocreatine content.

In heart failure, chronic changes of myocardial high-energy phosphate metabolism occur (see 10 for review). In residual intact myocardium of chronically infarcted rats two months after myocardial infarction (MI) we have recently demonstrated a decrease of about 35 % of both phosphocreatine and creatine, about a 50 % decrease of the mitochondrial creatine kinase isoenzyme, substantial increases of the fetal creatine kinase isoenzymes BB and MB, and significant reductions of total creatine content (17). Although increases of heart rate may be a weak acute metabolic stimulus, the effects of chronic heart rate reduction in heart failure may be substantial. In this context, we have recently demonstrated that in the chronic infarct (MI) rat heart failure model, chronic heart rate reduction by 20 % due to

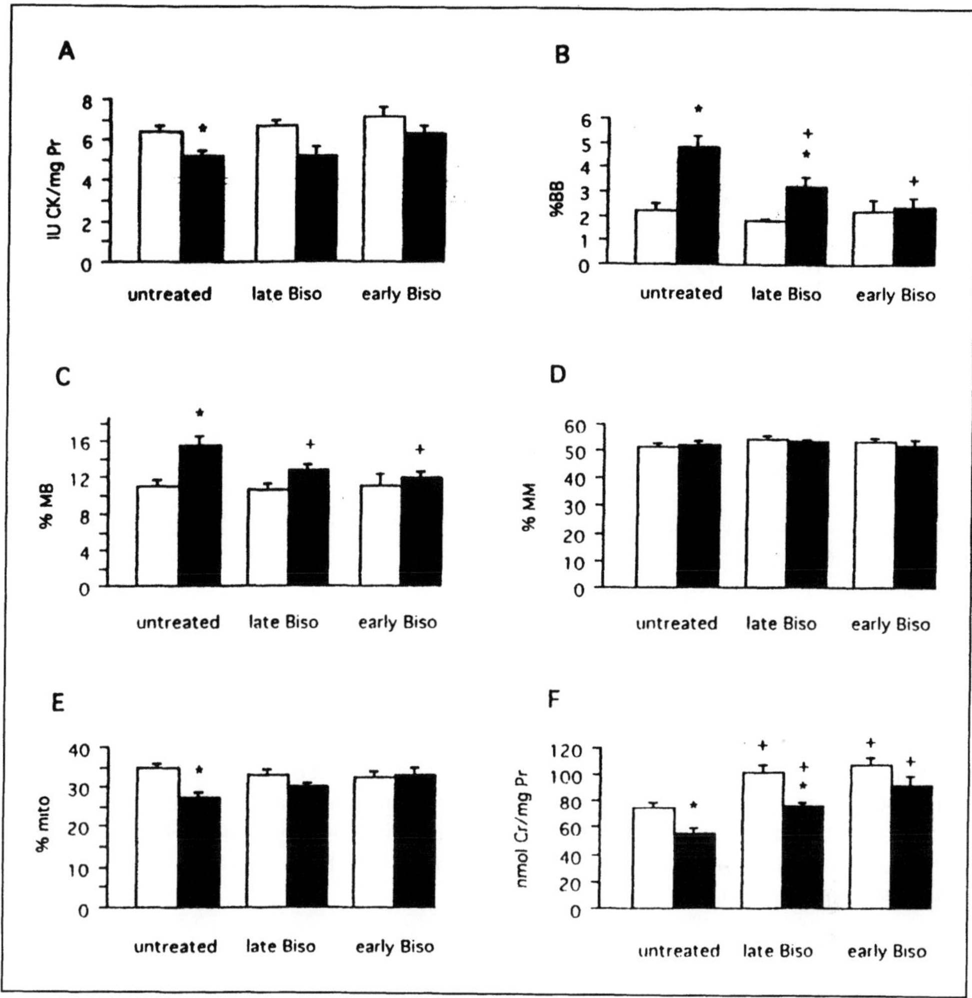

Fig. 6   Effects of late and early bisoprolol treatment on the creatine kinase system after myocardial infarction (light grey: sham hearts; dark grey: infarcted hearts). Changes of creatine kinase (CK) activity, CK isoenzyme distribution, and total creatine are shown in panels A-F. * $p < 0.05$ MI vs. sham; + $p < 0.05$ treated vs. untreated. Adapted from Laser A et al. (1996) J Am Coll Cardiol 27: 487–493. Reproduced with permission.

treatment with the beta-receptor blocker bisoprolol (13) has beneficial effects (Fig. 6). Early treatment was started immediately after, late treatment two weeks after MI. Two month after MI, bisoprolol (60 mg/kg/day) treatment prevented the decrease of total creatine kinase, the decrease of the mitochondrial creatine kinase isoenzyme, the increase of the fetal creatine kinase isoenzymes BB and MB, and the decrease of total creatine content. Early treatment was more effective than late treatment. In human failing myocardium, only anecdotal evidence exists concerning the energetic effects of chronic heart rate reduction. We have studied patients with heart failure due to dilated cardiomyopathy before and three months after medical therapy leading to clinical recompensation using repetitive 31P MR spectroscopy (19). In 4 out of 6 patients, therapy included 50 mg metoprolol/die. Heart rate

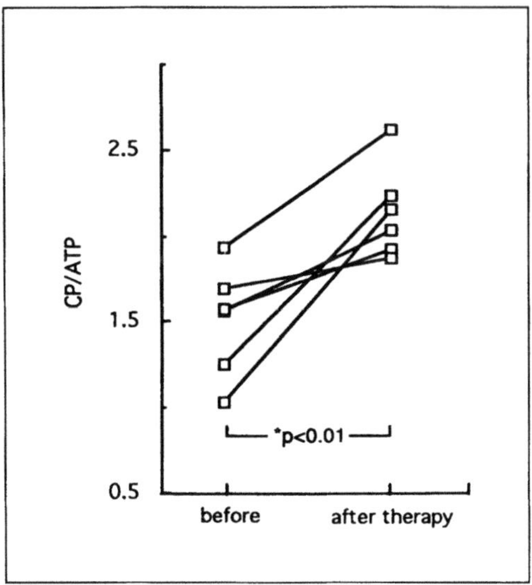

Fig. 7 PCr/ATP ratios before and after 12 ± 6 weeks of drug therapy in 6 patients with dilated cardiomyopathy. There was a significant increase of PCr/ATP from 1.51 ± 0.32 to 2.15 ± 0.27 (* $p < 0.01$). Adapted from Neubauer S et al. (1992) Circulation 86: 1810–1818. Reproduced with permission.

was about 10 % lower after treatment than before. In all patients, the phosphocreatine/ATP ratio improved during therapy (Fig. 7). We are currently planning systematic studies involving a large number of patients that will look at the long-term effects of heart rate reduction with beta-blocking agents in heart failure to further elucidate these points.

In summary, when myocardial workload is substantially increased, creatine kinase flux will increase markedly, phosphocreatine will show a small but detectable decrease, and ATP will not change. From the body of work reviewed here it is clear that heart rate is a much weaker acute metabolic stimulus than left ventricular developed pressure. However, in heart failure, chronic reduction of heart rate has beneficial effects on alterations of high-energy phosphate metabolism.

Acknowledgments The author would like to thank the following colleagues for their contributions over many years of collaboration: Joanne S. Ingwall, Ph. D., John A. Bittl, M.D., Harvard Medical School, Boston, USA; Kurt Kochsiek, M.D., Michael Horn, Ph.D., Helga Remkes, Medizinische Universitätsklinik Würzburg, Germany; Thomas Pabst, Ph.D., Meinrad Beer, M.D., Jörn Sandstede, M.D.,Thomas Krahe, M.D., Dietbert Hahn, M.D., Institut für Röntgendiagnostik, Würzburg University, Germany; Georg Ertl, M.D., Kai Hu, M.D., Anne Laser, Ph.D., Klinikum Mannheim, Universität Heidelberg, Germany.

References

1. Balaban RS (1990) Regulation of oxidative phosphorylation in the mammalian cell. Am J Physiol 258: C377–C389
2. Bittl JA, Ingwall JS (1985) Reaction rates of Creatine Kinase and ATP synthesis in the Isolated Rat Heart. A ^{31}P-NMR Magnetization transfer study. J Biol Chem 260, 6: 3512–3517
3. Bittl JA, Balschi JA, Ingwall JS (1987) Effects of norepinephrine infusion on myocardial high-energy phosphate content and turnover in the living rat. J Clin Invest 79: 1852–1859
4. Cain DF, Davies RE (1962) Breakdown of adenosine triphosphate during a single contraction of working muscle. Biochem Biophys Res Commun 8: 361–366
5. Field ML, Azzawi A, Unitt JF, Seymour AM, Henderson C, Radda GK (1996) Intracellular Ca^{2+} staircase in the isovolumic pressure-frequency relationship of Langendorff-perfused rat heart. J Mol Cell Cardiol 28: 65–77
6. Fiske CH, Subbarow Y (1927) The nature of the "inorganic phosphate" in voluntary muscle. Science 65: 401–403

7. Forsen S, Hofman RA (1963) Study of moderately rapid chemical exchange reactions by means of nuclear magnetic double resonance. J Chem Phys 39: 2892–2901

8. Gudbjarnason S, Mathes P, Ravens GK (1970) Functional compartmentation of ATP and creatine phosphate in heart muscle. J Mol Cell Cardiol 1: 325–339

9. Ingwall JS (1982) Phosphorus nuclear magnetic resonance spectroscopy of cardiac and skeletal muscles. Am J Physiol 242: H729–H744

10. Ingwall JS (1993) Is cardiac failure a consequence of decreased energy reserve? Circulation 87 (Suppl VII): 58–62

11. Kammermeier H (1973) Microassay of free and total creatine from tissue extracts by combination of chromatographic and fluorometric methods. Anal Biochem 56: 341–345

12. Kammermeier H, Schmidt P, Jüngling E (1982) Free energy change of ATP-hydrolysis: A causal factor of early hypoxic failure of the myocardium? J Mol Cell Cardiol 14: 267–277

13. Laser A, Neubauer S, Tian R, Hu K, Gaudron P, Ingwall J, Ertl G (1996) Long-term beta-blocker treatment prevent chronic creatine kinase and lactate dehydrogenase system changes in rat hearts post-myocardial infarction. J Am Coll Cardiol 27: 487–493

14. Lamb HJ, Beyerbacht HP, Doombos J, den Hollander JA, Pluim BM, van der Wall EE, de Roos A (1996) Metabolic response of human myocardium to atropine-dobutamine stress studied by 31P-MRS. Proc 4th int. meeting ISMRM 428 (Abstract)

15. Lawson JWR, Veech RL (1979) Effects of pH and free Mg^{2+} on the K_{eq} of the creatine kinase reaction and other phosphate hydrolyses and phosphate transfer reactions. J Biol Chem 254, 14: 6528–6537

16. Ligeti L, Osbakken MD, Clark BJ, Schnall M, Bolinger L, Subramanian H, Leigh JS, Chance B (1987) Cardiac transfer function relating energy metabolism to workload in different species as studied with 31P NMR. Magn Reson Med 4: 112–119

17. Neubauer S, Horn M, Naumann A, Tian R, Hu K, Laser M, Friedrich J, Gaudron P, Schnackerz K, Ingwall JS, Ertl G (1995) Impairment of energy metabolism in intact residual mycardium of rat hearts with chronic myocardial infarction. J Clin Invest 95: 1092–1100

18. Neubauer S, Hamman BL, Perry SB, Bittl JS, Ingwall JS (1988) Velocity of the creatine kinase reaction decreases in post-ischemic myocardium. A ^{31}P-NMR magnetization transfer study of the isolated ferret heart. Circ Res 63: 1–15

19. Neubauer S, Krahe T, Schindler R, Horn M, Hillenbrand H, Entzeroth C, Kromer EP, Riegger GAJ, Lackner K, Ertl G (1992) Cardiac ^{31}P-magnetic resonance spectroscopy of volunteers and patients with coronary artery disease and dilated cardiomyopathy – Altered cardiac high-energy phosphate metabolism in heart failure. Circulation 86: 1810–1818

20. Sellevold OFM, Jynge P, Aarstad K (1986) High performance liquid chromatography: A rapid isocratic method for determination of creatine compounds and adenine nucleotides in myocardial tissue. J Mol Cell Cardiol 18: 517–27

21. Wallimann T, Wyss M, Brdiczka D, Nicolay K, Eppenberger HM (1992) Intracellular compartmentation, structure and function of creatine kinase isoenzymes in tissues with high and fluctuating energy demands: The phosphocreatine circuit for cellular energy homeostasis. Biochem J 281: 21–40

22. Weiss RG, Bottomley PA, Hardy CJ, Gerstenblith G (1990) Regional myocardial metabolism of high-energy phosphates during isometric exercise in patients with coronary artery disease. New Engl J Med 323: 1593–1600

23. Zhang J, Duncker DJ, Xu Y, Zhang Y, Path G, Merkle H, Hendrich K, From AHL, Bache RJ, Ugurbil K (1995) Transmural bioenergetic responses of normal myocardium to high workstates. Am J Physiol 268: H1891–H1905

Author's address:
Stefan Neubauer, M.D.
Medizinische Universitätsklinik
Josef-Schneider-Strasse 2
97080 Würzburg
Germany

Force-frequency relation in patients with left ventricular hypertrophy and failure

D. A. Kass

Division of Cardiology, Johns Hopkins Medical Institutions, Baltimore, USA

Introduction

Genetic and acquired left ventricular hypertrophy are generally considered disorders of principally diastolic function (11, 13, 14, 27, 28). Reduced chamber compliance, delayed relaxation, and small and often deformed cavities all conspire to limit pump performance and reserve capacity while raising pulmonary venous pressures. Typically, patients have supranormal rest systolic function, intracavitary pressure gradients, dynamic obstruction, and ejection fractions well above 75 %. Clinical symptoms include angina-like chest discomfort, orthostatic intolerance, and exertional dyspnea. Both the chest pain and dyspnea have been linked to subendomyocardial hypoperfusion with worsened diastolic failure (2, 4, 5, 15, 16, 38).

Despite an appearance of preserved systolic function, limitations of systolic functional reserve may also contribute to exertional symptoms of patients with cardiac hypertrophy. Data measured in isolated muscle from failing or explanted hypertrophic hearts have revealed reduced expression and activity of excitation-contraction coupling proteins (notably the sarcoplasmic reticular ATPase) (6), and alterations of force-interval relations (13, 29, 30, 33). Quantification of abnormalties in force-frequency relations of intact patients has been more difficult to assess. This is primarily due to the substantial changes in chamber loading that accompany alterations in cycle length, which itself modifies most measures of ventricular function.

To circumvent this problem, we have employed continuous pressure-volume relation analysis to comprehensively examine the dependence of cardiac systolic and diastolic performance on varying steady-state and instantaneous cycle length in normal subjects, and patients with chronic symptomatic left ventricular hypertrophy (26). These data remain to date the most cardiac-specific detailed study of force-frequency behavior yet reported in conscious humans. This review discusses the major findings from this study, and their potential relevance for the exertional intolerance of patients with cardiac hypertrophy.

Results and discussion

Study population

The study population consisted of 18 patients, ten with chronic ventricular hypertrophy and 8 controls with normal hearts. Mean age in the hypertrophy group was slightly higher

(55 vs 38 y) and patients had a maximal mean wall thickness of 1.9 ± 0.4 cm (versus 0.96 ± 0.09 cm for controls). The majority of patients with hypertrophy had concentric disease, and their primary presenting symptom was congestive heart failure with either acute pulmonary edema (5 patients) or exertional dyspnea (2 patients). The remaining patients presented with atypical chest pain. Control subjects presented with either atypical chest pain or for evaluation of early hypertension. There was no objective evidence of ventricular abnormalities in this group. All patients had normal coronary arteries and valvular function. Studies were performed at the Johns Hopkins Medical Institutions, Baltimore, MD, (USA) or at the Veterans General Hospital, Taipei, Taiwan, and were approved by the respective Institutional Review Boards.

To assess force-frequency and force-interval relations, we employed pressure-volume relation analysis. Such methods were crucial, since varying heart rate markedly altered the filling volume to the heart as well as the effective afterload, and both could profoundly influence conventional indices of cardiac function such as pressures, mean flow, or rate of pressure rise (dP/dt_{mx}) (20). To obtain pressure-volume relations, a conductance-catheter method was used. An intracardiac catheter was placed along the longitudinal axis of the left ventricle to obtain a continuous analog signal proportional to cavity blood volume. Simultaneous display of this signal versus cavity pressure, the latter measured by micromanometer, provided real time pressure-volume loops. Cardiac loading was altered by transient obstruction of inferior vena cava inflow to yield sets of pressure-volume loops at varying preloads from which diastolic pressure-volume relations (yielding chamber compliance) and end-systolic pressure-volume and associated function relations (yielding contractile indexes) were derived. Details of these methods and catheterization procedure have been reviewed elsewhere (18, 21, 22).

Resting hemodynamic characteristics

Patients with LVH demonstrated significant resting diastolic abnormalities, but no differences in systolic parameters. End-diastolic pressure was signifcantly greater (20.2 ± 6.2 mmHg versus 12.3 ± 4.9 for controls), chamber compliance was lower (3.2 ± 0.7 ml/mmHg vs 5.1 ± 2.3), and isovolumic relaxation time constant was greater (52.6 ± 13.9 msec vs 40.8 ± 10.6) (all $p < 0.05$). There were no resting disparities in heart rate, cardiac output, arterial impedance, ejection fraction, systolic pressures or volumes, or systolic contractile function.

Effect of pacing rate on systolic cardiac function

The left-hand panels of Fig. 1 show mean systolic responses to incremental pacing. Data were recorded after at least two minutes of steady-state atrial pacing. Cardiac output (top left) was unchanged in both patient groups, as the decline in stroke volume (middle left) was matched by the rise in heart rate. Ejection fraction, however, decreased slightly more in the LVH patients at faster heart rates than in controls ($p < 0.05$). The statistical analysis used for these and other variables presented here was a 2-way analysis of covariance, based on the raw data.

More direct evidence to support reduced contractile reserve with elevated heart rate in LVH patients was revealed by pressure-volume relation analysis. Figure 2 displays example PV-loops and relations at gradually increasing heart rate from a control subject (panels a-d) and a patient with hypertrophic heart disease (HCM, e-h). The end-systolic pressure-

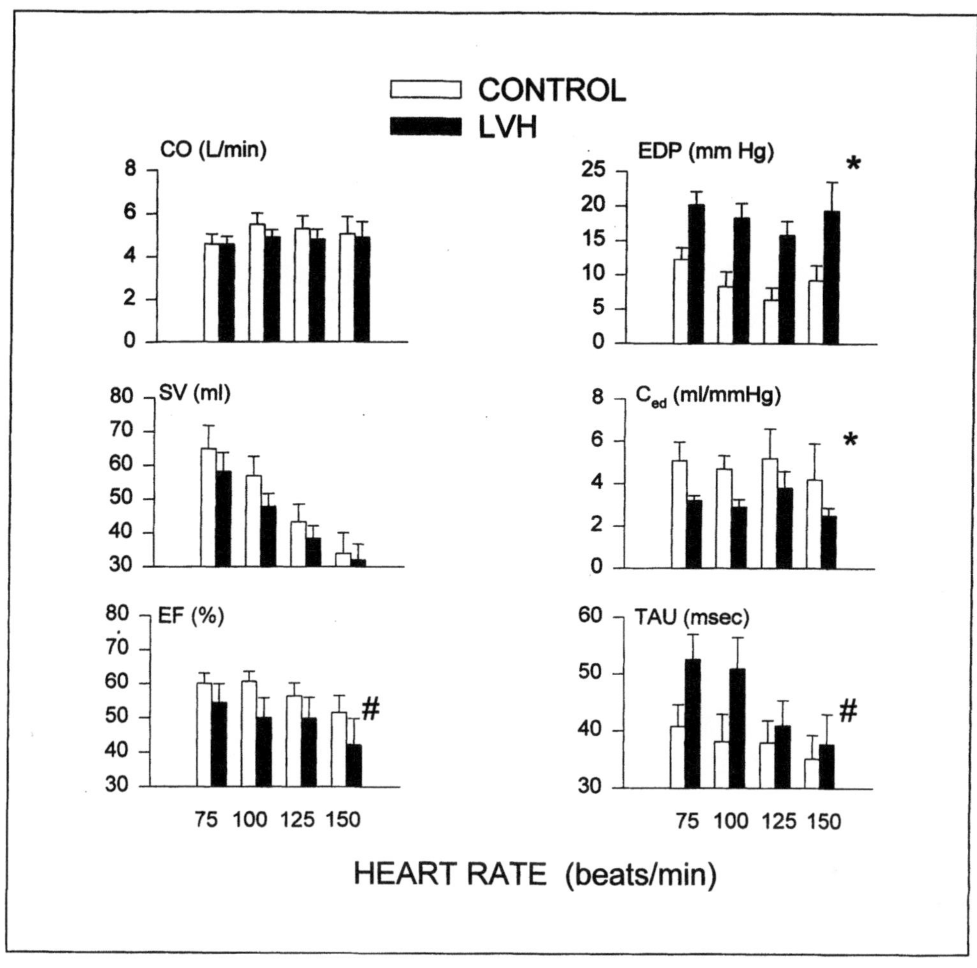

Fig. 1 Summary hemodynamic results of pacing in patients with normal (control) and hypertrophied (LVH) left ventricles. CO – cardiac output, SV – stroke volume, EF – ejection fraction, EDP – end-diastolic pressure, C_{ed} – chamber end-diastolic compliance, Tau – time constant of relaxation. * – $p < 0.05$ control versus LVH, # – $p < 0.05$ for ANOVA testing patient group effect on given variable's response to heart rate.

volume relation (ESPVR) is shown as a solid line linking the upper left corner of each set of pressure-volume loops, and the ESPVR at the lowest heart rate (~ 75 min^{-1}) from panels a and e are reproduced in the subsequent panels for comparison. As heart rate increased, there was gradual steepening of the ESPVR in the control subject, with maintenance or even a slight decline in the resting end-systolic volume. However, in the hypertrophied heart, increasing heart rate resulted in a rightward shift of the ESPVR from baseline, consistent with reduced contractile reserve. In this particular example, the volume axis intercept of the ESPVR (V_o) increased with faster heart rate. However, in the overall patient group, V_o did not change significantly, and this was also true for LVH subjects (Fig. 3A).

These pressure-volume relations were used to generate several function indices, including the slope of the ESPVR, or end-systolic elastance (E_{es}, 3B), the preload-adjusted maximal power index (PMX_{EDV}, 3E) (32), and the slope of the stroke work-end-diastolic

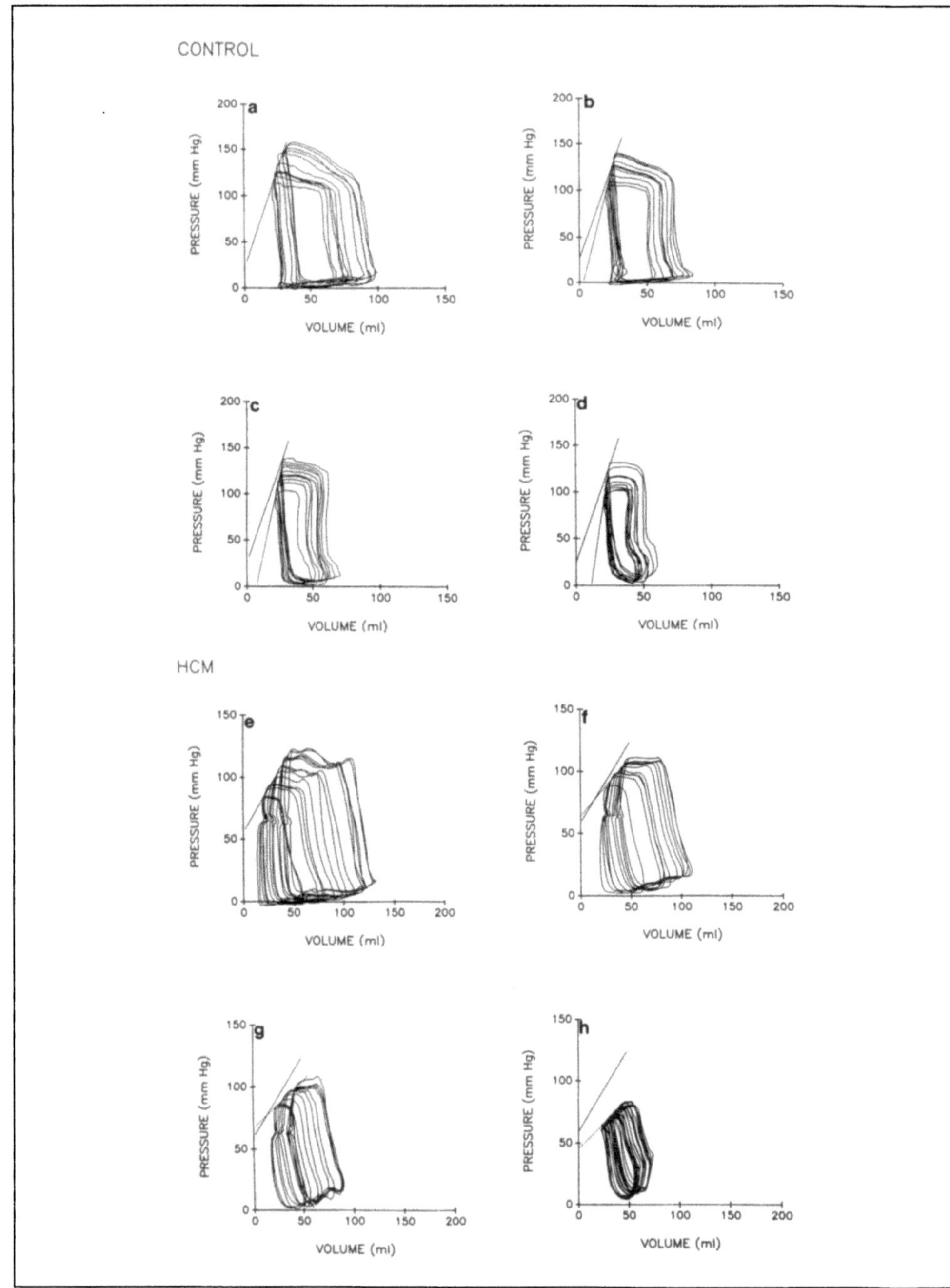

Fig. 2 Example pressure-volume loops and relations in a control and hypertrophied (HCM) patient. Each set of data reflects multiple cardiac cycles obtained during transient obstruction of inferior vena caval inflow. The end-systolic pressure-volume relation is identified by the lines connecting the upper left corners of these beats. Heart rate is increased from 75 (a,e), 100 (b,f), 125 (c,g), and 150 (d,h). Control patients displayed a rise in the slope of the ESPVR, with a slightly decline in end-systolic volume. In contrast, the HCM patients displayed an increase in end-systolic volume with a rightward shift and reduced slope of the ESPVR – consistent with reduced contractile reserve.

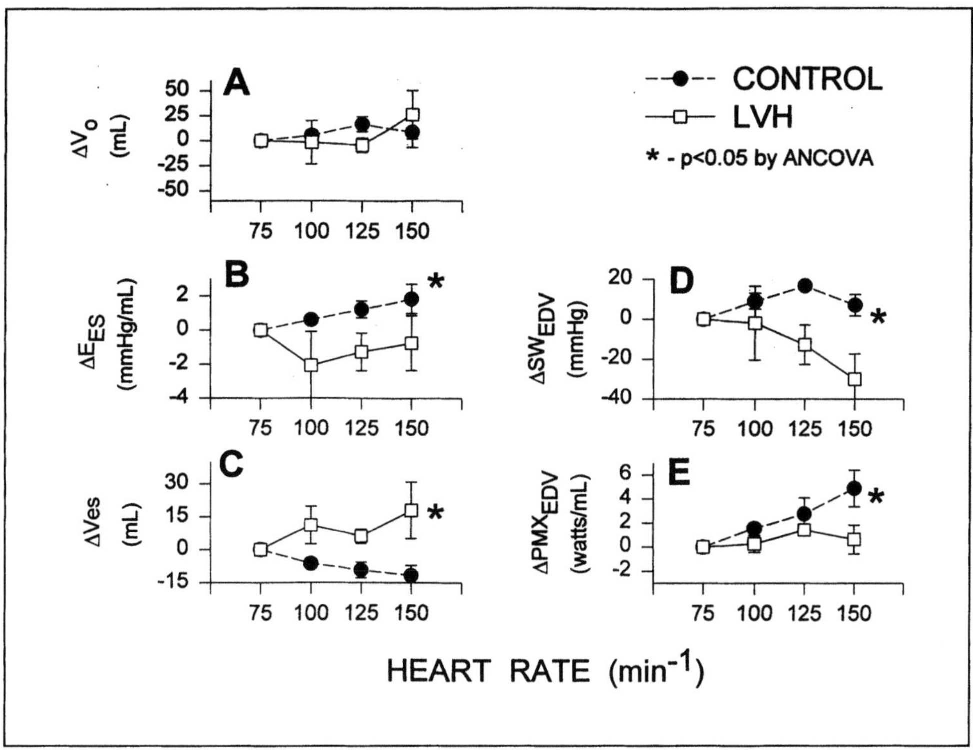

Fig. 3 Group data for contractile response to steady-state pacing rate. Data shown are absolute change from initial baseline for each group. V_o and E_{es} are the volume axis intercept and linear slope of the end-systolic pressure-volume relation, respectively, PMX_{EDV} is the ratio of maximal ventricular power divided by end-diastolic volume, SW_{EDV} is the slope of the relation between stroke work and end-diastolic volume, and Ves is end-systolic volume. There was a consistent reduction in contractile reserve in LVH subjects as compared with controls.

volume relation (SW_{EDV}, 3D) (12). With the exception of E_{es}, which was 2.1 ± 0.33 mm Hg/ml in controls versus 4.9 ± 1.5 mm Hg/ml in LVH patients, (p = 0.09), all the other indices were the same at rest in both groups. Each of these contractility indices was derived from ejection-phase measures, but was itself little influenced by chamber loading.

As shown in Fig. 3, all three contractile indices displayed a reduction in reserve with faster heart rate in LVH patients, whereas the control patients showed a positive dependence of contractile function with faster pacing rate. This is consistent with previous data based on velocity of circumferential fractional shortening in experimental LVH models (10). Figure 3C shows the cavity end-systolic volume, which was significantly reduced in controls, but not in LVH subjects. This further supports a differential effect on contractile reserve.

None of these indices are commonly used to assess contractile change with pacing rates in humans. Rather, the maximal first derivative of pressure (dP/dt_{max}) is the most common measure. Figure 4A displays results for this index, and they were just the opposite to that measured by the preceding less load-sensitive measures. LVH subjects by this analysis appear to have an enhanced contractile reserve with heart rate. However, as shown in Fig. 4B, ventricular diastolic volume declines markedly in both patient groups, but at the highest rates, continues to fall in controls but not in LVH subjects. The preload sensitivity of

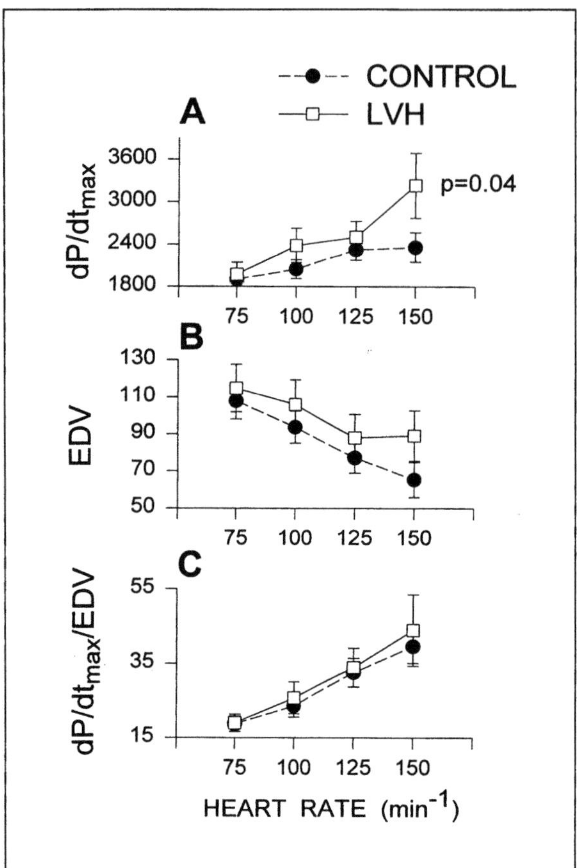

Fig. 4 [A] Effect of increasing heart rate on the maximal derivative of ventricular pressure (dP/dt_{max}). Unlike the ejection-phase indices of contractility (Fig. 3), dP/dt_{max} increased more in LVH subjects than in controls. However, there was a marked decline in end-diastolic volume (EDV) [panel B], which would offset dP/dt_{max} elevation (20, 23), and this was more pronounced at faster rates in controls than LVH subjects. Thus, when dP/dt_{max} is normalized by EDV [C], the two curves are superimposible.

dP/dt_{max} would therefore predict the higher value in LVH subjects that was observed at this rate. If one corrects for the preload change using the ratio of dP/dt_{max}/ EDV (20), the data now appear superimposible (Fig. 4C). This result still differs from that observed with the ejection-phase indices shown in Fig 3. This interesting disparity has indeed been previously reported in animal studies (10), but its underlying mechanism remains unclear. It may relate to increased viscosity of the hypertrophied heart that would make it more susceptible to contractile failure with elevated stimulation rate (37), or to alterations in calcium-myofilament interaction that principally manifest during sarcomere shortening.

Effects of pacing on diastolic cardiac function

The right hand panels of Fig. 1 show group mean diastolic parameter changes with incremental heart rate. As noted previously, left ventricular end-diastolic pressure, chamber compliance, and relaxation time constant were all abnormal at baseline in LVH patients. Unlike systolic function, however, increasing heart rate did not significantly worsen these abnormalities in these patients. LVEDP remained elevated by the same amount regardless of pacing rate, while chamber compliance was unchanged. Only the isovolumic relaxation time constant displayed a different response in the control and LVH group, becoming disproportionately faster in the LVH patients at higher heart rates. Relaxation was estimated using a monoexponential model assuming a non-zero pressure decay asymptote. Since end-systolic volume declined by 28 % in the control subjects, but was unchanged (+ 2 %) in LVH patients (Fig. 3C), this relaxation enhancement was unlikely to be due to increased restoring forces (i.e., diastolic suction) at faster rates. More likely, it reflected a greater adjustment of calcium removal from the cytosol and/or myofilaments with increasing heart rate in LVH patients. This may be a reflection of adaptive changes to reduced basal sarcoplasmic reticular function. Interestingly somewhat similar was reported in patients with heart failure due to dilated cardiomyopathy (8).

Effect of pacing-contractility limitation on ventricular-arterial coupling efficiency

Increasing steady-state heart rate had little direct influence on systemic arterial resistance (Fig. 5A), but significantly increased the effect of resistive load on the heart. Reducing the available time between cardiac cycles meant the heart had to generate higher pressures to achieve the same stroke volume for any given arterial impedance (35). This effective load can be described by the ratio of cardiac end-systolic pressure divided by stroke volume, known as the effective arterial elastance, E_a (36). E_a is approximately equal the product of mean systemic resistance times heart rate (34). Thus, as shown in Fig. 5B, while resistance

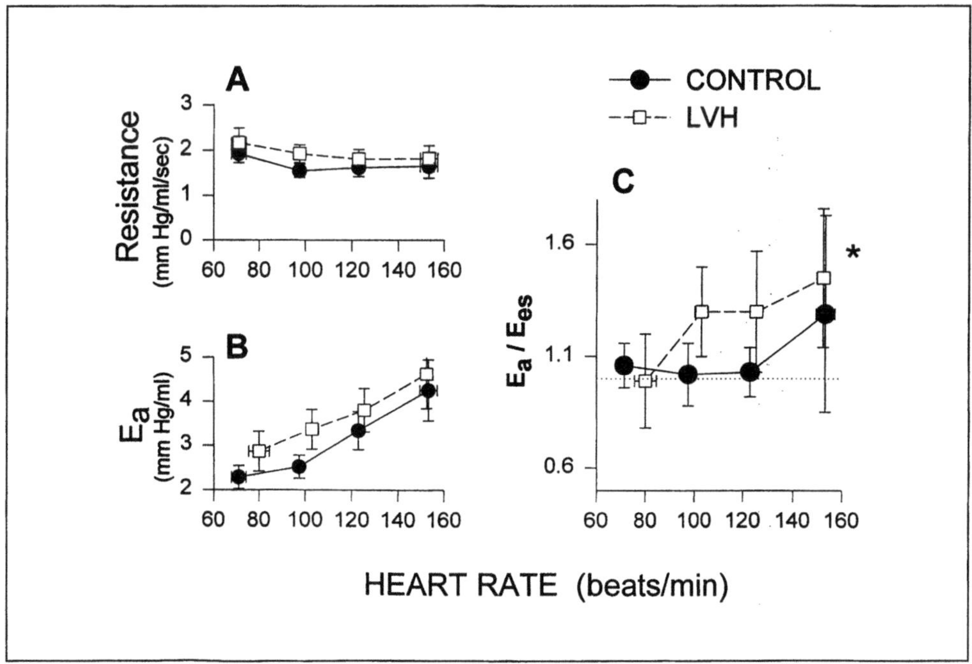

Fig. 5 Influence of reduced force-frequency relation on ventricular-arterial coupling. [A] – total vascular resistance, [B] effective arterial elastance (E_a) and [C] ratio of E_a/E_{es}, each as functions of heart rate. Resistance was unchanged whereas E_a increased with rate. Since cardiac inotropic response was blunted in LVH patients (i.e., reduced E_{es}) increase, the ratio of E_a/E_{es} rose in LVH, while it was better maintained at baseline levels in the control patients.

was little changed in either group with increased pacing rate, E_a rose proportionately with heart rate.

The change in E_a with pacing can be important, since coupling of the heart with the systemic arterial vasculature is related to the ratio of arterial and ventricular end-systolic elastances (E_a/E_{es} ratio) (34). Optimal cardiac efficiency and transfer of kinetic energy (power or stroke work) depends upon this ratio (7), which normally ranges between 0.5 to 1.0 (1, 19, 24, 25). In contrast, values of this ratio of 2.0 or more are associated with cardiac failure states (1, 17), in which systemic load is suboptimally coupled with the heart.

Both control and LVH groups had similar near optimal resting ratios of E_a/E_{es} (1.06 ± 0.1 CON, 0.99 ± 0.21 – LVH). However, as contractile reserve was limited with increased heart rates in LVH patients, (i.e., the E_{es} rise was blunted) whereas E_a rose proportiortally with rate, this ratio rose to 1.3 in LVH patients (at a heart rate of 125 min^{-1}). In contrast, corresponding increases in contractile state and load in control subjects maintained the ratio at baseline levels (1 .03 ± 0.11) at the same heart rate (p < 0.03) (Fig. 5C). At even faster rates, both patient groups displayed a slight further rise in the E_a/E_{es} ratio.

The results for control patients are consistent with prior data reported in normal exercising dogs (25). The disproportionate rise in E_a/E_{es} ratio in LVH patients meant that ventriculo-arterial interaction became suboptimal at faster heart rates, which could lower cardiac metabolic efficiency and limit power transfer from heart to vessels. The ratio change suggested a modest but nontrivial displacement of ventricular-arterial coupling from an optimal operating point and may have added to the etiology for limited cardiac reserve and exertional intolerance in the LVH patients.

Force-interval relations

In addition to the steady-state dependence of systolic and diastolic function on heart rate, the beat-to-beat dependence of contractility or cycle length can provide insight into the cycling kinetics of calcium. While admittedly not a direct measure of subcellular processes, analysis of post-rest potentiation, the decay of this potentiation, and the dependence of potentiation on the preceding cycle length, have all been used to probe abnormalities of excitation-contraction coupling in intact hearts.

To study post-rest potentiation, we examined cardiac contractions after sudden termination of rapid atrial pacing. The first beat after cessation of pacing was typically preceded by a pause of nearly 1 second (see example in Fig. 6A), associated with a marked rise in end-diastolic volume. The latter precluded use of maximal pressure derivative (dP/dt_{max}) to index potentiation, as often done in isolated muscle. However, we could use the end-systolic elastance derived from this beat or the measured stroke work for the potentiated beat at a matched preload so as to index contractile enhancement after the pause. Both indices revealed significantly greater potentiation in LVH hearts, as shown in Panel 6B, with nearly twice the rise in contractile function on this post-pacing beat in LVH versus control hearts. Increased potentiation has been demonstrated in some isolated muscle studies (29) and is consistent with the notion that a component of the steady-state decline in systolic function with LVH is related to delayed SR cycling and altered sarcolemmal calcium entry. By providing a longer intracycle period, there would be more time for calcium loading and release, which becomes manifest by enhanced potentiation.

The process of potentiation decay, or recirculation fraction, was used to index the component of intracellular calcium cycling mediated by SR re-uptake. If potentiation after pacing cessation reflects a given extent of extra cellular calcium available for contraction, then the decay over subsequent cycles can be viewed as a measure of how much of this extra

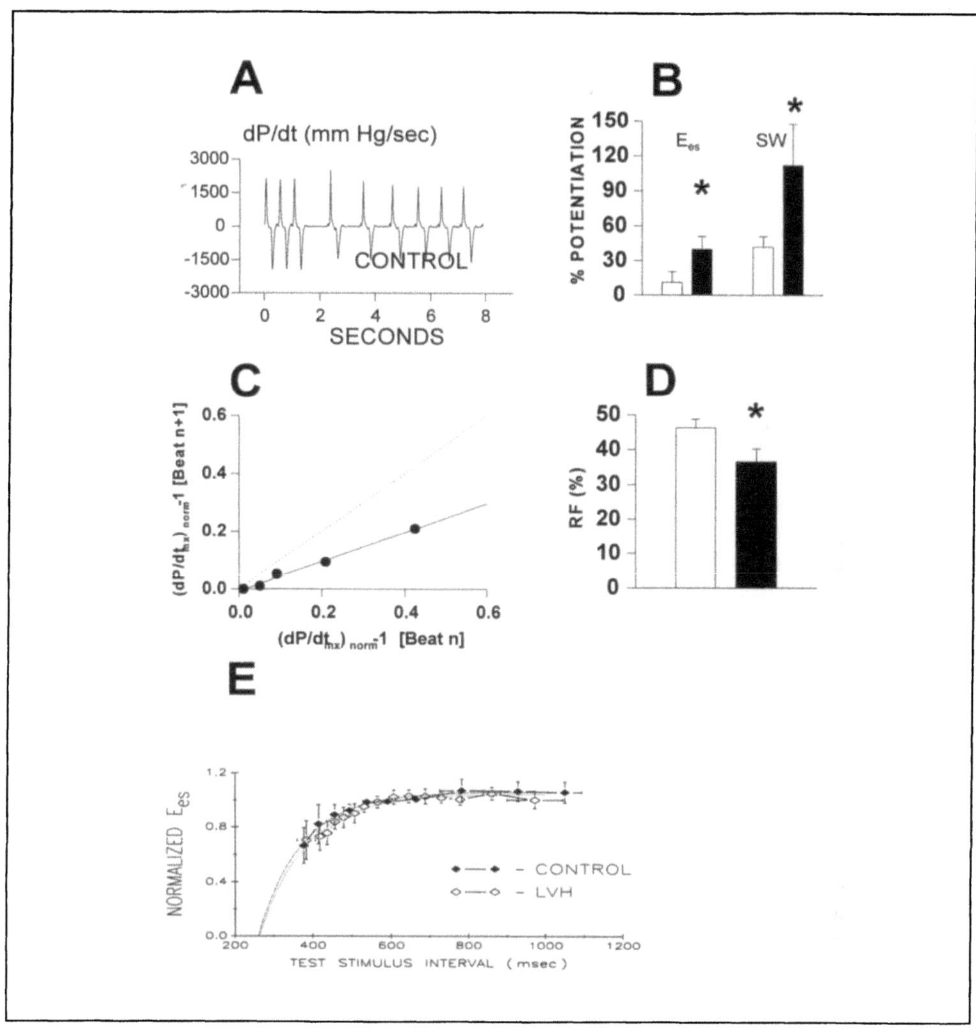

Fig. 6   Force-interval relations in control and LVH subjects. [A] – example of dP/dt data upon abrupt cessation of atrial pacing. After the initial 3 paced beats, the pacer is terminated, and the next series of beats recorded during sinus rhythm. The first potentiated contraction is evaluated for the magnitude of post rest potentiation, and the decay of potentiation is studied to determine the recirculation fraction. [B] – Post rest potentiation in control □ and LVH ■ hearts. There was significantly greater potentiation in the LVH ventricles. [C] Example of recirculation fraction calculation, with the decay of dP/dt_{max} examined to determine the percent reduction from beat to the consecutive beat. The slope provides the geometric decay percent. [D] Summary data for recirculation fraction shows a significant reduction in this value for LVH hearts. [E] Mechanical restitution curves from control and LVH patients. Data are superimposible, with no significant difference in time constant, intercept, or normalized amplitude.

Ca^{2+} is recirculated through the SR for release on the next beat. The greater the recirculation via the SR, the slower the decay of potentiation. Prior studies in heart failure had demonstrated that the fraction of recirculation is reduced in heart failure, consistent with abnormal SR uptake (31).

Figure 6A demonstrates a plot of dP/dt showing three initial beats at a rapid pacing rate followed by cessation of pacing with initial potentiation (beat #4) and subsequent geometric decay of potentiation (beats 5–9). The geometric decay constant can be derived by plotting dP/dt_{max} normalized to steady-state for beat n versus beat n+1 (e.g., Fig. 6C). Depicted in this manner, the data define a linear relation, and the slope of this relation is the recirculation fraction (expressed in percent). As shown in Fig. 6D, LVH patients had a significantly lower RF (36.5 ± 3.7 %) as compared to controls (46.3 ± 2.5 %, p < 0.001). These values are remarkably similar to those previously reported in patients with dilated heart failure (31).

Lastly, the relation between a given pre-test interval and subsequent developed contractile function was used to index the kinetics of Ca^{2+} release from the sarcoplasmic reticulum (3). This relation, known as the mechanical restitution curve, is characterized by a plateau amplitude (maximal potentiation), a monoexponential time constant (kinetics of SR cycling), and a t_o intercept (longest test interval with no mechanical response). We determined MRC relations in a subset of 4 control and 7 LVH patients, again using load-insensitive indices since varying cycle length has profound effects on cardiac filling. The results are displayed in Fig. 6E. Both curves yielded rapid time constants of restitution (104.6 ± 14.2 ms for controls, and 116.2 ± 16.4 ms for LVH) consistent with previously data measured in conscious animals (9), but there was no significant difference in the two relations as a function of cardiac disease. This suggests that the kinetics of SR calcium release, which is thought principally to reside in the ryanidine-sensitive Ca^{++} release channel, are not significantly altered in these patients with LVH.

Summary

Our study demonstrated a loss of normal systolic contractile enhancement with increasing heart rate in patients with ventricular hypertrophy and symptoms of congestive heart failure. This decline in systolic reserve was not accompanied by worsening of diastolic function, and would therefore not seem to reflect underlying ischemia. Rather, it was more likely related to abnormalities of excitation-contraction coupling, particularly in light of findings of both increased post-rest potentiation and a reduced recirculation fraction. In contrast, mechanical restitution was unchanged, suggesting that alterations in Ca^{2+} release from the SR did not play a major role. Finally, we showed that increasing heart rate adversely affects the efficiency of ventriculo-vascular coupling in LVH hearts. This suggested another explanation of how dysfunction of cardiac force-frequency behavior can lead to limited cardiovascular reserve and contribute to clinical symptoms of exertional intolerance. Future efforts aimed at enhancing the force-frequency response, perhaps by enhancing the SR-ATPase, or manipulating its regulation, should prove helpful in ameliorating the limitations of LVH patients associated with rapid heart rate.

References

1. Asanoi H, Sasayama S, Kameyama T (1989) Ventriculoarterial coupling in normal and failing heart in humans. Circ Res 65: 483–493
2. Bache RJ, Vrobel TR (1979) Effects of exercise on blood flow in the hypertrophied heart. Am J Cardiol 44: 1029–1033
3. Banijamali HS, Gao W, MacIntosh BR, ter Keurs HEDJ (1992) Force-interval relations of twitches and cold contractures in rat cardiac trabeculae. Effect of Ryanodine. Circ Res 69: 937–948

4. Cannon RO, III, Rosing DR, Maron BJ, Leon MB, Bonow RO, Watson RM, Epstein SE (1985) Myocardial ischemia in patients with hypertrophic cardiomyopathy: contribution of inadequate vasodilator reserve and elevated left ventricular filling pressures. Circulation 71: 234–243

5. Cannon ROI, Dilsizian V, O'Gara PT, Udelson JE, Tucker E, Panza JA, Fananapazir L, McIntosh CL, Wallace RB, Bonow RO (1992) Impact of surgical relief of outflow obstruction on thallium perfusion abnormalities in hypertrophic cardiomyopathy. Circulation 85: 1039–1045

6. de la Bastie D, Levitsky D, Rappaport L, Mercadier J, Marotte F, Wisnewsky C, Brovkovich V, Schwartz K, Lompre A (1990) Function of the sarcoplasmic reticulum and expression of its Ca^{2+}-ATPase gene in pressure overload-induced cardiac hypertrophy in the rat. Circ Res 66: 554– 564

7. de Tombe PP, Jones S, Burkhoff D, Hunter WC, Kass DA (1993) Ventricular stroke work and efficiency both remain nearly optimal despite altered vascular loading. Am J Physiol 264: H1817–1824

8. Feldman MD, Alderman JD, Aroesty JM, Royal HD, Ferguson JJ, Owen RM, Grossman W, McKay RG (1988) Depression of systolic and diastolic myocardial reserve during atrial pacing tachycardia in patients with dilated cardiomyopathy. J Clin Invest 82: 1661–1669

9. Freeman GL, Colston JT (1990) Evaluation of left ventricular mechanical restitution in closed-chest dogs based on single-beat elastance. Circ Res 67: 1437–1445

10. Fujii AM, Gelpi RJ, Mirsky I, Vatner SF (1988) Systolic and diastolic dysfunction during atrial pacing in conscious dogs with left ventricular hypertrophy. Circ Res 62: 462–470

11. Gaasch WH, Bing OHL, Mirsky I (1982) Chamber compliance and myocardial stiffness in left ventricular hypertrophy. Eur Heart J 3: 139–145

12. Glower DD, Spratt JA, Snow ND, Kabas JS, Davis JW, Olsen CO, Tyson GS, Sabiston DC, Rankin JS (1985) Linearity of the Frank-Starling relationship in the intact heart: the concept of preload recruitable stroke work. Circulation 71: 994–1009

13. Gwathmey JK, Warren SE, Briggs GM, Copelas L, Feldman MD, Phillips PJ, Callahan M Jr, Schoen FJ, Grossman W, Morgan JP (1991) Diastolic dysfunction in hypertrophic cardiomyopathy. J Clin Invest 87: 1023–1031

14. Hess OM, Schneider J, Koch R, Bamert C, Grimm J, Krayenbuehl HP (1981) Diastolic function and myocardial structure in patients with myocardial hypertrophy. Circulation 63: 360–371

15. Hittinger L, Shannon RP, Kohin S, Manders WT, Kelly P, Vatner SF (1990) Exercise-induced subendocardial dysfunction in dogs with left ventricular hypertrophy. Circ Res 66: 329–343

16. Hittinger L, She YT, Patrick TA, Hasebe N, Komamura K, Ihara T, Manders WT, Vatner SF (1992) Mechanisms of subendocardial dysfunction in response to exercise in dogs with severe left ventricular hypertrophy. Circ Res 71: 423–434

17. Ishihara H, Yokota M, Sobue T, Saito H (1994) Relation between ventriculoarterial coupling and myocardial energetios in patients with idiopathic dilated cardiomyopathy. J Am Coll Cardiol 23: 406–416

18. Kass DA (1992) Clinical evaluation of left heart function by conductance catheter technique. Eur Heart J 13 (Suppl E): 57–64

19. Kass DA, Kelly RP (1992) Ventriculo-arterial coupling: Concepts, assumptions, and applications. Ann Biomed Eng 20: 41–62

20. Kass DA, Maughan WL, Guo ZM, Kono A, Sunagawa K, Sagawa K (1987) Comparative influence of load versus inotropic states on indexes of ventricular contractility: Experimental and theoretical analysis based on pressure-volume relationships. Circulation 76: 1422–1436

21. Kass DA, Midei M, Graves W, Brinker JA, Maughan WL (1988) Use of a conductance (volume) catheter and transient inferior vena caval occlusion for rapid determination of pressure-volume relationships in man. Cath Cardiovasc Diag 15: 192–202

22. Kass DA, Yamazaki T, Burkhoff D, Maughan WL, Sagawa K (1986) Determination of left ventricular end-systolic pressure-volume relationships by the conductance (volume) catheter technique. Circulation 73: 586–595

23. Little WC (1985) The left ventricular dP/dt max end-diastolic volume relation in closed-chest dogs. Circ Res 56: 808–815

24. Little WC, Cheng C (1991) Left ventricular-arterial coupling in conscious dogs. Am J Physiol 261: H70–76

25. Little WC, Cheng CP (1993) Effect of exercise on left ventricular-vascular coupling assessed in the pressure-volume plane. Am J Physiol 264: H1629–1633

26. Liu CP, Ting CT, Lawrence W, Maughan WL, Chang MS, Kass DA (1993) Diminished contractile response to increased heart rate in intact human left ventricular hypertrophy: Systolic versus Diastolic Determinants. Circulation 88 (Pt. 1): 1893– 1906

27. Maron BJ, Bonow RO, Cannon RO, III, Leon MB, Epstein SE (1987) Hypertrophic cardiomyopathy: Interrelations of clinical manifestations, pathophysiology, and therapy. N Eng J Med 316: 780–789

28. Nihoyannopoulos P, Karatasakis G, Frenneaux MP, McKenna WJ, Oakley CM (1992) Diastolic function in hypertrophic cardiomyopathy: Relation to exercise capacity. J Am Coll Cardiol 19: 536–540

29. Schouten VJA, Vliegen HW, van der Larse A, Huysmans HA (1992) Altered calcium handling at normal contractility in hypertrophied rat heart. J Mol Cell Cardiol 22: 987–998

30. Schumacher C, Becker H, Sigmund M et al. (1992) Inversed Force-Frequency-Relationship in Hypertrophic Obstructive Cardiomyopathy. [Abstract] Circulation 86: I-839
31. Seed WA, Noble MIM, Walker JM, Miller GAH, Pidgeon J, Redwood D, Wanless R, Franz MR, Schoettler M, Schaefer J (1984) Relationships between beat-to-beat interval and the strength of contraction in the healthy and diseased human heart. Circulation 70: 799–805
32. Sharir T, Kass DA (1992) Load and inotropic sensitivity of maximal left ventricular power in humans. [Abstract] Circulation 86: I-2580
33. Siri FM, Krueger J, Nordin C, Ming Z, Aronson RS (1991) Depressed intracellular calcium transients and contraction in myocytes from hypertrophied and failing guinea pig hearts. Am J Physiol 261: H514–530
34. Sunagawa K, Maughan WL, Burkhoff D, Sagawa K (1983) Left ventricular interaction with arterial load studied in isolated canine ventricle. Am J Physiol 245: H773–780
35. Sunagawa K, Maughan WL, Sagawa K (1985) Stroke volume effect of changing arterial input impedance over selected frequency ranges. Am J Physiol 248: H477–484
36. Sunagawa K, Sagawa K, Maughan WL (1984) Ventricular interaction with the loading system. Ann Biomed Eng 12: 163–189
37. Tagawa H, Wang N, Narishige T, Ingber DE, Zile MR, Cooper G (1997) Cytoskeletal mechanics in pressure-overload cardiac hypertrophy. Circ Res 80: 281–289
38. Zhang J, Merkle H, Hendrich K, Garwood M, From AHL, Ugurbil K, Bache RJ (1993) Bioenergetic abnormalities associated with severe left ventricular hypertrophy. J Clin Invest 92: 993–1003

Author's address:
D. A. Kass M.D.
Halsted 500
Division of Cardiology
Johns Hopkins Medical Institutions
Baltimore, Maryland 21287
USA

Heart rate variability and electrical stability

Th. Fetsch, L. Reinhardt, Th. Wichter, M. Borggrefe, G. Breithardt

Westfälische Wilhelms-Universität, Department of Cardiology and Angiology, and Institute for Research in Arteriosclerosis, Münster

Heart rate variability

Heart rate is a dynamic parameter with wide-ranging changes over time. It is based on a basic periodic depolarization produced by pacemaker cells in the sinus node and a modulation of this basic rate by the autonomous nervous system. The pattern of heart rate reveals information about the sum of all apparent influences on sinus node activity at a given moment in time, but it cannot characterize the general impairment of the autonomous control or even the sympathetic or vagal imbalance in an individual patient. A large number of studies, however, has provided evidence that heart rate variability (HRV) measurements evaluate the autonomous nervous system. The variability of heart rate describes the pattern of beat-to-beat changes over time, commonly over 24 hours obtained from Holter tapes, including estimations of the total bandwidth of heart rate variations as well as averaged values for several time periods. In addition, frequency domain calculations of the heart beat tachogram are performed to identify periodic components and to estimate their frequency and power.

Time and frequency domain measures of HRV are defined in Table 1 according to the recommendations of a Task Force Committee (32). Time domain parameters are computed from the continuous electrogram, conventionally from 24 hour Holter tapes. The QRS complexes are interactively detected and the intervals between normal beats (NN intervals) are calculated. Time domain measures represent statistical calculations of NN intervals or numerical estimations of the geometrical shape of the NN distribution. Frequency parameters are obtained from a spectral analysis of the NN sequence. The instantaneous NN intervals, therefore, have to be resampled at fixed time periods to produce an equally spaced time series. Subsequently, the periodical components of the NN series are analyzed using either the classical Fast Fourier Transform (FFT) or an autoregressive model. The total frequency band derived from spectral analysis of NN intervals is divided into several frequency components of interest: the high frequency (HF) band at 0.15–0.4 Hz, the low frequency (LF) power at 0.04–0.15 Hz, the very low frequency (VLF) band at 0.003–0.04 Hz, and the ultra-low frequencies (ULF) below 0.003 Hz. Spectral analysis of heart rate variability was shown to provide distinct measures of the vagal as well as the sympathetic modulation of the heart. HF power represents the vagal control to the heart, modulated by breathing (1, 26, 27), whereas LF power has contribution from both, vagal and sympathetic modulation of the rhythm (1, 2, 21, 23). The ratio of LF/HF power is used as an index of the sympatho-vagal balance of the autonomous nervous influence on the heart (26).

A number of clinical studies have indicated the usefulness of heart rate variability measures for predicting death, especially for death of arrhythmic causes (4, 5, 16). Together

Table 1   Time and frequency domain measures of HRV (based on (32))

Variable	Statistical measures
time domain:	
SDNN [ms]	Standard deviation of all NN intervals
SDANN [ms]	Standard deviation of the average of NN intervals in all 5 min segments of the entire recording
RMSSD [ms]	Square root of the mean of the sum of the squares of differences between adjacent NN intervals
SDNN index [ms]	Mean of the standard deviations of all NN intervals for all 5 min segments of the entire recording
NN50 count	Number of pairs of adjacent NN intervals differing by > 50 ms in the entire recording
pNN50 [%]	NN50 count devided by the total number of all NN intervals
Triangular index	Total number of all NN intervals devided by the height of the histogram of all NN intervals measured on a discrete scale with bins of 1/128 s
frequency domain:	
Total power [ms^2]	Variance of all NN intervals
ULF [ms^2]	Power in the ultra low frequency range (≤ 0.003 Hz)
VLF [ms^2]	Power in the very low frequency range ($0.003 - 0.04$ Hz)
LF [ms^2]	Power in the low frequency range ($0.04–0.15$ Hz)
HF [ms^2]	Power in the high frequency range ($0.15–0.4$ Hz)

with other non-invasive parameters (analysis of the signal-averaged ECG, count of ventricular premature beats, calculation of baroreflex sensitivity, etc.) HRV has been widely used for risk stratification in patients after remote myocardial infarction (4, 5, 7, 17). Most results have shown HRV measure to be an independent risk factors, not correlated with impaired left ventricular function (25) and with the findings obtained from the analysis of the signal-averaged ECG (7, 15).

Electrical stability

The term 'electrical stability' is most frequently used for the description of a physiologic phenomenon: the ability of the beating heart to react to any kind of disturbance in a predefined way without loss of rhythm self-control – in consequence, the stabilization of the regular periodic rhythm and the prevention of arrhythmias. The frequent occurrence of ventricular premature beats or spontaneous episodes of ventricular runs are interpreted as markers of electrical instability presenting a susceptibility for life threatening ventricular tachyarrhythmias. Hence, for clinical use electrical stability can be defined as the absence of its opposite.

The heart is basically driven by the depolarization sequence of the sinus node spreading the electrical impulse via cell-to-cell conduction of the myocardial muscle cells or using the specific conduction system of the AV node, the bundle of His and the Purkinje fibers in a defined sequence over atria and ventricles. Habitually, disturbances of this regularity occur in the form of premature electrical impulses originating anywhere in both, atria and ventricles. Under physiologic conditions, self-control mechanisms of the heart are able to avoid the deterioration of the basic rhythm into arrhythmias – the electrical stability is preserved.

However, a variety of pathologic alterations of the heart potentially lead to arrhythmias as an expression of electrical instability involving different structural and functional levels of the myocardium. The cellular integrity of the myocytes represents the basic requirement for the stability of the total heart. This includes a sufficient energy metabolism as well as corresponding populations of ion channels in adequate distribution. Physiologic properties at the cellular level provide a normal level of the activation threshold, a regular pattern of the action potential, and consistent characteristics of cell-to-cell conduction. In addition, intact myocytes require an equilibrated environment of electrolytes and oxygen supply to operate properly. The subsequent anatomical and functional level, the myocardial syncytium, might be altered by structural changes, e.g., left ventricular enlargement, leading to slowing of cell-to-cell conduction. The homogeneity of the electrical wave front propagating through normal myocardial tissue as well as the anisotropic conduction properties are disordered in case of regionally scared or altered myocardium. Dissimilar conduction properties in neighbored regions will lead to inhomogenous electrical propagation with the consequence of electrical instability.

The heart is controlled by the autonomous nervous system, indirectly via adrenergic stimulating hormones delivered from the adrenal cortex, directly with efferent nerves innervating the myocardium. However, the autonomous nervous pathways are unequally distributed: sympathetic nerves mostly spread in the superficial subepicardium while vagal fibers are located in the subendocardium penetrating intramurally. In case of a non-transmural infarction, a regional imbalance of autonomous regulation might result if the degree of damage is grossly different in endocardial compared to epicardial regions. Consequently, electrical instability might follow.

It is obvious that electrical stability is a complex phenomenon presenting a dynamic behavior and depending on numerous factors. It became apparent that not one single test is able to characterize the total complexity of electrical stability. However, in clinical routine electrical stimulation of the heart via electrode catheters positioned in the right atrium and ventricle (electrophysiologic study [EPS]) represents a suitable method to verify susceptibility to electrical instability. Recently, some studies assessed the relation of heart rate variability and the inducibility as well as spontaneous occurrence of ventricular tachycardia – i.e., the association of HRV and electrical instability. Table 2 presents an overview of those five studies that will be discussed in detail.

HRV and electrical instability – clinical studies

Clinically, electrical instability can be characterized either on the basis of spontaneous arrhythmias or by the inducibility of sustained arrhythmias during electrophysiologic studies (Table 2). Huikuri et al. (10) analyzed 40 episodes of spontaneous ventricular tachycardia. In 18 consecutive patients, predominantly after remote myocardial infarction,

Table 2 Publications presenting findings about HRV and inducibility of ventricular tachycardia or HRV changes prior to spontaneous VT

Publication	Patients	Concepts and Methods	Results
Huikuri et al., Circulation 1993 (10)	18 pts., 16 post-MI, 11 pts. spontaneous sVT 7 pts. cardiac arrest	• Changes of HRV prior to VT – HRV (frequency domain) – arrhythmia scan – LHC – EPS	**Prior to spontaneous VT:** (12 sVTs, 28 ns VTS). ↑ LF/HF 16–60' prior to VT (↑) LF, ⟷ HF 15' prior to VT ↑ HR, 15' prior to sVT **sVT compared to nsVT:** ↓ of all frequency domain parameters 60' prior to sVT, (↑) prior to nsVT
Fei et al., JACC 1994 (8)	23 pts. with documented spontaneous idiopathic VT 15 pts. inducible for sVT	• Changes of HRV prior to VT • HRV and inducibility of VT – HRV (frequency domain) – arrhythmia scan – SAECG – LHC – EPS	**Prior to spontaneous VT:** (27 sVTs, 44 nsVTs). ↑ LF/HF 6–8' prior to VT ↓ HF, ⟷ LF 6–8' prior to VT ↑ HR, 6' prior to VT **no differences in HRV:** < 8' prior to VT prior to sVT vs. nsVT with vs. without inducible VT
Kjellegren et al., PACE 1994 (15)	59 pts. referred for EPS – 32 with CAD – 13 with other structural heart disease – 14 without structural heart disease 28 pts. inducible for sVT	• HRV and inducibility of VT – HRV (time + frequency domain) – arrhythmia scan – SAECG – LHC – EPS	**Pts. with inducible sVT:** ↓ PNN50 ↓ HF HRV independent of LVEF, SAECG, and VPBs
Valkama et al., JACC 1995 (33)	54 pts., all with CAD, 44 post-MI – 25 documented sVT – 29 cardiac arrest 30 pts. inducible for sVT	• Change of HRV prior to VT • HRV and inducibility of VT – HRV (SD; frequency domain) – arrhythmia scan – LHC – EPS	**Frequent vs. infrequent VPBs:** ↑ HR ↓ SDRR, SDTP, SDVLF, SDLF **With vs. without inducible sVT:** no significant differences of HRV parameters **Prior to spontaneous sVT:** (1h, 15', 5'; 21 episodes in 8 pts). no significant trends of HRV ↑ HR 5' prior to VT
Huikuri et al., Am J Cardiol 1995 (9)	60 pts., all post-MI – 30 sVT inducible – 30 matched controls	• HRV and inducibility of VT – HRV (SD, frequency domain) – LHC – EPS	**Pts. with inducible sVT:** ↓ SDNN, ULF, VLF, LF, LF/HF ⟷ HF ↓ circadian rhythm of LVF

MI = myocardial infarction, sVT = sustained monomorphic ventricular tachycardia, nsVT = nonsustained monomorphic ventricular tachycardia, CAD = coronary artery disease, LHC = left heart catheterization, EPS = electrophysiologic study, HR = heart rate, VPB = ventricular premature beat, SAECG = signal averaged ECG; HF = high frequency band, LF = low frequency band, VLF = very low frequency band, ULF = ultra low frequency band

28 episodes of nonsustained and 12 of sustained VTs were recorded in hospital on 24 h Holter tapes. The patients had been admitted for electrophysiological testing because of cardiac arrest (7 patients) or previously documented sustained VT (11 patients). HRV parameters in the frequency domain were analyzed in 15 min segments starting one hour before the onset of the arrhythmia. The authors found a significant increase in the total power of HRV one hour prior to the onset of nonsustained ventricular tachycardia, while the same parameter remained unchanged before sustained VTs or even showed a tendency toward decreasing values in patients presenting both types of arrhythmias in the same recording. Average heart rate tended to increase in the 15 min segment preceding sustained VTs only. In contrast, most obvious alterations of frequency domain measures were apparent prior to the onset of nonsustained ventricular tachycardia, presenting an increase in LF power without changes in HF power, hence, leading to a significant increase of the LF/HF ratio. LF power did not significantly increase during the hour preceding the appearance of sustained ventricular tachycardia, and HF power remained unchanged or tended to decrease. All parameters of frequency domain measures were significantly lower one hour prior to sustained compared to nonsustained VTs. In conclusion, HRV measurements tended to increase one hour before episodes of nonsustained VT compared to the average values of the total 24 h period while lower values appeared preceding sustained VTs. However, LF and HF power did not change significantly during the hour before the onset of sustained ventricular tachycardia and the LF/HF ratio just reached the level of significance in the 15 min prior to VT, only.

Fei et al. (8) also assessed HRV changes prior to the onset of spontaneous ventricular tachycardia. In 23 patients without structural heart disease, they analyzed frequency domain parameters of HRV in 2 min segments obtained from Holter tapes with 71 episodes of sustained and nonsustained idiopathic VT. No significant differences could be observed between HRV parameters during one hour preceding the arrhythmias and the corresponding 24 h period. In contrast, 6–8 min before the onset of all ventricular tachycardia the LF/HF ratio was significantly higher. This alteration was due to a notable decrease of the HF component whereas the LF segment remained unchanged. Mean heart rate also increased significantly during the last 6 min preceding ventricular tachycardia. In contrast to the results of Huikuri et al. (10), the parameters of HRV showed no differences comparing the time period prior to sustained versus nonsustained VTs. The authors also investigated the relationship between inducibility of sustained ventricular tachycardia at electrophysiologic studies and corresponding HRV findings. However, no significant differences of HRV parameters could be found comparing 15 inducible with the 8 noninducible patients.

The relation between inducibility of ventricular tachycardia and measures of HRV as well as presence of ventricular late potentials was investigated by Kjellgren et al. (15). They analyzed a heterogeneous group of 59 patients admitted for electrophysiologic studies. Most of them had documented sustained or nonsustained VTs but there were also some patients included presenting a history of supraventricular tachycardia or unexplained syncope. Coronary heart disease was present in 32 patients whereas 13 subjects had other forms of structural heart disease, and 14 patients were without evidence of structural heart disease. Numerous parameters of HRV in time and frequency domain were calculated from 24 h Holter recordings. All patients underwent invasive electrophysiologic studies. Left ventricular ejection fraction was obtained in 47 patients. Sustained monomorphic ventricular tachycardia were inducible during invasive electrophysiologic study in 28 patients. Most of the clinical parameters including age, gender, LVEF, and diagnostic category did not differ with respect to the outcome of the electrophysiologic study. Results of the conventional arrhythmia scan (ventricular premature counts, etc.) obtained from Holter tapes did not predict inducibility either. However, the presence of ventricular late potentials strongly correlated with inducible VTs. Of the HRV time domain parameters, only PNN50 was significantly decreased in patients with compared to those without inducible ventricular tachycardia. The HF power of the 24 h period was additionally found to be significantly lower in those subjects, whereas the one hour measures of maximal and minimal HF power as well as LF and total power showed no significant differences with respect to the outcome of the electrophysiologic study. HRV parameters were found to be independent of age, impaired left ventricular function, findings of the Holter arrhythmia scan, and the presence of ventricular late potentials.

Valkama et al. (33) retrospectively studied 54 patients with coronary artery disease who were admitted to the hospital because of documented sustained ventricular arrhythmias (25 patients) or cardiac arrest (29 patients) not related to acute myocardial infarction. Fourty-four patients had a history of previous MI. In addition to the assessment of frequency domain parameters of HRV, the frequency of ventricular premature beats was obtained from the 24 h Holter recordings of all patients. Sustained ventricular tachycardia occurred in 8 patients during Holter recordings. Electrophysiologic and angiographic studies were performed in the majority of the patients. The authors did not find any significant trends or alterations in HRV during 1 h, 15 min, and 5 min before the onset of 21 spontaneous sustained ventricular tachycardia in 8 patients. In concordance to previous findings (8, 10) the average heart rate was significantly higher in a 5 min period prior to the tachycardia. LF and VLF components of HRV in the entire 24 h period were significantly lower in patients with spontaneous VTs compared to the rest of the study population. In addition, patients presenting frequent ventricular premature beats (> 30/h) in the 24 h Holter recording revealed significantly lower total, LF and VLF power. Remarkably, there were no differences of HRV measures comparing the group of 30 patients with and those without inducible monomorphic ventricular tachycardia.

From the same group, Huikuri et al. (9) reported a case-control study on inducibility of ventricular tachycardia and its relation to HRV findings. Sixty patients with a history of Q-wave infarction were included, 30 subjects with inducible monomorphic VT at the electrophysiologic study and previous cardiac arrest or documented spontaneous VT and 30 matched controls without inducibility of VT and no history of arrhythmias. The control group was matched with respect to age, sex, number of previous infarctions, left ventricular ejection fraction, number of diseased coronary arteries, and β-blocker therapy. Measures of frequency domain HRV were obtained from 24 h Holter tapes recorded a few days before the electrophysiologic study. Results showed significantly reduced LF, VFL, and ULF power in patients rendered inducible compared to the non-inducible matched controls. The HF power did not differ; consequently, the LF/HF ratio was also significantly lower in the VT group. In addition, the circadian rhythm of the VLF power was reduced in those patients throughout the 24 h period.

Table 3 Summary of HRV findings prior to spontaneous VT (8, 10, 33)

subjects	concordant findings	discordant findings
26 pts. with CAD 23 pts. without structural heart disease 60 episodes of sVT 72 episodes of nsVT	↑ HR prior to VT	– ↑ LF/HF ratio 15–60' prior to VT (10) – ↑ LF/HF ratio 6–8' prior to VT, but no significant trend of HRV > 8' prior to VT (8) – no significant trend of HRV 60', 15' or 5' prior to VT (33) – ⟷ HF + (↑) LF prior to VT (10) – ↓ HF + ⟷ LF prior to VT (8)

Table 4   Summary of HRV relations to inducible VTs (8, 9, 15, 33)

subject	concordant findings	discordant findings

146 pts. with CAD
13 pts. with other structural
   heart disease (15)
37 pts. without structural
   heart disease (8, 15)
 	
103 pts. inducible for VT
	none	– ↓ PNN50 + HF (15)
		– ↓ SDNN, ULF, VLF, LF, LF/HF (9)
		– no significant differences of HRV comparing
		   pts with and without inducible VT (8, 33)

In conclusion, 4 of the 5 studies included patients with severe coronary artery disease, most of them after remote myocardial infarction. Together, 164 patients with CAD have been studied including 120 patients post-MI. In addition, 37 patients without structural heart disease and 13 subjects with types of heart diseases other than CAD have been included. The results can be divided in two major categories: changes in HRV prior to spontaneous episodes of ventricular tachycardia (Table 3) and differences in HRV findings in patients with and without inducible (Table 4).

Before spontaneous VT, only Valkama et al. (33) found no alterations of HRV in the 60, 15, and 5 min before the onset. Both other studies consistently demonstrated a significant increase in the average heart rate. Additionally, both found an obvious increase in the LF/HF ratio prior to VT episodes. However, while Huikuri et al. (10) observed this increase 60 to 15 min preceding VT, Fei et al. (8) noted similar effects in the 6–8 min intervals prior to VT onset only. The extension of the time period to more than 8 min preceding the ventricular tachycardia showed no changes in HRV parameters. The concordant increase in LF/HF ratio was based on different mechanisms: Huikuri et al. demonstrated a moderate increase in LF power and no changes in the HF component, whereas Fei et al. found a significant decrease in HF power without any changes in the LF frequency band.

Analysis of HRV parameters in subjects with inducible and non-inducible VTs also provided controversial results. Fei et al. (8) and Valkama et al. (33) did not find any significant difference in heart rate variability between both subgroups. In contrast, Kjellgren et al. (15) observed a decreased power in all frequency domain parameters of HRV, most significantly in the HF segment, in patients rendered inducible compared to non-inducible subjects. Consistent with these findings, Huikuri et al. (9) could demonstrate a significantly decreased power in the ULF, VLF, and LF bands leading to a reduced LF/HF ratio in the subgroup of inducible patients. The HF power, in contrast, did not differ in their findings between both subgroups.

HRV and electrical instability – considerations

There is no hesitation about the concept that heart rate variability reflects the modulation of an existing potentially arrhythmogenic substrate. However, it is still controversial whether it is more a reflection of the sympatho-vagal balance of autonomous nervous control or predominantly of the parasympathetic efference to the heart. There is some evidence for the latter observation because the sinus and atrioventricular nodes and the atria are richly innervated by parasympathetic fibers, whereas the vagal innervation of the ventricles is relatively sparse (31). It is important to note that heart rate variability is not a direct measure of the autonomous influence of the autonomous nervous system to all structures of the heart. It purely reflects the nervous control of the sinus and, to some extent, of the atrioventricular node. The sympatho-vagal input to the tissue directly involved in the establishment and perpetuation of a ventricular tachycardia – the ventricular myocardium – can only indirectly be estimated from the effects on sinus node regulation. Differences in autonomous nervous contribution to the sinus node and the ventricular muscle, especially in case of regional abnormalities following myocardial infarction or chronic ischemia, makes it questionable whether measures of heart rate variability are able to characterize specific pathophysiologic mechanisms leading to ventricular arrhythmias.

From several experimental and clinical studies, it is known that vagal hyperactivity prevents ventricular arrhythmias especially in the presence of ischemic heart disease (14, 24). Experimental studies have demonstrated that the heart rate response to coronary artery occlusion is markedly different in dogs susceptible to ventricular arrhythmias compared to resistant dogs (12, 29, 35, 36). In susceptible dogs, the physiologically elevated heart rate was further increased whereas the resistant dogs tended to decrease heart rate during exercise. Significantly reduced vagal tone was found to be responsible for these findings (11). These differences in autonomous nervous input to the heart were apparently not present before the myocardial infarction.

Kjellgren et al. (15) assumed their findings of a clear association between low HF power and the ability to induce sustained ventricular tachycardia to reflect reduced vagal tone in patients prone to life threatening ventricular tachycardia. In addition, this conclusion was confirmed by the observation that the peak vagal activity during 24 h recording also differed between patients rendered inducible versus non-inducible subjects, but not the minimal vagal tone during the same period. They, therefore, speculated that the ability to modulate vagal tone is protective against the emergence of sustained ventricular tachycardia, i.e., it preserves electrical stability. In contrast, Huikuri et al. (9) considered impaired LF power to be specifically related to arrhythmia susceptibility, consistent with another retrospective study (5) demonstrating reduced LF power as a predictor of future arrhythmic mortality. Subsequently, the same authors (9) mentioned that due to some overlap in the LF power between both, inducible and non-inducible patients, reduced HRV seemed not to be a sole requirement for the development of ventricular tachycardia and none of the frequency domain parameters of HRV appeared to be a very sensitive marker of arrhythmic suscepti-bility. In two other studies (8, 33) no correlation between HRV measures and inducibility of VT could be demonstrated which, thus, do not substantiate any association between sympatho-vagal impairment and electrical instability. Thus, whether parasympathetic activation has a direct electrophysiological effect on the ventricular level in parallel to changes in adrenergic activity remains unclear. Most studies have indicated that the effects of vagal activity are the direct consequence of opposition to the effects of sympathetic activity. These effects, however, depend on the presence of an arrhythmogenic substrate, in ischemic heart disease as well as in other underlying structural heart diseases. There is con-sensus that even in idiopathic ventricular tachycardia, an arrhythmogenic substrate exists on the cellular level with a high grade of sensitivity to the autonomous nervous control sys-tem. There is no evidence that the autonomous nervous system constitutes an arrhythmo-genic substrate on its own.

Does the assessment of heart rate variability reflect a measure of an acute trigger mechanism as evidenced from of impaired HRV parameters prior to the onset of ventricu-lar tachycardia? Huikuri et al. (10) observed temporal relations between impaired HRV and the onset of ventricular tachycardia. The LF/HF ratio increased 60 to 15 min before the occurrence of ventricular tachycardia. They considered these fluctuations of HRV to reflect changes in factors that may lead to electrical instability and facilitate the initiation or perpetuation of arrhythmias. They concluded that under such circumstances, impaired HRV may actively participate in the pathophysiological process. However, since all four components of HRV frequency domain measurements were reduced, the pathophysiological mechanisms how the autonomous nervous system might contribut to the development of ventricular tachycardia remains unclear. Fei et al. (8) consistently observed significant changes in HRV parameters prior to the onset of VT, however, in a short time segment only. In this study reduced HF power was the major responsible parameter. The HF component is known to represent almost exclusively vagal activity, while the LF segment is mediated by sympathetic activity with some influence from vagal control. The LF/HF ratio consequently characterizes the sympatho-vagel balance of cardiac innervation. The authors assumed that there is an abnormality of autonomous nervous activity preceding the onset of ventricular tachycardia that mainly results from reduced vagal activity, because only the high frequency power was significantly decreased. In contrast, Valkama et al. (33) found no significant trends or alterations preceding episodes of ventricular tachycardia. They were not able to confirm previous observations of the same research group (10). They concluded that it remains uncertain whether a temporal relation exists between impaired HRV and the spontaneous onset of ventricular tachycardia.

However, a consistent increase in heart rate before spontaneous episodes of ventricular tachycardia was noted in most of the observation (6, 8, 10, 33). There is evidence from experimental as well as clinical studies than an elevated heart rate may greatly favor the occurrence of a re-entrant tachycardia (3, 30). Increased heart rate is followed by several consequences supporting the establishment and perpetuation of ventricular tachycardia, including shortening and increased inhomogeneity of refractory periods and decrease of conduction velocity accompanied by the development of unidirectional block (13).

It is incontestable that heart rate modulation does play a role in the development of ventricular arrhythmias, but nevertheless other mechanisms are also important. The susceptibility to electrical instability detected by means of impaired heart rate variability rather reflects the modulation of the underlying disease than a direct participation in the basic pathophysiological process. However, experimental studies using a well-defined model of sympatho-vagal interactions on different substrates and their contributions to alterations in heart rate variability are still missing. There is evidence that measures of impaired heart rate variability shortly prior to the onset of ventricular tachycardia are able to predict episodes of arrhythmias, but only adequate prospective studies will be able to verify the clinical usefulness of these findings.

Electrical stability remains a complex phenomenon involving multiple mechanisms at different structural and functional levels. Heart rate variability, however, describes the potential contribution of the autonomic nervous system to electrical stability in the context of an underlying arrhythmogenic substrate only. It should always be remembered that heart rate variability is a marker and not a mechanism.

References

1. Akselrod S, Gordon D, Ubel FA, Shannon DC, Berger AC, Cohen RJ (1981) Power spectrum of heart rate fluctuation: A quantitative probe of beat-to-beat cardiovascular control. Science 213: 220–222
2. Appel ML, Berger RD, Saul JP, Smith JM, Cohen RJ (1989) Beta to beat variability in cardiovascular variables: Noise or music? J Am Coll Cardiol 14: 1139–1148
3. Bayés de Luna A, Coumel P, Leclerq JF (1989) Ambulatory sudden cardiac death: Mechanisms of productin of fatal arrhythmia on the basis of data from 157 cases. Am Heart J 117: 151–159

4. Bigger JT, Fleiss JL, Rolnitzki LM, Steinman RC (1993) Frequency domain measures of heart period variability to assess risk late after myocardial infarction. J Am Coll Cardiol 14: 215–230

5. Bigger JT, Fleiss JL, Steinman RC, Rolnitzky LM, Kleiger RE, Rottman JN (1992) Frequency domain measures of heart period variability and mortality after myocardial infarction. Circulation 85: 164–171

6. Coumel P (1989) Rate dependence and adrenergic dependence of arrhythmias. Am J Cardiol 59: 41J–45J

7. Farrell TG, Bashir Y, Cripps T, Malik M, Poloniecki J, Bennett ED, Ward DE, Camm AJ (1991) Risk stratification for arrhythmic events in postinfarction patients based on heart rate variability, ambulatory electrocardiographic variables and the signal-averaged electrocardiogram. J Am Coll Cardiol 18: 687–697

8. Fei L, Statters DJ, Hnatkova K, Poloniecki J, Malik M, Camm AJ (1994) Change of autonomous influence on the heart immediately before the onset of spontaneous idiopathic ventricular tachycardia. J Am Coll Cardiol 24: 1515–1522

9. Huikuri HV, Koistinen J, Ylie-Mäyry S, Airaksinen KEJ, Seppänen T, Ikäheimo M, Myerburg RJ (1995) Impaired low-frequency oscillations of heart rate in patients with prior acute myocardial infarction and life-threatening arrhythmias. Am J Cardiol 76: 56–60

10. Huikuri HV, Valkama OV, Airaksinen J, Seppänen T, Kessler KM, Takkunen JT, Myerburg RJ (1993) Frequency domain measures of heart rate variability before the onset of nonsustained and sustained ventricular tachycardia in patients with coronary artery disease. Circulation 87: 1220–1228

11. Hull SS, Evans AR, Vanoli E, Adamson PB, Stramba Badiale M, Albert DE, Foreman RD, Schwartz PJ (1990) Heart rate variability before and after myocardial infarction in conscious dogs at high and low risk of sudden death. J Am Coll Cardiol 16: 978–985

12. Inoue H, Zipes DP (1987) Results of sympathetic denervation in the canine heart: Supersensitivity that may be arrhythmogenic. Circulation 75: 877–887

13. Janse MJ (1987) Frequency dependency of experimental arrhythmias. J Electrophysiol 1: 12–16

14. Kent KM, Smith ER, Redwood DR et al. (1973) Electrical stability of acutely ischemic myocardium: Influences of heart rate and vagal stimulation. Circulation 47: 291–302

15. Kjellgren O, IP J, Suh K, Gomes JA (1994) The role of parasympathetic modulation of the reentrant arrhythmic substrate in the genesis of sustained ventricular tachycardia. PACE 17: 1276–1287

16. Kleiger RE, Miller JP, Bigger JT et al. (1987) Decreased heart rate variability and its association with increased mortality after acute myocardial infarction. Am J Cardiol 59: 256–262

17. La Rovere MT, Bigger JT Jr, Marcus FI, Mortara A, Schwartz PJ (1998) Baroreflex sensitivity and heart-rate variability in prediction of total cardiac mortality after myocardial infarction. ATRAMI (Autonomic Tone and Reflexes After Myocardial Infarction) Investigators. Lancet 351 (9101): 478–484

18. Lombardi F, Sandrone G, Pernpruner S, Sala R, Garimoldi M, Cerutti S, Baselli G, Pagani M, Malliani A (1987) Heart rate variability as an index of sympathovagal interaction after acute myocardial infarction. Am J Cardiol 60: 1239–1245

19. Malik M, Camm AJ (1990) Significance of long term components of heart rate variability for the further prognosis after acute myocardial infarction. Cardiovasc Res 24: 793–803

20. Malliani A, Lombardi F, Pagani M (1994) Power spectrum analysis of heart rate variability: A tool to explore neural regulatory mechanisms. Br Heart J 71: 1–2

21. Malliani A, Pagani M, Lombardi F, Cerutti S (1991) Cardiovascular neural regulation explored in the frequency domain. Circulation 84: 1482–1492

22. Martin GJ, Magid NM, Myers G, Barnett PS, Schaad JW, Weiss JS, Lesch M, Singer DH (1987) Heart rate variability and sudden death secondary to coronary artery disease during ambulatory electrocardiographic monitoring. Am J Cardiol 60: 86–89

23. Mantano N, Gnecchi Ruscone T, Porta A, Lombardi F, Pagani M, Malliani A (1994) Power spectrum analysis of heart rate variability to assess the changes in sympathovagal balance durcin graded ortzhostatic tilt. Circulation 90: 1826–1831

24. Myers RW, Pearlman AS, Hyman RM et al. (1974) Beneficial effects of vagal stimulation and bradycardia during experimental acute myocardial ischemia. Circulation 49: 943–952

25. Odemuyiwa O, Malik M, Farrell T, Bashir Y, Poloniecki J, Camm J (1991) Comparison of the predictive characteristics of heart rate variability index and left ventricular ejection fraction for all-cause mortality, arrhythmic events and sudden death after acute myocardial infarction. Am J Cardiol 68: 434–439

26. Pagani M, Lombardi F, Guzzetti S et al. (1986) Power spectral analysis of heart rate and arterial pressure variabilities as a marker of sympathovagal interactions in man and conscious dog. Circ Res 59: 178–193

27. Pomeranz B, Macaulay RJB, Caudill MA et al. (1985) Assessment of autonomous function in humans by heart rate spectral analysis. Am J Physiol 248: H151–H153

28. Rich MW, Saini JS, Kleiger RE, Carney RM, TeVelde A, Freedland KE (1988) Correlation of heart rate variability with clinical and angiographic variables and late mortality after coronary angiography. Am J Cardiol 62: 714–717

29. Schwartz PJ, Billman GE, Stone HL (1984) Autonomous mechanisms in ventricular fibrillation induced by myocardial ischemia during exercise in dogs with a heald myocardial infarction. Circulation 69: 780–792

30. Smeets JL, Allessie MA, Lammers WJ et al. (1986) The wavelength of the cardiac impulse and reentrant arrhythmias in isolated rabbit atrium: The role of heart rate, autonomous transmitters, temperature and potassium. Circ Res 58: 96–109
31. Takahashi N, Barber MJ, Zipes DP (1985) Efferent vagal innervation of the canine left ventricle. Am J Physiol 248: H89–H97
32. Task Force of the European Society of Cardiology and The North American Society of Pacing and Electrophysiology (1996) Heart rate variability. Standards of measurement, physiological interpretation, and clinical use. Eur Heart J 17: 354–381
33. Valkama JO, Huikuri HV, Koistinen MJ, Yli-Mäyry S, Airaksinen KEJ, Myerburg RJ (1995) Relation between heart rate variability and spontaneous and induced ventricular arrhythmias in patients with coronary artery disease. J Am Coll Cardiol 25: 437–443
34. Vybiral T, Glaeser DH, Goldberger AL, Rigney DR, Hess KR, Mietus J, Skinner JE, Francis M, Pratt CM (1993) Conventional heart rate variability analysis of ambulatory electrocardiographic recordings fails to predict imminent ventricular fibrillation. J Am Coll Cardiol 22: 557–565
35. Warner MR, Wisler PL, Hodges TD, Watanabe AM, Zipes DP (1993) Mechanisms of denervation supersensitivity in regionally denervated canine hearts. Am J Physiol 264: H815–H820
36. Zipes DP (1990) Influence of myocardial ischemia and infarction on autonomic innervation of heart. Circulation 82: 1095–1105

Author's address:
Th. Fetsch
Westfälische Wilhelms-Universität
Department of Cardiology and Angiology
and Institute for Research in Arteriosclerosis
48129 Münster
Germany

Rate-dependence of antiarrhythmic and proarrhythmic properties of class I and class III antiarrhythmic drugs

J. Weirich, H. Antoni

Physiologisches Institut, Universität Freiburg

Abstract

Rate or frequency-dependence is a characteristic property of antiarrhythmic drugs belonging to the Vaughan William classes I and III. The rate-dependence of class I drugs (i.e., increasing blockade of fast Na^+-channels with faster rates) results from periodical drug binding to Na^+-channel sites which are preferably available in the activated and/or inactivated channel states (use-dependence). With respect to their binding and unbinding kinetics, class I drugs can be subdivided into three groups (group 1 – group 3) which differ in their block-frequency relations as well as in their onset kinetics of channel blockade. These properties can serve as predictors of the anti- and proarrhythmic potential of class I drugs. Class III drugs (blockers of potassium channels) are mostly characterized by reverse rate-dependence (loss of class III action at faster rates). However, this property cannot be attributed to reverse use-dependence, i.e., binding to channels in the rested state. It is more likely due to different rate-dependent contributions of the two components of the delayed rectifier potassium current to repolarization, when the rapidly activating, the rectifying component I_{Kr} is specifically blocked by class III drugs, while the slowly activating component I_{Ks} remains unchanged. In spite of their reverse rate-dependence, class III drugs exert an antifibrillatory effect when fibrillation is induced by frequent stimulation. This can be attributed to the slow time course of the decline (offset kinetics) of the class III effect accompanying a sudden increase in frequency. Proarrhythmic effects of class III drugs result from the delay in repolarization that may favor the development of early afterdepolarizations. The proarrhythmic potential of class III drugs is species dependent and is favored if the contribution of I_{Kr} to the repolarization phase of the action potential is comparatively large.

Key words Antiarrhythmic class I and class III drugs – rate-dependence – frequency-dependence – block-frequency relation – onset kinetics – offset kinetics – proarrhythmic effects – early afterdepolarization

General characteristics of class I and class III drugs

Antiarrhythmic agents characterized as class I drugs according to the Vaughan Williams classification (25) are the well-known local anaesthetics which exert their effects by more or less specifically blocking the fast cardiac Na^+-channels. Their antiarrhythmic influence can be attributed to prolongation of the functional refractory period but may also be due to conversion of unidirectional into bidirectional block of conduction (1, 2). Both actions are mainly effective in preventing re-entry arrhythmias. However, there are also proarrhythmic influences of class I drugs, for instance, due to their slowing of impulse conduction as well as to their negative inotropic side effects (21).

Class III agents increase the duration of the cardiac action potential, mainly by blocking certain potassium channels and in this way prolong the refractory period (6). As distinguished from class I drugs, they exert no inhibitory influence on impulse conduction. However, there is also some proarrhythmic potency due to the delay in repolarization that may favor the development of triggered activity due to early afterdepolarizations (11).

Rate-dependence of class I drugs due to periodical ligand binding

Class I antiarrhythmics include a great number of different substances which show different drugs-specific, rate-dependent properties (7, 27). In the past, this aspect had been hardly considered when attempts were made to divide the class I drugs into different subclasses (3, 26). As will be shown, a more complete description of the frequency-dependence of class I action must include the kinetics of rate-dependent changes in drug activity as well as the saturation behavior of drug action at faster rates (28, 29).

Concerning the rate- or frequency-dependence of the action of class I drugs, there is now good evidence to suggest that this property results from changes of the drug binding affinity of the channel receptor in the course of a cardiac cycle (8). Instead of true temporal changes of the affinity of the receptor site, changes of the accessibility of the receptor may exert a similar influence (22). For instance, if the drug receptor is located within the channel pore, its binding potency may depend on whether the receptor is accessible by the drug when the channel is open, or is not accessible when it is closed. This has been expressed in a general way by the term "use-dependence". However, it should be taken into account that use-dependence and rate- or frequency-dependence are not identical. As will be shown for class III drugs, use-dependence is only one possible mechanism among others which may be responsible for the rate- or frequency-dependence.

In general, with class I drugs the affinity (or accessibility) of drug binding sites seems to be linked to open and/or inactivated channel states (23). Thus, Na^+-channel blockade, measured by the reduction of the fast sodium current, increases during systole when the drug binding sites are available, and decreases during diastole as a result of drug unbinding.

This is illustrated in Fig. 1. The kinetics of drug binding and unbinding are drug specific and can be described by corresponding time constants τ_{on} and τ_{off}. This simple concept explains why class I drugs with fast unbinding time constants such as lidocaine cause virtually no Na^+-channel blockade at comparatively low frequencies, but will increase their efficacy when the frequency increases and drug unbinding during diastole becomes incomplete. Then – after several activation cycles – the end-diastolic Na^+-channel blockade will attain a new steady state, which is characterised by an equal amount of blockade acquired during systole and lost during diastole. Plotting this steady state blockade against the corresponding frequency gives the drug-specific block-frequency relation, which is shown in the lower panel of Fig. 1.

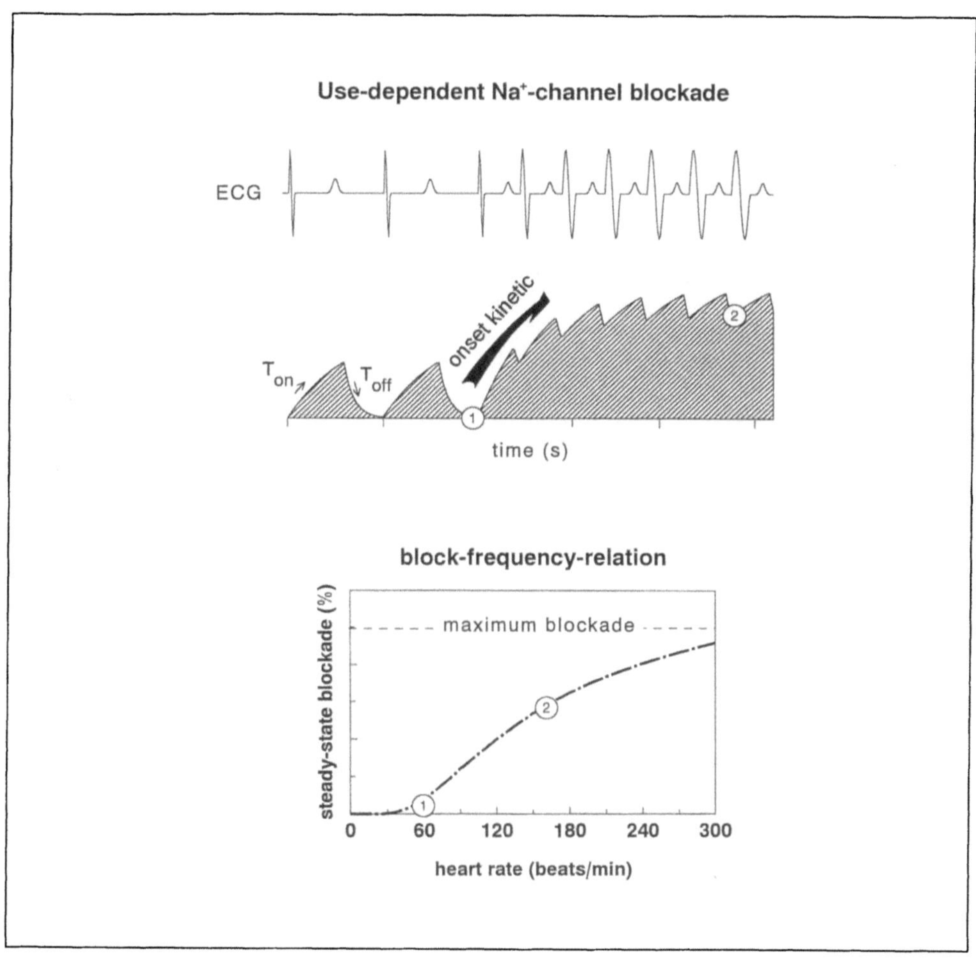

Fig. 1 *Upper panel:* rate-dependent variation of Na⁺-channel blockade (shaded area) induced by class I anti-arrhythmic drugs according to periodical drug binding to Na⁺-channels. With class I agents drug binding occurs during activity (systole) and drug unbinding during rest (diastole). Hence, the Na⁺-channel blockade increases during systole and decreases during diastole with the drug-specific time constants for drug binding (τ_{on}) and unbinding (τ_{off}). Long diastolic intervals allow complete drug unbinding, i.e., recovery from block and, therefore, the end-diastolic steady state blockade (point 1) is minimal, as is apparent from the narrow QRS complexes of the corresponding ECG traces. Shortening of the diastolic intervals results in accumulation of the end-diastolic blockade that – after several beats – attains a new steady state (point 2). The exponential onset kinetics can be quantitatively expressed by the onset rate, r_{onset} (beat⁻¹), i.e., the percentage increase in blockade per beat. *Lower panel:* relation between heart rate and rate-dependent steady state blockade of Na⁺-channels, i.e., levels of end-diastolic blockade (point 1 and 2 corresponds to the end-diastolic block levels in the upper panel). At high heart rates the block-frequency relation approaches the concentration dependent maximum blockade due to continuous drug binding.

Onset kinetics and saturation behavior of class I drugs

If the drug binding sides were continuously available, the block-frequency relation would approach a maximal value that does only dependent on the drug concentration. Such a condition is approached at higher rates, and from this it becomes clear that at higher rates the block-frequency relation will show a saturation behavior. In general, saturation will appear at low frequencies, if the time constant for unbinding of the drug is slow, and will be shifted to higher frequencies, if it is fast (see equation 7 in ref. 27).

In a comprehensive analysis of class I drugs in view of their steady state block-frequency relation as well as of their onset kinetics, we could clearly separate three different drug groups from one another (27). The block-frequency relations reflecting the main characteristics of the drugs of a group are represented in Fig. 2 by the continuous lines. Accordingly, group 1 of class I drugs is of little effect at low frequencies, but shows a steep rise of its block-frequency relation at higher rates with a half maximal frequency at about 150 beats/min and with saturation being not yet attained even at 300 beats/min. By contrast, group 3 drugs are already effective in the low frequency range, because saturation of the Na$^+$-channel blockade is almost complete at slow rates. Group 2 drugs show an intermediate block-frequency relation, but clearly separate from group 1 and group 3.

However, there are additional differences between the three groups concerning their onset kinetics – that is the time required to attain a new steady state blockade upon a sudden change in frequency. In Fig. 2 these kinetics are indicated by the arrows and are character-ized by the annotations "fast" and "slow". With group 1 the onset kinetics are fairly fast which means that upon a change in frequency a new steady state is attained within a few beats (average rate constant: 0.6/beat; compare also Fig. 1).With group 2 this adaptation to a new frequency lasts about 10 times longer. The onset kinetics of group 3 drugs are of less

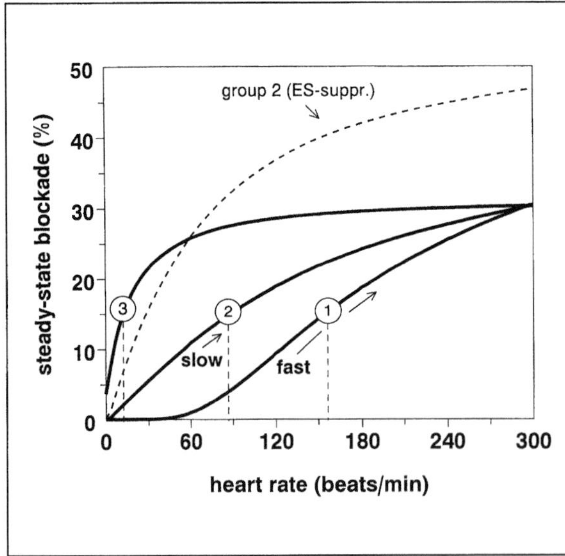

Fig. 2   Different block-frequency relations (indicated by numbers) based on an analysis of frequency-dependent Na$^+$-channel blockade induced by 13 different class I antiarrhythmic drugs (adapted from ref. 27). The class I drugs cluster into three groups with regard to their respective half-maximal frequency (frequency at which half of the maximal channel blockade is attained, indicated by the vertical dashed lines). With group 1 drugs (lidocaine, mexiletine, tocainide) the half maximal frequency is well above 150 beats/min, with group 2 drugs (encainide, flecainide, lorcainide, pro-cainamide, quinidine) it is in the range of resting sinus rhythm, and with group 3 drugs disopyramide, ethmozine, nicaino-prol, prajmaline, propafenon) well below 30 beats/min. The dashed curve is the hypothetical block-frequency relation for group 2 drugs in order to suppress extrasystoles effectively.

significance since the Na^+-channel blockade induced by these drugs is already saturating at such low rates.

Comparison of these groups with those of the subclassification proposed by Vaughan Williams (26) reveals a clear correspondence between class Ib drugs and our group 1. However, Ia and Ic drugs show little correlation to our grouping and are evenly distributed over our groups 2 and 3.

Clinical aspects concerning the different kinetics of class I drugs

Are there possible clinical consequences of the described kinetic differences between various class I drugs? An answer to this question may be given by comparison of drugs belonging to groups 2 and 3. Let us assume a condition where both groups of drugs may have caused an equal widening of QRS at resting sinus rhythm. As can be derived from Fig. 2, this QRS widening as a marker of a possible overdosage has a very different meaning in view of the strongly different saturation behavior with the two groups: In the case of the group 3, it represents the almost maximally available frequency-dependent Na^+-channel blockade which is already approached at resting sinus rhythm. Thus, a further increase in frequency will not change very much. By contrast, in the case of the group 2 drugs, an increase in heart rate (for any given reason) would cause a substantial – and perhaps pro-arrhythmic – additional widening of QRS. This appears still more important since in the classification of Vaughan Williams, drugs from both groups may belong to the same subclass.

Another example may illustrate the special significance of the differences in the onset kinetics between the three groups. Assumed that a Na^+-channel blockade of about 25 % might be sufficient to suppress extrasystoles or tachycardias effectively, then, in case of a sudden increase in heart rate due to tachycardia or to salvos of extrasystoles, drugs of group 1 will rapidly achieve this required effect due to their fast onset kinetics. With drugs of group 3 the antiarrhythmic efficacy might be in the required range already at sinus rhythm and the onset kinetics are of no further relevance. Those drugs may be very effective in suppressing extrasystoles, but in order to produce a measurable Na^+-channel blockade, the drug concentration has to be in the range of the Kd value for drug binding. Hence, with group 3 drugs the frequency dependent blockade is very sensitive to variations in the drug's plasma level and precise adjustment of the dosage is required. In the case of group 2 drugs, because of their slow onset kinetics, the antiarrhythmic efficacy may not be increased in due time during a sudden increase in frequency. Thus, in order to be effective, such drugs have to be applied at relatively high concentrations. Then, the block frequency relation is within the antiarrhythmic range already at resting sinus rhythm and extrasystoles can be suppressed effectively (see Fig. 2, dashed curve). However, this is achieved only with the risk that a moderate but long-lasting increase in heart rate should lead to a possibly pro-arrhythmic conduction delay as has been shown by Ranger and colleagues under clinical conditions (18). Moreover, one would expect that this risk could be reversed by limitations of the heart rate for instance due to beta-adrenergic blockade, and this again has been found with patients as reported by Myerburg and coworkers (17).

Rate dependence of class III drugs

What are the freqency-dependent aspects of class III drugs? Ideally, such an agent should selectively prolong the action potential at high frequencies. However, the class III drugs so far studied show a pattern of frequency-dependence just opposite to that typically observed with class I drugs (9, 24). Such an influence is exemplarily shown in Fig. 3 for the class III drug d-sotalol and its prolongation of the action potential duration in the ventricular myocardium of the guinea pig.

As a seemingly convincing explanation of the reverse rate-dependence of class III drugs, it was suggested that – just opposite to class I drugs – these agents may preferably bind to closed potassium channels (i.e., during diastole) and may unbind, when the channels are open (i.e., during systole). In other words, the class III effects were assumed to be governed by reverse use-dependence (9). However, this assumption was disproved by experimental findings showing that the potassium channel blockade does obey classical use-dependence (4, 5) with a block-frequency relation saturating at very low frequencies which is comparable to the behavior found with certain class I drugs (see group 3 in Fig. 2). But nevertheless in their overall behavior these class III drugs exhibit reverse rate-dependence (5, 6, 9, 24).

Hence, there must be another mechanism responsible for this discrepancy, and this has been attributed to the existence of two components of the delayed rectifier potassium current: I_{Kr} (rapidly activating, rectifying) and I_{Ks} (slowly activating) (19). According to Sanguinetti and coworkers, class III drugs like d-sotalol, dofetilide, structurally related to the methanesulfonanilde compound E-4031, selectively block the I_{Kr} component leaving the I_{Ks} component unchanged (13, 19). The reverse rate-dependence is then the consequence of a different rate-dependent contribution of the components to the repolarization phase.

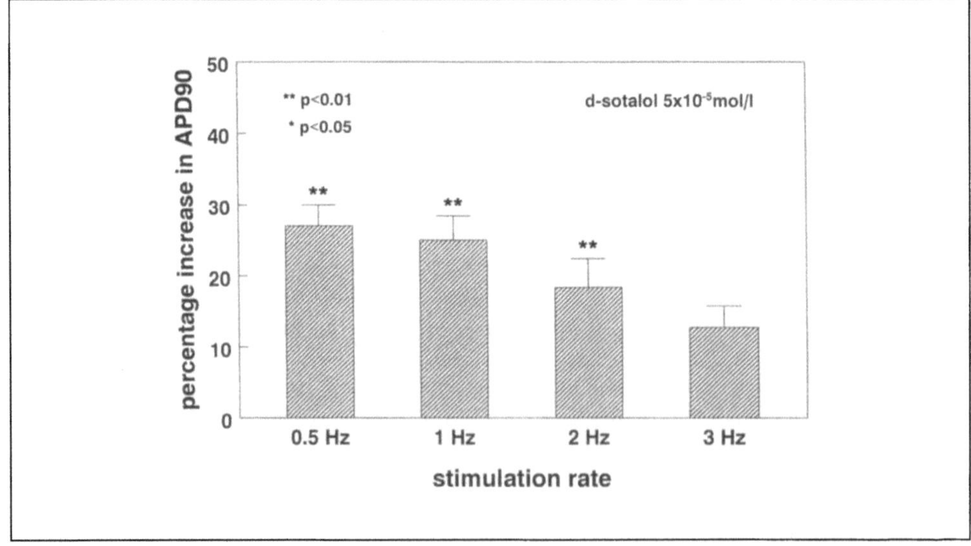

Fig. 3 Reverse rate-dependence of the action potential prolongation induced by the class III drug d-sotalol in the ventricular myocardium of the guinea pig. The action potential duration was measured at the level of 90 % repolarization (APD90). Values are expressed as mean ± SE of 4 preparations at each frequency.

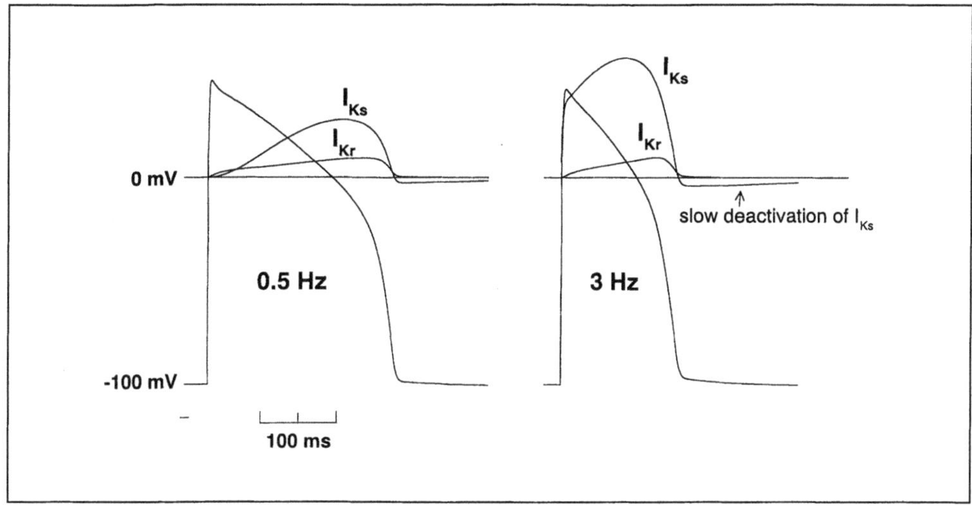

Fig. 4 Action potentials computed according to the model for the guinea pig action potential proposed by Rudy et al. (16, 33). The figure shows in addition to the shape of the action potentials the behavior of the two components I_{Kr} and I_{Ks} of the delayed rectifier K$^+$ current for two given stimulation rates. At the faster excitation rate of 3 Hz, I_{Ks} becomes the predominant current during repolarization since only this current accumulates due to incomplete deactivation within the shorter diastolic intervals.

In order to illustrate this point further, we computed by means of the Luo-Rudy-model for the guinea pig action potential (16, 33) the contribution of the I_{Kr} and of the I_{Ks} component to the repolarization phase at a slow (0.5 Hz) and a fast (3 Hz) stimulation rate. The results are depicted in Fig. 4, which shows the simulated action potentials together with the respective current traces for the two stimulation rates. As can be readily seen, the magnitude of I_{Kr} is about the same at both stimulation rates, whereas I_{Ks} becomes almost doubled at the faster rate. The latter is due to accumulation of the I_{Ks} component at faster rates because the relatively slow kinetics of this current does not permit the current to completely deactivate during the short diastolic intervals. Thus, after, for instance, complete blockade of I_{Kr} by class III drugs, a relatively large fraction of the delayed rectifier current (sum of I_{Ks} and I_{Kr}) is blocked at the slow stimulation rate, but only a relatively small fraction at the faster rate. This will result in a substantial class III action at slow rates, but in a less pronouncd drug effect at faster rates, i.e., in reverse rate-dependence of class III drugs.

However, from more recent findings (10, 32) its again seems questionable, whether this explanation may fully account for any condition. Notably, reverse rate-dependence has been also observed on rabbit myocardium (5, 31) which seems to be devoid of a substantial I_{Ks} component (4).

Antiarrhythmic effects of class III drugs in spite of their reverse rate-dependence

Of course, independent of its proper mechanism, reverse rate-dependence has to be accepted as a real phenomenon and as a possible limiting factor of the antifibrillatory efficacy of class

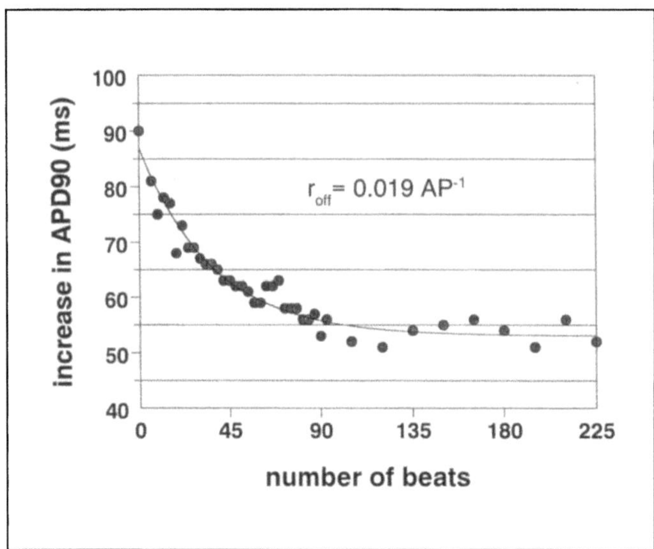

Fig. 5 Offset kinetics of the class III effect (i.e., time course of the rate-dependent decline of the action potential prolongation) of d-sotalol (50 μM) upon a sudden increase of the stimulation rate from 30 to 180/min on guinea pig papillary muscle. For the sake of clarity, during the first 20 s the respective prolongation of every third action potential is shown, afterwards only every 12th value is represented. The time course of the decrease in action potential prolongation can be fitted by a mono-exponential (continuous line) with an offset rate (r_{off}) of 0.019 AP^{-1}.

III drugs (6, 9). Hence, it must be asked, whether class III drugs can be antiarrhythmic at higher heart rates at all. The answer to this question has to consider another property of these drugs that may partly compensate for their reverse rate-dependence mainly when sudden changes in frequency are considered. This property is given by comparatively slow offset kinetics of the drugs (28). An example for this temporal behavior of the class III action (action potential prolongation) caused by d-sotalol in the guinea pig ventricular myocardium during a sudden change in frequency (from 30 to 180/min) is given in Fig. 5. As can be seen from this figure, there is a slow exponential decline of the class III action that attains a new steady state only within about half a minute. This comparatively slow

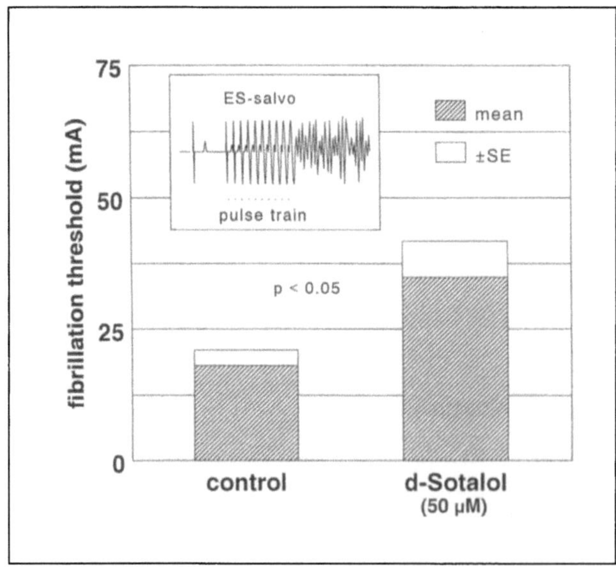

Fig. 6 Influence of d-sotalol on the ventricular fibrillation threshold (VFT) determined by train pulses (pulse duration 5 ms at 40 Hz for 1 s). As illustrated by the inset figure, the pulse train started 70 ms after the R-wave analogue of the electrogram. With this stimulation protocol 10 closely coupled extrasystoles are elicited which eventually merge into fibrillation. Despite this maximal increase in heart rate, the VFT is still significantly increased by the drug ($p < 0.05$) provided the protocol is applied during a slow basic heart rate of about 60/min.

offset kinetics may preserve the antiarrhythmic class III action for some time during a sudden increase in heart rate and may, thus, exert a favorable influence which has not been considered in the past. This influence should become obvious when ventricular fibrillation is induced by a salvos of closely coupled extrasystoles. In order to examine such a condition, we measured the ventricular fibrillation threshold in the isolated guinea pig heart using d-sotalol (50 μM) as class III drug (Fig. 6).

In order to induce fibrillation, a train of 5 ms pulses was applied at 40 Hz for 1 s. With this maneuver, fibrillation is usually initiated after a run of up to 12 extrasystoles – that is after a maximal increase of the excitation rate. Hence, in view of the reverse rate-dependence of class III action, one might expect that such a condition should minimize the antifibrillatory efficacy of the drug. Buth nevertheless, at the slow basic rhythm of 60/min, the class III drug still increased the ventricular fibrillation threshold significantly by about 90 %. However, if the same protocol was used after the hearts had been beating at the faster rate of 240/min for several minutes, the drug did no longer alter the ventricular fibrillation threshold significantly (not shown in Fig. 6). From the persistent antifibrillatory efficacy of the class III drug during a salvo of extrasystoles, it can be assumed that the slow offset kinetics does counteract the reverse rate-dependence during a sudden increase in excitation rate for some time.

Proarrhythmic effects of class III drugs: Significance of the I_{Ks} component

On the cellular level proarrhythmic effects of class III drugs become manifest as disturbances of the repolarization phase at the end of the action potential plateau, known as early afterdepolarizations (EADs), an example of which is given in Fig. 7. Early afterdepolarizations mainly arise from an excessively prolonged action potential and are thus favored by slow stimulation because of the reverse rate-dependence of the class III activity. The excessive prolongation of the action potential plateau may permit the slow Ca^{++} inward

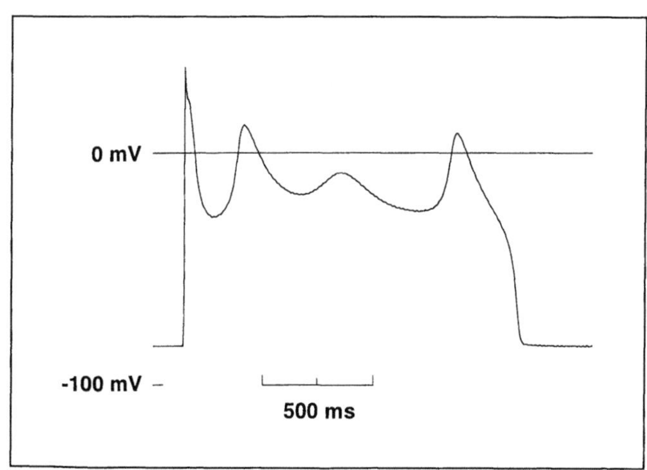

Fig. 7 Example for repeated afterdepolarizations in rabbit ventricular myocardium due to an excessive prolongation of the action potential at a slow stimulation rate of 0.2 Hz in the presence of dofetilide (0.1 μM).

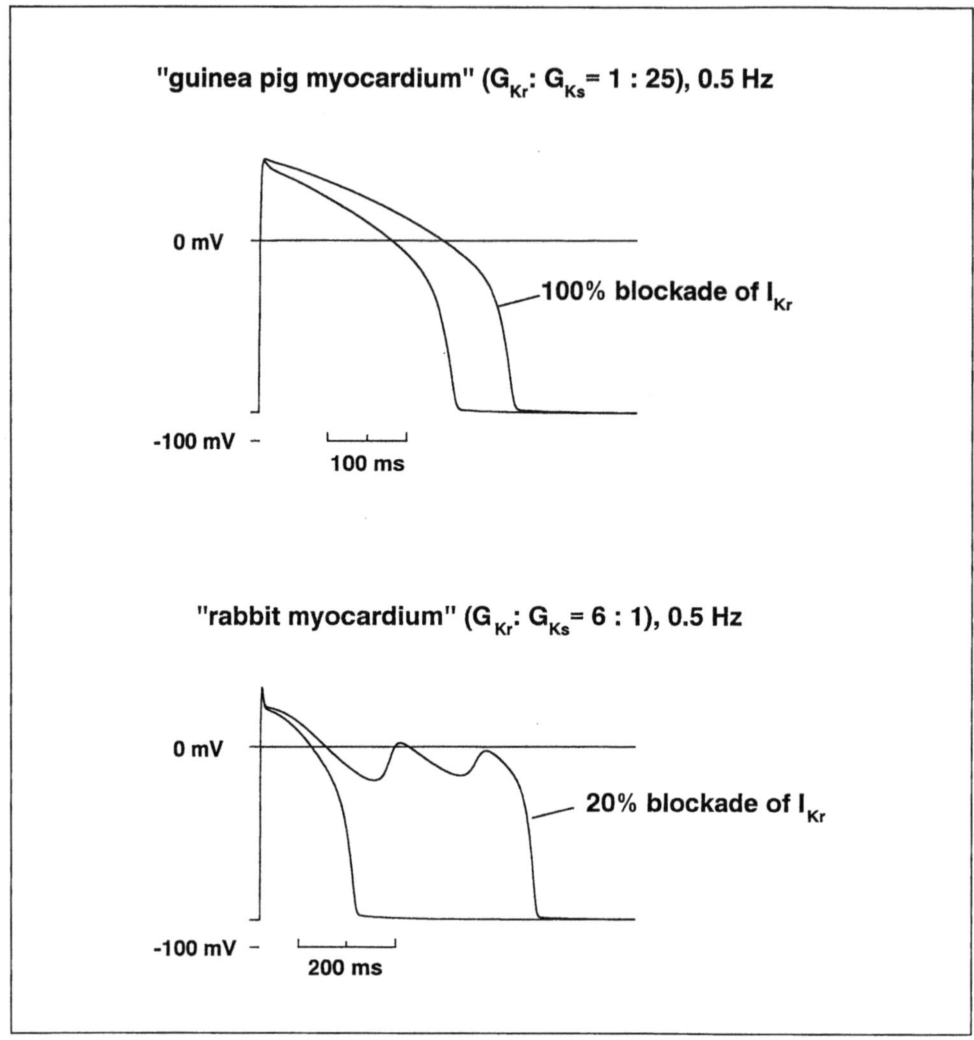

Fig. 8 Computed myocardial action potentials of different species (top panel: guinea pig; bottom panel: rabbit) by means of modifications of the Luo-Rudy model for the guinea pig action potential (16, 33). G_{Kr} and G_{Ks} are the conductances of the respective components of the delayed rectifier potassium curent, I_{Kr} and I_{Ks}. Please note the different time scales of the panels.

current to reactivate and to generate the secondary depolarizations (12). Early afterdepolarizations are discussed as one possible mechanism underlying triggered activity or Torsade de pointes arrhythmias which can be observed in patients with an acquired long QT-syndrome (11).

Interestingly, we could never observe early afterdepolarizations in multicellular preparations of guinea pig myocardium, even at high concentrations of class III antiarrhythmic drugs. Thus, prolongation of the action potential by about 30 % (see Fig. 3), which is enough to produce a substantial increase in the fibrillation threshold, seems to be the maximum extend of class III action achievable on guinea pig myocardium (13, 19, 31) under normal conditions ($[K^+]_e = 5.4$ mmol/l) and hardly results in early afterdepolarizations. Hence, in guinea pig the I_{Ks} component myocardium obviously ensures normal repolarization even after full blockade of the I_{Kr} component by class III antiarrhythmics.

This is very different from what can be observed in rabbit ventricular myocardium, which may be devoid from a substantial I_{Ks} component (4). In this species, relatively low drug concentrations, which produce only half-maximal prolongation in guinea pig myocardium, can be sufficient to increase the action potential duration to such an extend that the conditions for the development of early afterdepolarizations are given (Fig. 7). Thus, due to the lack of a substantial I_{Ks} component in rabbit myocardium, the occurrence of early afterdepolarizations is a rather common phenomenon at slow rates and at higher drug concentrations (31). In multicellular preparations of failing human myocardium, we observed early afterdepolarizations very rarely and, again, this might be attributed to the existence of an I_{Ks} component of the delayed rectifier potassium current or to alterations of other ionic currents (14).

Presumably, the incidence of early afterdepolarizations in the presence of class III antiarrhythmic drugs strongly depends on the extend to which the I_{Ks} component is expressed in the myocardium of a certain species to compensate for the block of the I_{Kr} component by class III drugs. We made an attempt to substantiate this hypothesis by simulating the cardiac action potential of the guinea pig and of the rabbit by introducing some modifications into the Luo-Rudy model (Fig. 8).

In short, the quite convincing results are as follows: the behavior of the guinea pig myocardium could be simulated by introducing a maximal conductance (G_{Ks}) for the slow component I_{Ks}, which was considerably larger than the maximal conductance (G_{Kr}) of the rapidly activating component, I_{Kr} (Fig. 8, top). In order to simulate the rabbit myocardium, besides the introduction of an additional transient outward current, G_{Kr} was enlarged and G_{Ks} substantially reduced ensuring the I_{Kr} component to be the predominant repolarizing current during the action potential plateau and the consecutive repolarization phase (Fig. 8, lower). Under these conditions blockade of only about 20 % of the I_{Kr} was sufficient to induce repeated early afterdepolarizations in rabbit myocardium, whereas a 100 % blockade of this current in guinea pig myocardium only results in a maximum prolongation of the action potential by about 30 %.

In human myocardium, alterations of the gene (HERG) encoding for potassium channels which produce a current likely to be I_{Kr} have been identified as the possible cause of the long QT-syndrome (20). Hence, in human myocardium, normal repolarization may be strongly dependent on the I_{Kr} component despite of an I_{Ks} component which has been identified only recently (14).

Different contributions of the two components of the delayed rectifier potassium current to repolarization may be also responsible for regional differences in the class III effects on ventricular myocardium. Thus, a weeker I_{Ks} component in the midwall region of the ventricular myocardium may cause a prominent class III action and a higher incidence of proarrhythmic responses in this myocardial layer (15, 31).

References

1. Antoni H (1971) Electrophysiological mechanisms underlying pharmacological models of cardiac fibrillation. Pflügers Arch 269: 171–199
2. Antoni H, Weirich J (1990) Neue Aspekte der elektrophysiologischen Wirkung von Antiarrhythmika. Herz 15: 61–69
3. Campbell TJ (1983) Kinetics of onset of rate-dependent effects of class I antiarrhythmic drugs are important in determining their effects on refractoriness in guinea pig ventricle and provide a theoretical basis for their subclassification. Cardiovasc Res 17: 344–352

4. Carmeliet E (1992) Voltage- and time-dependent block of the delayed K^+ current in cardiac myocytes by dofetilide. J Pharmacol Exp Ther 262: 809–817

5. Carmeliet E (1993) Use-dependent block of the delayed K^+ current in rabbit ventricular myocytes. Cardiovascular Drugs and Therapy 7: 599–604

6. Colatsky TJ, Follmer CH, Starmer CF (1990) Channel specificity in antiarrhythmic drug action. Mechanism of potassium channel block and its role in suppressing and aggravating cardiac arrhythmias. Circulation 82: 2235–2242

7. Heistracher P (1971) Mechanisms of action of antifibrillatory drugs. Naunyn-Schmiedeberg's Arch Pharmacol 269: 199–212

8. Hondeghem LM, Katzung BG (1977) Time- and voltage-dependent interactions of antiarrhythmic drugs with cardiac sodium-channels. Biochim Biophys Acta 472: 373–398

9. Hondeghem LM, Snyders DJ (1990) Class III antiarrhythmic agents have a lot of potential but a long way to go. Circulation 81: 686–690

10. Gintant GA (1996) Two components of delayed rectifier current in canine atrium and ventricle. Does IKs play a role in the reverse rate dependence of class III agents? Circ Res 78: 26–37

11. Jackman WM, Friday KJ, Anderson JL, Aliot EM, Clark M (1988) The long QT syndromes: a critical review, new clinical observations and unifying hypothesis. Prog Cardiovas Dis 31: 115–172

12. January CT, Riddle JM, Salata JJ (1988) A model for early afterdepolarizations: Induction with Ca-channel antagonist Bay K 8644. Circ Res 72: 75–83

13. Jurkiewicz NK, Sanguinetti MC (1993) Rate-dependent prolongation of cardiac action potentials by a methanesulfonanilide class III antiarrhythmic agent. Specific block of rapidly activating delayed rectifier K^+ current by dofetilide. Circ Res 72: 75–83

14. Li GR, Feng J, Yue L, Carrier M, Nattel S (1996) Evidence for Two Components of the Delayed Rectifier K^+ Current in Human Ventricular Myocytes. Circ Res 78: 689–696

15. Liu D, Antzelevitch C (1995) Characteristics of the delayed rectifier current (I_{Kr} and I_{Ks}) in canine venticular epicardial, midmyocardial, and endocardial myocytes. A weeker Iks contributes to the longer action potential of the M cell. Cir Res 76: 351–365

16. Luo CH, Rudy Y (1991) A model of the ventricular cardiac action potential. Depolarization, repolarization, and their interaction. Circ Res 68: 1501–1526

17. Myerburg RJ, Kessler KM, Cox MM, Huikuri H, Terracall E, Interian A, Fernandaz P, Castellanos A (1989) Reversal of proarrhythmic effects of flecainide acetate and encainide hydrochloride by propranolol. Circulation 80: 1571–1579

18. Ranger S, Talajic M, Lemery R, Roy D, Nattel S (1989) Amplification of flecainide-induced ventricular conduction slowing by exercise. Circulation 79: 1000–1006

19. Sanguinetti MC, Jurkiewicz NK (1990) Two components of cardiac delayed rectifier K^+ current. Differential sensitivity to block by class III antiarrhythmic agents. J Gen Physiol 96: 195–215

20. Schwartz PJ, Priori SG, Locati EH, Napolitano C, Cantu F, Towbin JA, Keating MT, Hammoude H, Brown AM, Chen L-S, Colatsky TJ (1995) Long QT-syndrome patients with mutations of the SCN5A and HERG genes have differential responses to Na^+ channel blockade and to increases in heart rate. Implications for gene-specific therapy. Circulation 92: 3381-3386

21. Singh BN (1990) Controlling cardiac arrhythmias: To delay conduction or to prolong refractoriness. Cardiovasc Drugs Ther 3: 671–674

22. Starmer CF (1986) Theoretical characterization of ion channel blockade: Ligand binding to periodically accessible receptors. J of Theor Biol 119: 235–249

23. Starmer CF, Grant AO, Strauss HC (1984) Mechanisms of use-dependent block of sodium channels in excitable membranes by local anesthetics. Biophys J 46: 15–27

24. Tande PM, Bjornstad H, Yang T, Refsum H (1990) Rate-dependent class III antiarrhythmic action, negative chronotropy, and positive inotropy of a novel Ik blocking drug, UK-68-798: potent in guinea pig but no effect in rat myocardium. J Cardiovasc Pharmacol 16: 401–410

25. Vaughan Williams EM (1989) Classification of Anti-arrhythmic Agents. Springer, Berlin Heidelberg New York

26. Vaughan Willams EM (1984) Subgroups of class 1 antiarrhythmic drugs. Eur Heart J 5: 96–98

27. Weirich J, Antoni H (1990) Differential analysis of the frequency-dependent effects of class-I-antiarrhythmic drugs according to periodical ligand binding: Implications on antiarrhythmic and proarrhythmic efficacy. J Cardiovasc Pharmacol 15: 998–1009

28. Weirich J, Hohnloser SH, Antoni H (1992) Differential analysis of frequency-dependent effects of antiarrhythmic drugs: Importance of the saturation behavior of frequency-dependent sodium-channel blockade. J of Cardiovasc Pharmacol 20 Suppl 2: 8–16

29. Weirich J (1992) Frequency-dependent action of antiarrhythmic drugs: The useful concept of periodical ligand binding. Basic Res Cardiol 8: 205–214

30. Weirich J. Hohnloser A, Antoni H (1994) D-Sotalol and Dofetilide Exhibits Slow Offset Kinetics: Significance for Their Antifibrillatory efficacy. Pace 17 II: 332

31. Weirich J, Bernhardt R, Lowen N, Wenzel W, Antoni H (1996) Regional- and Species-Dependent Effects of K+-Channel Blocking Agents on Subendocardium and Mid-Wall Slices of Human, Rabbit and Guinea Pig Myocardium. Pflugers Arch 431 Supp: 328
32. Yang T, Roden DM (1996) Extracellular potassium modulation of drug block of IKr. Implications for torsades de pointes and reverse use-dependence. Circulation 93: 407–411
33. Zeng J, Laurita KR, Rosenbaum DS, Rudy J (1995) Two components of the delayed rectifier K+ current in ventricular myocytes of the guinea pig type. Circ Res 77: 140–152

Author's address:
PD Dr. med. Jörg Weirich
Physiologisches Institut
Universität Freiburg i. Br.
Hermann Herder Str. 7
79104 Freiburg
Germany

Autonomic control of heart rate: Pharmacological and nonpharmacological modulation

E. Vanoli[1], D. Cerati[2], R. F. E. Pedretti[3]

[1] Dipartimento di Cardiologia, IRCCS San Matteo, Università di Pavia, Italy
[2] Istituto di Clinica Medica Generale e Terapia Medica, Università di Milano, Italy
[3] Divisione di Cardiologia, Fondazione Salvatore Maugeri, IRCCS Clinica del Lavoro e della Riabilitazione, Centro Medico di Riabilitazione, Tradate, Italy

Abstract

The evidence of the predictive value of autonomic markers has generated a growing interest for interventions able to influence autonomic control of heart rate. The hypothesis is that an increase in cardiac vagal activity as detected by an increase in heart rate variability (HRV) or baroreflex sensitivity (BRS) may be beneficial in the ischemic heart. Numerous experimental data support the hypothesis that augmenting vagal activity might be protective against lethal ischemic arrhythmias. Among them is the evidence that ventricular fibrillation during acute myocardial ischemia may be largely prevented by electrical stimulation of the right cervical vagus or by pharmacological stimulation of cholinergic receptors with oxotremorine. There is an inherent danger in the so far unwarranted assumption that modification of HRV or BRS translates directly in cardiac protection. This may or may not be the case. It should be remembered that the true target is the improvement in cardiac electrical stability and that BRS or HRV are just markers of autonomic activity. Low dose scopolamine increases HRV in patients with a prior myocardial infarction. This observation, combined with the evidence that elevated cardiac vagal activity during acute myocardial ischemia is antifibrillatory, has generated the hypothesis that scopolamine might be protective after MI. We tested low dose scopolamine in a clinically relevant experimental preparation for sudden death in which other vagomimetic interventions are effective and found that this intervention does indeed increase cardiac vagal markers but has minimal antifibrillatory effects. This is in contrast to exercise training that in the same experimental model had a marked effect on both BRS and HRV and at the same time provided strong protection from ischemic ventricular fibrillation. Thus, based on the current knowledge it seems appropriate to call for caution before attributing excessive importance to changes in „markers" of vagal activity in the absence of clear-cut evidence for a causal relation with an antifibrillatory effect.

Key words Vagal activity – ventricular fibrillation – myocardial infarction

Introduction

Experimental and clinical evidence have established and have described the existence of a dose relationship between the autonomic nervous system, acute myocardial ischemia, and occurrence of lethal cardiac arrhythmias (6, 25, 40, 41, 49). Specifically, dominance of sympathetic or vagal reflexes during acute myocardial ischemia markedly increases or decreases, respectively, the risk for developing lethal arrhythmias and sudden death.

Almost two decades ago, our group developed an experimental preparation for sudden death in conscious dogs with a prior myocardial infarction (38). This animal model provided the first experimental evidence that the likelihood of having predominant sympathetic reflexes, and thus a greater risk of dying, or vagal reflexes, and a greater chance of surviving, during acute myocardial ischemia could be predicted by analyzing autonomic control of heart rate prior to the occurrence of the ischemic event. Baroreflex sensitivity (BRS) was used to analyze autonomic control of heart rate and correctly identified a large number of post-myocardial infarction animals at high risk of having arrhythmic death at the time of a new and brief ischemic episode (42). This represented a strong rationale to test the potential of autonomic markers to identify among post-myocardial infarction patients those at higher risk of dying of lethal arrhythmic events. The clinical relevance of this information was initially suggested by some pilot studies (16, 23). More recently the multi-center international trial ATRAMI (Autonomic Tone and Reflexes After Myocardial Infarction) has prospectively shown in 1284 post-myocardial infarction patients that both BRS and heart rate variability (HRV) have strong and independent predictive value for cardiac mortality (22).

The evidence of the predictive value of autonomic markers has generated a growing interest for interventions able to influence autonomic control of heart rate. The thought underlying this interest is that an increase in cardiac vagal activity as detected by an increase in HRV or BRS may be beneficial in the ischemic heart. As matter of fact the concept that interventions augmenting vagal activity might be protective against lethal ischemic arrhythmias is supported by numerous experimental data (11). Among them, the evidence that ventricular fibrillation during acute myocardial ischemia may be largely prevented by electrical stimulation of the right cervical vagus (48) or by pharmacological stimulation of cholinergic receptors with oxotremorine (9, 10).

There is, however, an inherent danger in the so far unwarranted assumption that modification of HRV or BRS translates directly in cardiac protection.This may or may not be the case. It should be remembered that the true target is the improvement in cardiac electrical stability and that BRS or HRV are just markers of autonomic activity.

Hereafter, a brief summary of experimental and clinical data concerning the predictive value of autonomic markers and the potential mechanisms involved in autonomic derangements in the ischemic heart will be presented. Subsequently, the influences on cardiac electrical stability of pharmacological and nonpharmacological interventions able to modulate autonomic markers will be discussed.

The predictive value of autonomic markers

Autonomic markers and risk for ventricular fibrillation

Much information on the mechanisms involved in the genesis of sudden cardiac death had been obtained in an experimental model in which ventricular fibrillation could be reproducibly induced by clinically relevant stimuli (38). This conscious animal preparation, already described in several circumstances, combines three elements highly relevant to the genesis of malignant arrhythmias in man: a healed myocardial infarction, acute myocardial ischemia, and physiologically elevated sympathetic activity. In brief, 30 days after an anterior wall myocardial infarction, chronically instrumented dogs perform a submaximal exercise stress test. When heart rate reaches approximately 210–220 b/min, a 2 minute occlusion of the circumflex coronary artery is performed by means of a pneumatic occluder previously positioned around the vessel. After 1 minute exercise stops while the occlusion

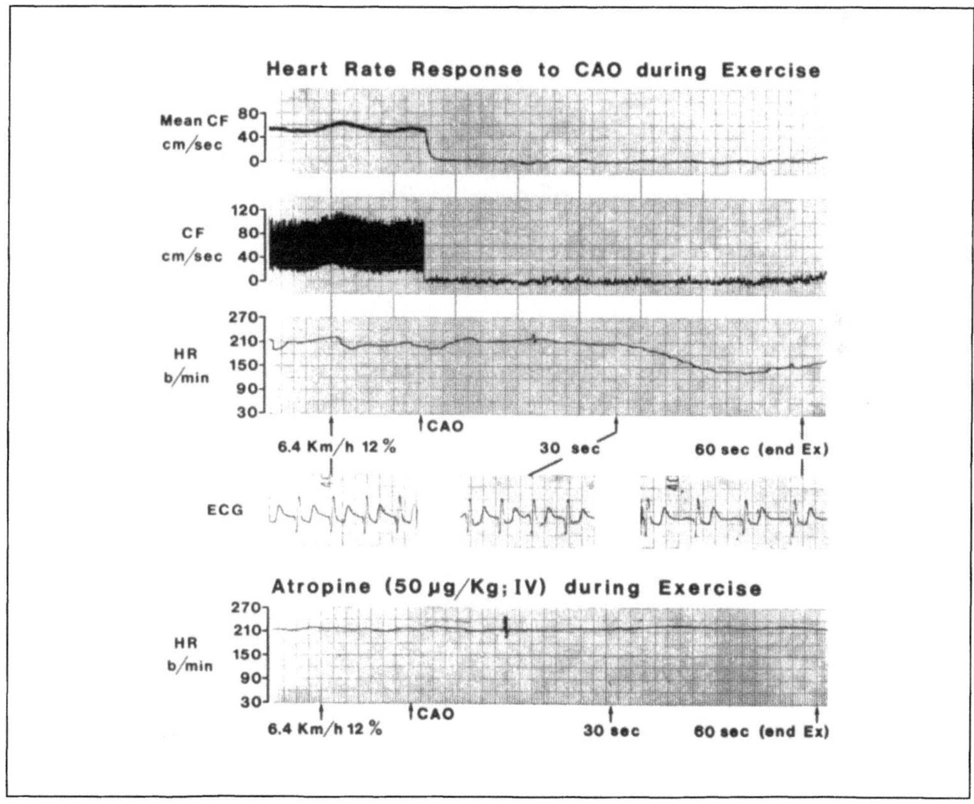

Fig. 1 Heart rate response to acute myocardial ischemia in a dog resistant to ventricular fibrillation. From top to bottom, mean and actual coronary flow (CF), the tachogram, and the electrocardiogram (ECG) before and at 30 and 60 seconds of acute ischemia. Within 30 seconds of ischemia, a marked bradycardia occurs despite the ongoing exercise and the animal is protected from lethal events. Atropine completely prevents the reflex heart rate reduction during ischemia.

continues for another minute. This "exercise and ischemia test" triggers ventricular fibrillation in almost 50 % of the animals. The dogs run with steel paddles ligated to their chest so that an effective defibrillation can be accomplished within seconds from the onset of the lethal arrhythmia. The outcome of the test is highly reproducible over time in the same animal and allows for to the clear separation of two groups: 1) animals that develop ventricular fibrillation and are defined "susceptible" to sudden death; 2) dogs that survive and are defined "resistant". A critical difference between the two groups of dogs was that "resistant" dogs very often had marked reduction in heart rate during acute myocardial ischemia despite the ongoing exercise, while susceptible dogs had an opposite response, i.e., an increase in heart rate (38). The reflex heart rate increase during ischemia could have been readily explained by the combination of the baroreflex response to the decline in arterial blood pressure and of the excitatory cardio-cardiac sympathetic reflex (28). However, in the susceptible dogs the reflex tachycardia could not be attributed to a greater hemodynamic impairment, since mean blood pressure and dp/dt max just before the occurrence of ventricular fibrillation was not different from that of resistant dogs at the same moment (7). The unexpected heart rate reduction induced by myocardial ischemia in the resistant dogs was clearly dependent on a vagal reflex, as it could be prevented by atropine (Fig. 1; 12).

Based on this evidence it became rational to try to measure cardiac vagal reflexes to test whether such a measure could identify those individuals more likely to activate the vagus during acute myocardial ischemia and, thus, more likely to survive. A simple approach was to measure BRS specifically looking to the vagally mediated reflex bradycardia consequent to blood pressure rise. The method used was the one described by Sleight's group (43): BRS was measured by the slope of the regression line correlating consecutive R-R intervals with the increasing values of systolic blood pressure due to the bolus injection of phenylephrine. The changes at the sinus node level after injection of phenylephrine reflect primarily vagal reflex activity but are significantly influenced by the concomitant level of sympathetic activity (5, 17). The main finding of this study was that in the 86 dogs resistant to sudden death BRS was markedly and significantly higher than in the 106 dogs at high risk for ventricular fibrillation (17.7 ± 6.0 vs. 9.1 ± 6.5 ms/mmHg p < 0.001). This indicated that the capability of reflexly increasing vagal activity was significantly depressed in those dogs that were at higher risk for developing ventricular fibrillation.

The link between altered autonomic control of heart rate and risk for lethal arrhythmias was further described by the use of HRV (18, 47). The predictive value of this marker has been extensively described (46).

Mechanisms of autonomic imbalance after myocardial infarction

The comprehension of the potential factors involved in autonomic imbalance after myocardial infarction is critical for the use of autonomic markers for post-myocardial infarction risk stratification and for the interpretation of the effects of autonomic interventions. Such mechanisms are not yet fully understood, but neural reflexes of cardiac origin are likely involved. Among the various possibilities (40), cardio-cardiac sympatho-vagal reflexes may play an important role (27). The changes in the geometry of a beating heart secondary to the presence of a necrotic and noncontracting segment may quite conceivably increase beyond the normal firing of sympathetic afferent fibers by mechanical distortion of their sensory endings. Such a sympathetic excitation affects and impairs the baroreceptor reflex, i.e., interferes with the physiological increase in the activity of vagal fibers directed to the sinus node (5, 17). This hypothesis is supported by experimental evidence obtained by recording vagal efferent activity prior to and after removal of the left sided afferent and

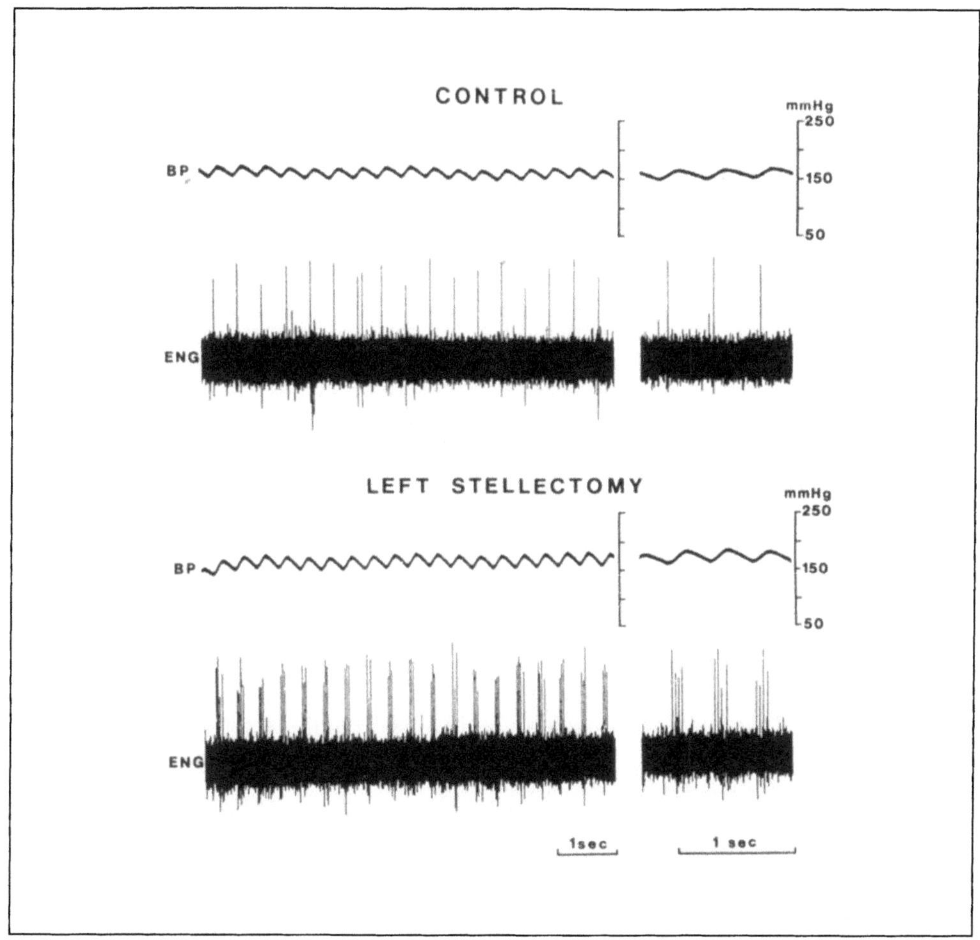

Fig. 2 Tracings showing the activity of a single cardiac vagal efferent fiber at the same blood pressure level before and after (bottom panel) left stellectomy. The fiber shows a pulse-synchronous activity that is clearly increased after left stellectomy.

efferent cardiac sympathetic fibers by left stellectomy in anesthetized cats (5). Both tonic and reflex vagal activity (following the rise in blood pressure) were significantly higher after left stellectomy. In 16 anesthetized cats removal of the left stellate ganglion increased resting level of vagal activity from 1.2 ± 0.2 to 2.1 ± 0.3 imp/sec ($+ 75 \%$, $p < 0.01$, Fig. 2). In the same cats, vagal activity during similar blood pressure rises induced by phenylephrine was also higher after left stellectomy (4.7 ± 0.7 vs. 2.2 ± 0.4 imp/sec, $p < 0.001$), with an increment of 134 ± 24 vs. $86 \pm 18 \%$ ($p < 0.05$) versus the resting level. These data indicate that the presence of cardiac afferent sympathetic activity produces a tonic constraint on vagal efferent activity and blunts the reflex increases secondary to blood pressure rises. They also support the hypothesis that the depression in vagal control of heart rate observed often after myocardial infarction may depend largely on an increase in afferent sympathetic traffic of cardiac origin.

Modulation of autonomic control of heart rate

Nonpharmacological interventions: Exercise training

A physiologic way to achieve an increase in vagal control of heart rate is represented by exercise training. It is a common knowledge that exercise training produces a lower resting and exercising heart rate (37). This typical response has been interpreted as the consequence of a combined effect of exercise training on both limbs of the autonomic nervous system.

The exercise training-induced changes in cardiac vagal activity are the results of several significant modifications on the heart and on the autonomic nervous system. Specifically, clinical and experimental findings indicate that exercise training increases myocardial contractility (44), maximal oxygen uptake (14), and cardiac oxygen consumption. In trained individuals total heart catecholamine content is decreased (13). An attenuated adrenergic, alpha mediated, vasoconstrictor activity on coronary vessels has been observed in trained dogs (24). Surprisingly, there is very little information of the effects of exercise training on autonomic markers. An increase in HRV and BRS after exercise training has been described in normal and in mild hypertensive subjects (1, 32). One of the potential accepted mechanisms for the reduction in cardiac sympathetic activity is the documented reduction in beta-adrenergic receptors density after exercise training (45). The increase in vagal activity could be due to a greater baroreceptorial stimulation consequent to the increase in contractility (50). Independently from the mechanisms involved, the net outcome of these combined effects is that exercise training shifts the autonomic control of heart rate toward a predominance of the vagal component. A critical aspect of this informations is related to the fact that exercise training has been associated with increased health benefits, and specifically with reduced cardiovascular mortality (15, 31, 36).

The availability of the experimental model in conscious dogs where occurrence or prevention of lethal arrhythmias primarily depends upon autonomic reflexes allowed us to investigate the relation between autonomic modifications induced by exercise training and risk for sudden cardiac death. In a first study (2), we observed that 6 weeks of exercise training significantly increased the depressed BRS of 8 dogs with a healed myocardial infarction susceptible to ventricular fibrillation (from 5.4 ± 1.2 to 13.2 ± 4 msec/mmHg). At the same time, another group of susceptible dogs was kept for six weeks in cage rest and did not show any autonomic change. The main finding of the study was that, concomitant with the increase in BRS, all 8 trained dogs became resistant to lethal arrhythmias during the exercise and ischemia test while all but one cage-rested dogs had no change in BRS and had recurrence of ventricular fibrillation. The one dog that behaved differently in this latter group had an increase in its BRS and became resistant to sudden cardiac death. The advantage of the experimental preparation is that, in contrast to clinical trials, by definition no changes in lifestyle other than exercise training occurred in the subjects under study. In this controlled environment this was the first documentation that training could be an independent factor able to concomitantly modify a marker of cardiac vagal activity and to reduce risk for ventricular fibrillation.

Two studies by Hopie and colleagues supports the concept that exercise training increases electrical stability of the ventricle. In the first study (30) it was found that isolated hearts from trained rats had a higher ventricular fibrillation threshold and a lower increase in cAMP in the ischemic area when compared to hearts from untrained rats. In the second study (35), in a similar preparation ventricular fibrillation threshold was higher in rats treated with exercise training after a first myocardial infarction than in untrained rats both prior to and after the onset of a second acute myocardial infarction.

Our initial observation in conscious dogs was interpreted as potentially dependent upon an increased cardiac performance in hearts damaged by the anterior wall myocardial infarction. We recently extended the initial observation to dogs without myocardial infarction to test whether exercise training prior to an ischemic event could be of benefit at the time of its occurrence (19). Seven healthy dogs that developed ventricular fibrillation during a control exercise and ischemia test were exposed to six weeks of exercise training. After this treatment, the low to high frequency ratio in the spectral analysis of HRV was decreased by 52 % BRS by 69 % from 16 ± 8 to 27 ± 14 msec/mmHg. Electrical threshold for ventricular repetitive responses was increased by 44 %, from 32 ± 6 to 46 ± 4 mA. At the same time, none of the dogs developed again ventricular fibrillation during a second exercise and ischemia test (Fig. 3). A likely mechanism involved in this antifibrillatory effect involves the fact that exercise training increases metabolic efficiency during ischemia. However, the fact that repetitive extrasystole threshold was also significantly increased after training strongly supports the hypothesis that this intervention, by modulating autonomic balance, significantly improves the electrical stability of the ventricles.

In conclusion, exercise training is a very effective tool, able to significantly increase vagal contribution to the autonomic control of heart rate. This results in an improvement of cardiac electrical stability and, ultimately, in a reduced risk for arrhythmic events in the ischemic heart as the consequence of several concomitant actions on ventricular performance, metabolic activity, and cardiac reflexes. Indeed, exercise training seems to be able to specifically act at various sites and on various mechanisms involved in genesis of ischemia-dependent ventricular tachyarrhythmias.

Exercise training appears to be an inexpensive non-pharmacological intervention, available for mass program that can reduce risk for cardiovascular mortality in coronary artery disease patients and may have the potential to significantly influence risk for lethal events even when performed prior to the development of ischemic heart disease.

Fig. 3   Effect of exercise training on baroreflex sensitivity (BRS) heart rate variability (HRV), repetitive extrasystole threshold (RET), and on risk for ventricular fibrillation during the exercise and ischemia test.

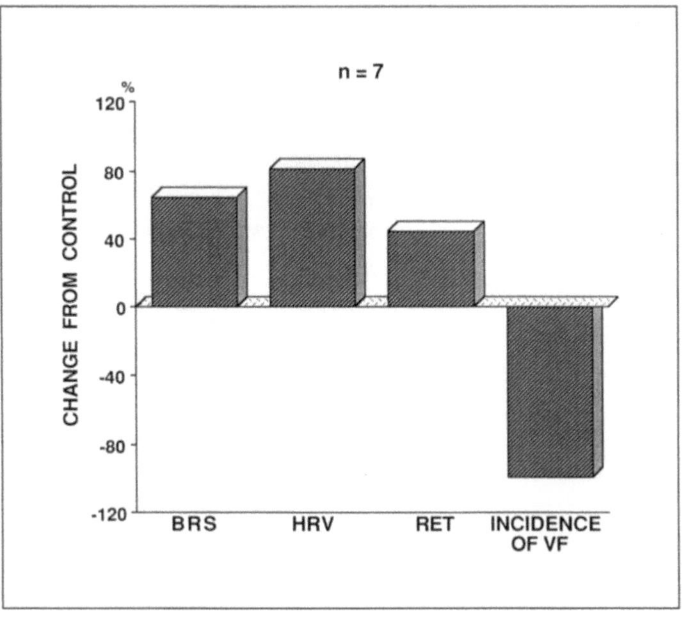

Pharmacological interventions:
Low dose of muscarinic receptors blocking agents

Low dose of muscarinic receptors blockers may produce a paradoxical increase in vagal efferent activity. Atropine is known to induce bradycardia (as a "paradoxical" vagomimetic effect) at low doses and the expected heart rate increase (as the typical antimuscarinic effect) at higher doses (52). For atropine this effect has been recognized since the beginning of the century (54), but the precise mechanisms have not yet been fully clarified. There has been indeed a proliferation of publications reporting the "positive" effect of a variety of interventions on HRV and BRS (4, 8, 34, 51).

In 1993 four different studies from independent groups reported similar findings using transdermal administration of scopolamine. The main finding common to the four studies was that in patients with a healed myocardial infarction low dose scopolamine was able to significantly increase various measures of HRV both in time and frequency domain. The conclusion derived from the HRV results were also strengthened by the study of BRS performed in three of these four studies (4, 8, 34). BRS was increased by scopolamine by an extent ranging from 42 to 98 %.

In one of these studies (34) the influences of transdermal scopolamine on cardiac electrical properties were also evaluated. Effective refractory periods of right atrium, atrioventricular node, and right ventricle were assessed before and after scopolamine in 20 patients with a recent myocardial infarction. After wearing one patch of transdermal scopolamine for 24 hours, right atrium refractory period decreased from 242 ± 44 to 223 ± 41 msec (p < 0.01), atrioventricular node refractory period increased from 320 ± 65

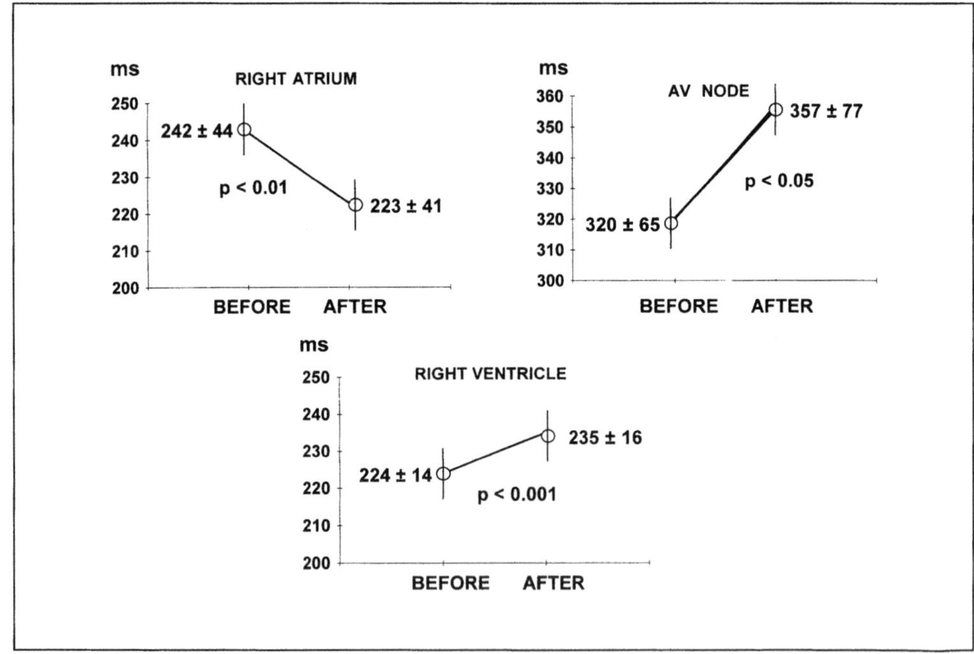

Fig. 4 Effect of low dose scopolamine on refractoriness in the right atrium and ventricle and on the atrioventricular node (av node). The increase in cardiac vagal activity after scopolamine results in an increased refractoriness of the av node and of the right ventricle and in reduced refractoriness at the atrial level.

to 357 ± 77 msec (p < 0.05) and right ventricle refractory period increased from 224 ± 14 to 235 ± 16 msec (p < 0.001) (Fig. 4).

More recently attention has been devoted to pirenzepine, an antimuscarinic agent widely used for peptic ulcer therapy. Low doses of intravenous pirenzepine have been found to increase the standard deviation of the RR intervals by 58 % in 6 normal volunteers (52). Pirenzepine in contrast to scopolamine does not have central action, and more importantly can be used orally for long time with minimal side effects. As matter of fact preliminary attempts of chronic therapy with transdermal scopolamine had failed because of a large incidence of side effects. Recently, at our institution, a study aimed to assess efficacy and safety of transdermal scopolamine after MI on a middle-term treatment was interrupted owing to the high incidence of adverse effects (RFE Pedretti unpublished data). Of five patients randomized to transdermal scopolamine, four (80 %) had to withdraw the therapy within the first month of treatment. Two patients developed an intractable cutaneous erythema at the site of patch application, and the two other complained of blurred vision and drowsiness.

In a single-blind, placebo-controlled crossover trial (33), 20 patients underwent evaluation of short-term HRV and BRS 19 ± 6 days after the infarction. Analysis was performed under control conditions and during placebo, oral pirenzepine, and transdermal scopolamine administration. In an initial dose-response study 5 of 8 post-myocardial infarction patients showed a significant increase in BRS and were considered responders to pirenzepine. BRS was reassessed after 2 days of therapy for each oral dose tested. If a BRS increase >4ms/mmHg occurred, the patient was considered responder to pirenzepine and that dose was defined effective. All responder patients underwent treatment with a higher dose to assess the possibility of a further increase of vagal activity. In all responder patients administration of a pirenzepine dose higher than the effective one did not induce a further increase in BRS value.

During treatment with 25 mg b.i.d., pirenzepine increased BRS by 58 % (9.16 ± 3.96 vs. 5.71 ± 3.74 msec/mmHg in control condition, p = 0.007). Compared with placebo, at the dose of 25 mg b.i.d. pirenzepine significantly increased all time and frequency domain measures of HRV and augmented by 60 % BRS (10.37 ± 6.82 vs. 6.47 ± 3.22 msec/mmHg, p = 0.0025). Pirenzepine showed a vagomimetic effect that was comparable with that observed with scopolamine; nevertheless, the overall incidence of adverse effects was significantly lower during pirenzepine than during scopolamine condition (1 [5 %] of 20 vs. 10 [50 %] of 20). Thus, oral pirenzepine appeared to have a greater therapeutic potential for the long term treatment of post-myocardial infarction patients than what observed with scopolamine.

Marracini et al. recently found that intravenous pirenzepine may significantly increase exercise tolerance in patients with effort myocardial ischemia compared with saline (26). Time to ischemia and rate-pressure product of ischemia were significantly improved by pirenzepine and the antiischemic effect of pirenzepine was similar to that induced by intravenous isosorbide dinitrate, the reference drug used in the study. Whether the oral dose of pirenzepine used to modulate the cardiac autonomic function could also induce an anti-ischemic effect still has to be demonstrated.

Overall these data combined with the experimental evidence of the antifibrillatory effect of vagal stimulation fostered the idea that low dose scopolamine could have been an effective tool to reduce arrhythmic risk after myocardial infarction. However, confirmatory data were necessary to prove that such a change in autonomic markers would indeed result in a significant increase in the electrical stability of the ischemic heart.

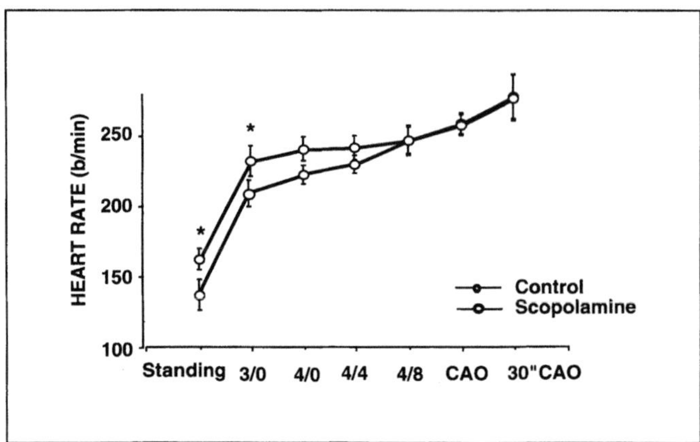

Fig. 5 Heart rate response to exercise and acute myocardial ischemia in control conditions and after scopolamine.

Experimental evidence: The effect of scopolamine on autonomic markers and on ventricular fibrillation

In order to investigate whether a relation exists between changes in markers of cardiac vagal activity and changes in cardiac electrical stability an experimental study was designed with the specific goal to verify if an intervention known for its ability to increase HRV and BRS would, at the same time, be effective in reducing the incidence of ischemia-induced ventricular fibrillation in the clinically relevant animal preparation (38) in which the capability of BRS and, later, of HRV of predicting risk for arrhythmic death was first described (see above). The effects of low dose scopolamine i.v. on HRV and cardiac electrical stability were studied in dogs with a prior MI that had or did not have ventricular fibrillation during an exercise and ischemia test (20).

Prior to scopolamine, susceptible animals had an average StD of the mean R-R interval lower than that of the resistant ones (136 ± 30 vs. 224 ± 33 msec, – 65 %, p < 0.01). This difference was progressively reduced by increasing doses of scopolamine and at 1 and 3 µg/kg the values among the two groups became similar: 322 ± 35 vs. 223 ± 31 msec (NS). At higher dose, 10 µg/kg, StD decreased. The coefficient of variance (i.e., the StD of RR interval corrected for heart rate) showed the same pattern observed for the StD. Prior to scopolamine, it was lower by 45 % in the susceptible dogs when compared with the resistant dogs (203 ± 40 vs. 294 ± 33, P < 0.01). This difference was reduced to 2 % after administration of 3 µg/kg of scopolamine (224 ± 23 vs. 198 ± 43; NS).

Thus, the effect of scopolamine in autonomic markers in this experimental study paralleled the clinical findings observed in the 4 studies in post-myocardial infarction patients. Additionally, 3.0 µg/kg of scopolamine reduced heart rate at rest and during the lower levels of exercise and ischemia test. However, the chronotropic effect of scopolamine disappeared at higher levels of exercise. During the exercise and ischemia test just prior to the occlusion of the circumflex coronary artery, heart rate was 227 ± 8 b/min in the control test and 226 ± 7 b/min with scopolamine. The reflex response to acute myocardial ischemia was also, in this setting, unaffected by scopolamine. Heart rate at 30 seconds of ischemia was 245 ± 15 b/min in the control tests and 244 ± 15 b/min with scopolamine (Fig. 5).

The critical finding of the study was that scopolamine had minimal antifibrillatory effect. Ventricular fibrillation was indeed prevented in only 1 (14 %) of the 7 susceptible dogs in which it was tested (Fig. 6).

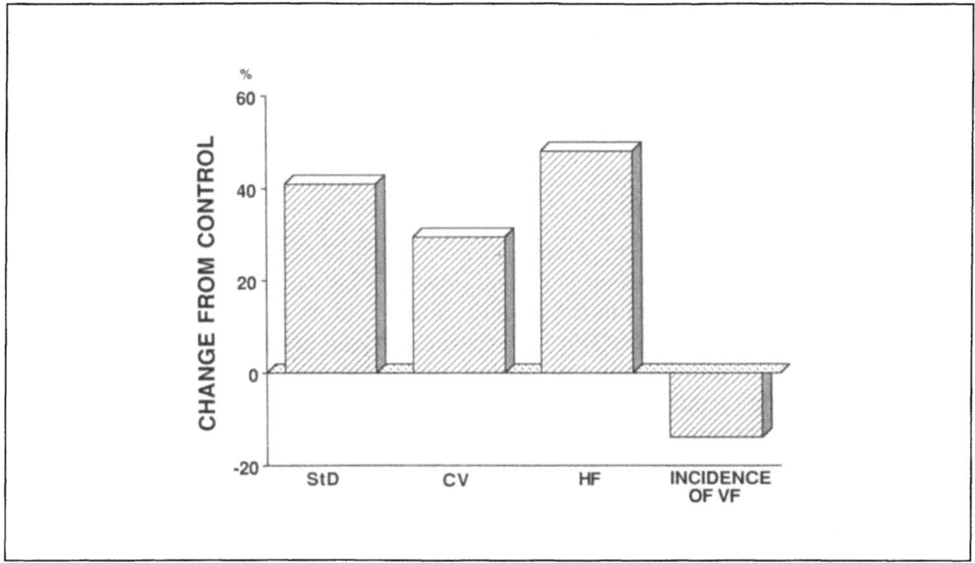

Fig. 6 Effect of low dose scopolamine on different measures of heart rate variability and on risk for ventricular fibrillation during the exercise and ischemia test. Std = standard deviation of RR intervals; CV = coefficient of variance; HF = power in the high frequency band of spectral analysis of heart rate variability.

Mechanisms of action of low dose muscarinic receptors blockers and possible explanation of the observed failure

Low dose atropine increases neural activity directly recorded in the vagus (21). Acetylcholine mediates the effects of inhibitory fibers projecting from the ventrolateral respiratory reticular formation on the vagal motoneurons (29). Specifically, during inspiration acetylcholine released from these fibers causes a hyperpolarization of vagal motoneurons and, consequently, a reduction in their firing rate. Atropine, by blocking these inhibitory mechanisms may increase the activity of vagal motoneurons. This hypothesis is supported by the fact that iontophoretic administration of atropine in the area of the nucleus ambiguous increases the activity of vagal-cardiac motoneurons (29). In addition to central actions, peripheral mechanisms, notably blockade of the presynaptic muscarinic modulation of acetylcholine release (53), may contribute to the effect of low dose scopolamine on HRV. This is suggested by the evidence that pirenzepine, the analog of scopolamine that does not seem to have central actions, increases HRV (33).

The chronotropic effects of scopolamine progressively decreased with exercise and were largely lost at the highest workload of the submaximal test. The reflex response to acute myocardial ischemia was also unaffected by scopolamine. Overall, the vagal antagonism of the detrimental electrophysiologic effects of adrenergic activation (22) was absent when mostly needed. Based on these findings, the failure of scopolamine in preventing ventricular fibrillation is no longer surprising, particularly in a preparation in which sympathetic reflexes are major contributors to the occurrence of lethal arrhythmias.

The dose of scopolamine may represent a possible mechanism involved in the apparent discrepancy between effects on autonomic markers and effects on lethal arrhythmias. At doses higher than 3 μg/kg it produces two opposite effects, as it markedly increases efferent vagal activity, while simultaneously blocking the vagal effects on heart rate. Thus, the prevalence of the cardiac post-synaptic vagolytic effect of scopolamine at higher doses limits its use to doses probably inadequate to counteract the elevated adrenergic activation due to exercise and ischemia-dependent reflexes.

Clinical implications

The clinical implications of the present data are that low dose of muscarinic receptors blockers have a positive effect on autonomic markers but seems to be of little effect in reducing risk for lethal events in the acutely ischemic heart specifically at a time when sympathetic activity is elevated. This is in sharp contrast to what has been observed with exercise training, which by affecting several aspects of the cardiovascular system and regulation significantly increases autonomic markers and also provides a striking protection from ventricular fibrillation.

On the other hand the potential importance of a chronic (as with exercise training) versus an acute (as with scopolamine) modulation of the autonomic activity shold not be underestimated. From this prospective the use of pirenzepine, a muscarinic antagonist, that as just described increases autonomic markers and can be chronically used may open the prospective of long term treatment. The possibility of a chronic modulation of cardiac vagal activity in high risk post-myocardial infarction patients deserves attention. A multicenter pilot study involving the Fondazione Maugeri and the University of Pavia is currently ongoing in Italy. This study is aimed at testing the effects of long term therapy with oral pirenzepine in post-myocardial infarction patients with a depressed left ventricular function and markers suggestive of a depressed cardiac vagal activity. The two main issues to be addressed are the persistence over time of the autonomic effects of pirenzepine and its tolerability. If a chronic modulation of cardiac vagal activity appears feasible, this will open the prospective of testing such an intervention in a large post-myocardial infarction population. The experimental evidence that acute administration of these compounds does not reduce risk for ventricular fibrillation in the setting of a new acute ischemic episode after a recent myocardial infarction does not exclude the possibility that chronic vagal stimulation may favorably influence the recovery from a myocardial infarction and ultimately reduce the risk for lethal events.

Conclusions

The rationale for the attempts to increase autonomic markers in post-myocardial infarction patients rests on the multiple evidende that the risk for cardiac mortality and sudden death is higher among individuals with signs of decreased vagal activity. Contrasting scatter data exists about the effects of beta-blockers, which so far represent one of the most effective treatment after myocardial infarction, on autonomic markers (39). ACE inhibitors, which are also effective in reducing mortality after myocardial infarction, probably exert an useful action on sympathovagal balance (3).

A major limitation to the use of autonomic markers to predict efficacy is represented by the fact the degree of increase in vagal activity that may produce antifibillatory effects is still unknown. Exercise training acts on several aspects of cardiovascular regulation and function, shifts the autonomic balance toward a vagal dominance, and significantly increases cardiac electrical stability. On the other hand, low dose of muscarinic antagonists, while positively affecting autonomic markers, seem to have little effect on cardiac electrical stability specifically in condition of elevated sympathetic activity. A possible explanation for this failure is that acute administrations of these compounds looses efficacy when mostly needed, i.e., in the condition of elevated sympathetic activity. The possibility that chronic treatment with low dose muscarinic antagonists may be beneficial deserves further investigation. However, based on the current knowledge it seems appropriate to call for caution before attributing excessive importance to changes in "markers" of vagal activity in the absence of clearcut evidence for a causal relation with an antifibrillatory effect.

References

1. Bedford GB,Tipton CM (1987) Exercise training and arterial baroreflex. J Appl Physiol 63: 1926–1932
2. Billman GE, Schwartz PJ, Stone HL (1984) The effects of daily exercise on susceptibility to sudden cardiac death. Circulation 69 (6): 1182–1189
3. Bonaduce D, Petretta M, Morgano G et al. (1992) Effects of converting enzyme inhibition on baroreflex sensitivity in patients with myocardial infarction. J Am Coll Cardiol 20: 587–93
4. Casadei B, Pipilis A, Sessa F, Conway J, Sleight P (1993) Low doses of scopolamine increases cardiac vagal tone in the acute phase of myocardial infarction. Circulation 88: 335–357
5. Cerati D, Schwartz PJ (1991) Single cardiac vagal fiber activity, acute myocardial ischemia, and risk for sudden death. Circ Res 69: 1389–1401
6. Corr PB, Yamada KA, Witkowski FX (1986) Mechanisms controlling cardiac autonomic function and their relation to arrhythmogenesis. In: The heart and cardiovascular system. Vol II (Fozzard HA, Haber E, Jennings RB, Katz AM, Morgan HE (Eds) Raven Press, New York, pp 1343–1403
7. De Ferrari GM, Grossoni M, Salvati P, Patrono C, Schwartz PJ (1993) Reflex response to acute myocardial ischemia in conscious dogs susceptible to ventricular fibrillation. Eur Heart J 14 (Abstr Suppl): 41
8. De Ferrari GM, Mantica M, Vanoli E, Hull SS Jr, Schwartz PJ (1993) Scopolamine increases vagal tone and vagal reflexes in patients after myocardial infarction. J Am Coll Cardiol 22: 1327–1334
9. De Ferrari GM, Salvati P, Grossoni M, Ukmar G, Vaga L, Patrono C, Schwartz PJ (1993) Pharmacologic modulation of the autonomic nervous system in the prevention of sudden cardiac death. A study with propranolol, methacholine and oxotremorine in conscious dogs with a healed myocardial infarction. J Am Coll Cardiol 21: 283–290
10. De Ferrari GM, Vanoli E, Curcuruto P, Tommasini G, Schwartz PJ (1992) Prevention of life-threatening arrhythmias by pharmacologic stimulation of the muscarinic receptors with oxotremorine. Am Heart J 124: 883–890
11. De Ferrari GM, Vanoli E, Schwarz PJ (1995) Cardiac vagal activity, myocardial ischemia and sudden death. In: Cardiac electrophysiology. From cell to bedside. II edition (Zipes DP and Jalife J, Eds) WB Saunders Co, Philadelphia, pp 422–434
12. De Ferrari GM Vanoli E, Stramba-Badiale M, Hull SS Jr, Foreman RD, Schwartz PJ (1991) Vagal reflexes and survival during acute myocardial ischemia in conscious dogs with healed myocardial infarction. Am J Physiol 261: H63–H69
13. De Schryver C, De Herdt P, Lammerant J (1967) Effect of physical training on cardiac catecholamine concentrations. Nature (London) 214: 907–912
14. Detry JR, Rousseau M, Vanderbrouke G, Kusumi F, Brasseur LA, Bruce RA (1971) Increased arteriovenous oxygen difference after physical training in coronary artery disease. Circulation 44: 109–118
15. Ekelund GL, Haskell WL, Johnson JL, Whaley FS, Criqui MH, Sheps DS (1988) Physical fitness as a predictor of cardiovascular mortality in asymptomatic North American men: the Lipid Research Clinics Mortality Follow-up Study. N Engl J Med 319: 1379–1384
16. Farrell TG, Paul V, Cripps TR et al. (1991) Baroreflex sensitivity and electrophysiological correlates in patients after acute myocardial infarction. Circulation 83: 945–952
17. Gnecchi Ruscone T, Lombardi F, Malfatto G, Malliani A (1987) Attenuation of baroreceptive mechanisms by cardiovascular sympathetic afferent fibers. Am J Physiol 253: H787–H791
18. Hull SS, Evans AR, Vanoli E, Adamson PB, Stramba-Badiale M, Albert DE, Foreman RD, Schwartz PJ (1990) Heart rate variability before and after myocardial infarction in conscious dogs at high and low risk of sudden death. J Am Coll Cardiol 16: 978–985
19. Hull SS Jr, Vanoli E, Adamson PB, Verrier RL, Foreman RD, Schwartz PJ (1994) Exercise training confers anticipatory protection from sudden death during acute myocardial ischemia. Circulation 89: 548–552

20. Hull SS Jr, Vanoli E, Adamson PB, De Ferrari GM, Foreman RD, Schwartz PJ (1995) Do increases in markers of vagal activity imply protection from sudden death? The case of scopolamine. Circulation 91: 2516–2519
21. Katona PG, Lipson D, Dauchot PJ (1977) Opposing central and peripheral effects of atropine on parasympathetic cardiac control. Am J Physiol 232: H146–H151
22. La Rovere MT, Bigger JT Jr, Marcus FI, Mortara A, Camm AJ, Hohnloser SH, Nohara R, Schwartz PJ (1995) Prognostic value of depressed baroreflex sensitivity. The ATRAMI study. (Abstr.) Circulation 92: 676
23. La Rovere MT, Specchia G, Mortara A, Schwartz PJ (1988) Baroreflex sensitivity, clinical correlates and cardiovascular mortality among patients with a first myocardial infarction. A prospective study. Circulation 78: 816–824
24. Liang IYS, Stone HL (1983) Changes in diastolic coronary resistance during submaximal exercise in conditioned dogs. J Appl Physiol 54: 1057–1962
25. Lown B, Verrier RL (1976) Neural activity and ventricular fibrillation. New England J Medicine 294 (21): 1165–1170
26. Marracini P, Orsini E, Nassi G, Michelassi C, L'Abbate A (1992) Usefulness of pirenzepine, an M_1 antimuscarinic agent, for effort myocardial ischemia. Am J Cardiol 69: 1407–11
27. Malliani A, Recordati G, Schwartz PJ (1973) Nervous activity of afferent cardiac sympathetic fibres with atrial and ventricular endings. J Physiol 229: 457–469
28. Malliani A, Schwartz PJ, Zanchetti A (1969) A sympathetic reflex elicited by experimental coronary occlusion. Am J Physiol 217: 703–709
29. McCloskey DI (1994) Cardiorespiratory integration. In: Vagal control of the heart: Experimental basis and clinical implications (Levy MN and Schwartz PJ eds) Futura Publishing Co, Armonk, NY, pp 481-508
30. Noakes TD, Higginson L, Opie LH (1983) Physical training increases the ventricular fibrillation threshold of isolated hearts during normoxia, hypoxia and regional ischemia. Circulation 67: 24–30
31. O'Connor GT, Buring JE, Yusuf S, Goldhaber SZ, Olmstead M, Paffenbarger RS Jr, Hennekens CH (1989) An overview of randomized trials of rehabilitation with exercise after myocardial infarction. Circulation 80: 234–244
32. Pagani M, Somers V, Furlan R, Dell'Orto S, Conway J, Baselli G, Cerutti S, Sleight P (1988) Changes in autonomic regulation induced by physical training in mild hypertension. Hypertension 12: 600–610
33. Pedretti RFE, Colombo E, Sarzi Braga S, Ballardini L, Carù B (1995) Effects of oral pirenzepine on heart rate variability and baroreceptor reflex sensitivity after acute myocardial infarction. J Am Coll Cardiol 25: 915–921
34. Pedretti R, Colombo E, Sarzi Braga S, Carù B (1993) Influence of transdermal scopolamine on cardiac sympathovagal interaction after acute myocardial infarction. Am J Cardiol 72: 384–392
35. Posel D, Noakes T, Kantor P, Lambert M, Opie LH (1989) Exercise training after experimental myocardial infarction increases the ventricular fibrillation threshold before and after the onset of reinfarction in the isolated rat heart. Circulation 80: 138–145
36. Sandvik L, Erikssen J, Thaulow E, Erikssen G, Mundal R, Rodahl K (1993) Physical fitness as a predictor of cardiovascular mortality among healthy, middle-aged norwegian man. N Engl J Med 328: 533–537
37. Scheuer J, Tipton CM (1977) Cardiovascular adaptations to physical training. Ann Rev Physiol 39: 221–251
38. Schwartz PJ, Billman GE, Stone HL (1984) Autonomic mechanisms in ventricular fibrillation induced by myocardial ischemia during exercise in dogs with a healed myocardial infarction. An experimental preparation for sudden cardiac death. Circulation 69: 780–790
39. Schwartz PJ, De Ferrari GM (1995) Interventions changing heart rate variability after acute myocardial infarction. In: Heart rate variability (Malik M, Camm AJ eds) Futura Publishing Company Inc, Armonk, NY pp 407–420
40. Schwartz PJ, La Rovere MT, Vanoli E (1982) Autonomic nervous system and sudden cardiac death. Circulation 85 (suppl I): 77–91
41. Schwartz PJ, Priori SG (1990) Sympathetic nervous system and cardiac arrhythmias. In: Cardiac electrophysiology. From cell to bedside (Zipes DP, Jalife J (eds) WB Saunders Co, Philadelphia, pp 330–343
42. Schwartz PJ, Vanoli E, Stramba-Badiale M, De Ferrari GM, Billman GE, Foreman RD (1988) Autonomic mechanisms and sudden death. New insights from the analysis of baroreceptor reflexes in conscious dogs with and without a myocardial infarction. Circulation 78: 969–979
43. Smyth HS, Sleight P, Pickering GW (1969) Reflex regulation of arterial pressure during sleep in man. Circ Res 24: 109–121
44. Stone HL (1977) Cardiac function and exercise training in conscious dogs. J Appl Physiol 42: 824–832
45. Sylvestre-Gervais L, Nadeau A, Nguyen MH, Tancrede G, Rousseau-Migneron S (1982) Effects of physical training on beta-adrenergic receptors in rat myocardial tissue. Cardiovasc Res 16: 530–534
46. Task Force of the European Society of Cardiology and the North American Society of Pacing and Electrophysiology (Bigger JT Jr, Breithardt G, Camm AJ, Cerutti S, Cohen RJ, Coumel P, Fallen EL, Kennedy HL, Kleiger RE, Lombardi F, Malik M, Malliani A, Moss AJ, Rottman JN, Schmidt G, Schwartz PJ, Singer DH): Heart rate variability (1996) Standards of measurement, physiological interpretation, and clinical use. Circulation 93: 1043–1065, and Eur Heart J 17: 354–381

47. Vanoli E, Adamson PB, Cerati D, Hull SS (1995) Heart rate variability and risk stratification post-myocardial infarction. In: Heart rate variability (Malik M, Camm AJ eds) Futura publishing. Armonk NY, pp 347–361
48. Vanoli E, De Ferrari GM, Stramba-Badiale M, Hull SS Jr, Foreman RD, Schwartz PJ (1991) Vagal stimulation and prevention of sudden death in conscious dogs with a healed myocardial infarction. Circ Res 68: 1471–1481
49. Vanoli E, Schwartz PJ (1990) Sympathetic-parasympathetic interaction and sudden death. Basic Res in Cardiol 85 (Suppl 1): 305–321
50. Verani MS, Hartung GH, Hoepfel-Harris J, Wellon DE, Pratt CM, Miller RR (1981) Effects of exercise training on left ventricular performance and myocardial perfusion in patients with coronary artery disease. Am J Cardiol 47: 797–786
51. Vybiral T, Glaeser DH, Morris G, Hess KR, Yang K, Francis M, Pratt CM (1993) Effects of low doses scopolamine on heart rate variability in acute myocardial infarction. J Am Coll Cardiol 22: 1320–1326
52. Wellstein A, Pitschner HF. Complex dose-response curves of atropine in man explained by different functions of M1- and M2-cholinoceptors (1988). Naunyn-Schmiedeberg's Arch Pharmacol 338: 19–27
53. Wetzel GT, Brown JH (1985) Presynaptic modulation of acetylcholine release from cardiac parasympathetic neurons. Am J Physiol 248: H33
54. Wilson FN (1915) The production of atrioventricular rhythm in man after the administration of atropine. Arch Intern Med 16: 989–1007

Author's address:
Emilio Vanoli, MD
Dipartimento di Cardiologia
Università di Pavia
IRCCS San Matteo
Piazza Golgi 2
Pavia
Italy

Left ventricular restoring forces:
Modulation by heart rate and contractility

M. M. LeWinter, J. Fabian, S. P. Bell

Cardiology Unit, Fletcher Allen Health Care, MCHV Campus, Burlington, USA

Abstract

We used a servomotor system in open-chest dogs to rapidly clamp left atrial pressure below left ventricular (LV) diastolic pressure in order to produce nonfilling diastoles during which the LV fully relaxed at its end-systolic volume (ESV). Restoring forces (RFs) generated during contraction which result in LV filling by suction were considered to be present when the fully relaxed pressure (FRP) was negative. We characterized RFs in terms of the fully relaxed pressure-volume relation (FRPV relation, FRP plotted vs ESV), which has negative and positive portions and an equilibrium volume (FRP = 0 mmHg). A negative FRP is ordinarily present over the lower half of the physiologic filling range. Increased contractility (systemic dobutamine) shifts the FRPV relation downward, indicating greater RFs at any ESV. Intracoronary dobutamine administered via the left anterior descending coronary artery has the same effect. Acute increases in heart rate from about 100 to 150 beats/min did not alter the FRPV relation. In contrast, chronic tachycardia heart failure resulted in marked depression of the ability to generate RFs, even at very low volumes. Thus, RFs normally contribute to LV filling. They are augmented by acute increases in global and anterior wall contractility but not heart rate, within the range specified above. Chronic tachycardia heart failure markedly attenuated RFs. The latter may constitute a previously unappreciated mechanism of diastolic dysfunction in heart failure.

Key words Restoring forces – left ventricle – diastolic function – suction

Introduction

When the left ventricle (LV) contracts below its equilibrium volume (Veq) in the end-systolic (ES) configuration, the chamber may be considered to be under compression, meaning that restoring forces (RFs) have been generated during contraction. The magnitude of RFs is inversely related to ES volume (ESV). When dissipated, the energy of these forces returns LV volume to the equilibrium value, resulting in filling by suction (19). Although physiologists have been aware of suction for many years (3, 6, 12), quantitative study of RFs which cause suction has been difficult, especially in the intact heart, because the process of filling obscures the presence of RFs. To help delineate the presence and magnitude of RFs, Yellin, Nikolic, and co-workers replaced the mitral valve with an electronically controlled prosthesis in open-chest dogs (15, 20). The prosthesis was maintained in the closed position following a ventricular systole, resulting in a non-filling diastole during which the LV fully relaxed at its ES volume. Under these conditions, a negative fully relaxed pressure (FRP) indicates that RFs are present (i.e., LV volume is below Veq) and is a measure of their magnitude. These investigators measured very substantially negative FRPs (–5 to –10 mmHg) at LV volumes thought to be within the physiologic range (15). Recently, we reported the use of a servomotor system connected to the left atrium (LA) which rapidly clamps LA pressure at a value below LV diastolic pressure (2), eliminating the pressure gradient for LV filling and resulting in a nonfilling diastole. This system was based on a modification of that originally reported by Ingels et al. (10). This approach allows us to measure the FRP without disrupting the mitral valve and apparatus, a potential drawback of the prosthetic valve method. In this chapter, we will review selected results using this method, with an emphasis on effects of changes in heart rate and global and regional contractility on RFs.

Methods

All experiments were performed in open-chest mongrel dogs (median sternotomy and bilateral thoracotomy), anesthetized with either i.v. pentobarbital or halothane. Instrumen-

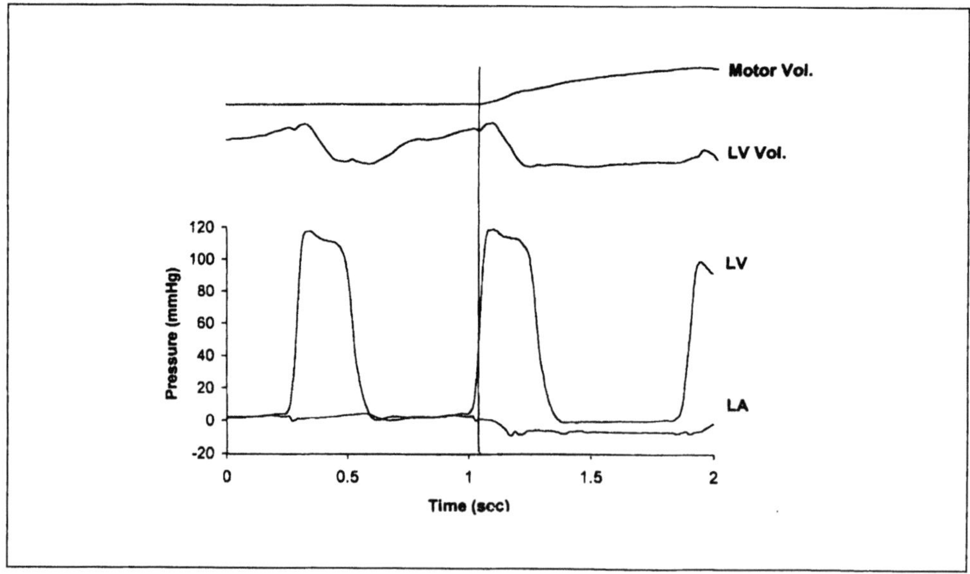

Fig. 1 Example of a nonfilling diastole during which the left ventricle (LV) fully relaxes at its end-systolic volume. Vertical cursor indicates time at which servomotor begins to withdraw volume from left atrium (LA) to clamp LA pressure below LV pressure. (Reprinted by permission from Bell SP, Fabian J, Higashiyama A, Chen Z, Tischler MD, Watkins MW, LeWinter MM (1996) Restoring forces assessed with left atrial pressure clamps. Am J Physiol 270: H1015–1020.)

tation consisted of Millar micromanometer pressure sensors in the LV and LA, a volume conductance catheter inserted into the LV through the apical dimple and, in some cases, sonomicrometer crystals implanted in the anterior midwall of the LV. The servomotor system has recently been described (2) and consists of a computer controlled linear motor-syringe assembly connected to the LA which either withdraws or adds blood in order to change and then clamp LA pressure (P) at a specified value through the succeeding diastole. To produce a non-filling diastole, the LAP was clamped at less than LV diastolic pressure. To verify the absence of filling, we required that the LV volume not change beyond the time when the LVP reached the LA-LV crossover pressure (determined from the preceding beat) and that the LVP decline monotonically to its fully relaxed value. We also confirmed absence of transmitral flow using color Doppler echocardiography when these criteria were met (2). Examples of typical tracings obtained during a non-filling diastole are shown in Fig. 1. Timing of hemodynamic events (end-diastole, end-systole, etc) was accomplished with standard algorithms (2).

In order to delineate the relation between ESV and FRP (the FRPV relation), ESV was varied with brief, steady-state constrictions of the caval vessels or the descending thoracic aorta, and volume infusion. The sinus node specific calcium channel antagonist zatebradine (Boehringer Ingelheim, Ridgefield, CT), 1 mg/kg iv, was employed to lower the native rate to < 90 beats/min. The LA was then electronically paced throughout to maintain a constant rate (90–100 beats/min). LA pacing was briefly discontinued coincident with each LAP clamp. Global contractility was augmented with intravenous dobutamine at a dose sufficient to increase steady-state LV peak + dP/dt by 30–40 %. Regional contractility was augmented by administration of dobutamine via a cannula inserted in the left anterior descending (LAD) coronary artery just distal to its first diagonal branch. The dose of intracoronary dobutamine was set at 10 % of the intravenous dose.

Tachycardia heart failure was produced by implantation of an epicardial right ventricular pacemaker lead and pulse generator under sterile conditions and pacing the right ventricle at 240 beats/min for two weeks. At that time, open chest studies as described above were undertaken after cessation of ventricular pacing.

Results

Results from individual experiments relating LV end-diastolic pressure (EDP) to the FRP as cardiac filling is varied solely by altering venous return (caval constriction, volume infusion) are shown in Fig. 2. On average, at a LVEDP of 4.0 ± 1.5 (± SD) FRP was –2.1 ± 1.9 mmHg, at LVEDP 8.1 ± 0.9 mmHg FRP was –0.2 mmHg, and at LVEDP 12.8 ± 2.1 mmHg FRP was 1.1 ± 3.2 mmHg. ESV progressively increased as LVEDP increased. Thus, in the open chest dog, Veq occurs at about the midphysiologic filling range and RFs are present over roughly the lower half of physiologic LV filling pressures. Typical results relating ESV to FRP, the FRPV relation, are shown in Fig. 3. This relation was derived from sequential caval and aortic constrictions. Note the inverse relationship between ESV and the FRP. The effects of systemic and regional dobutamine administration on the FRPV relation are displayed in Fig. 4. Both interventions result in a downward shift of this relation, i.e., RFs were increased at any ESV in this range. Increasing heart rate from baseline levels (typically 90–100 beats/min) to 140–150 beats/min had no measurable effect on the FRPV relation. In contrast, preliminary results indicate that chronic tachycardia has striking

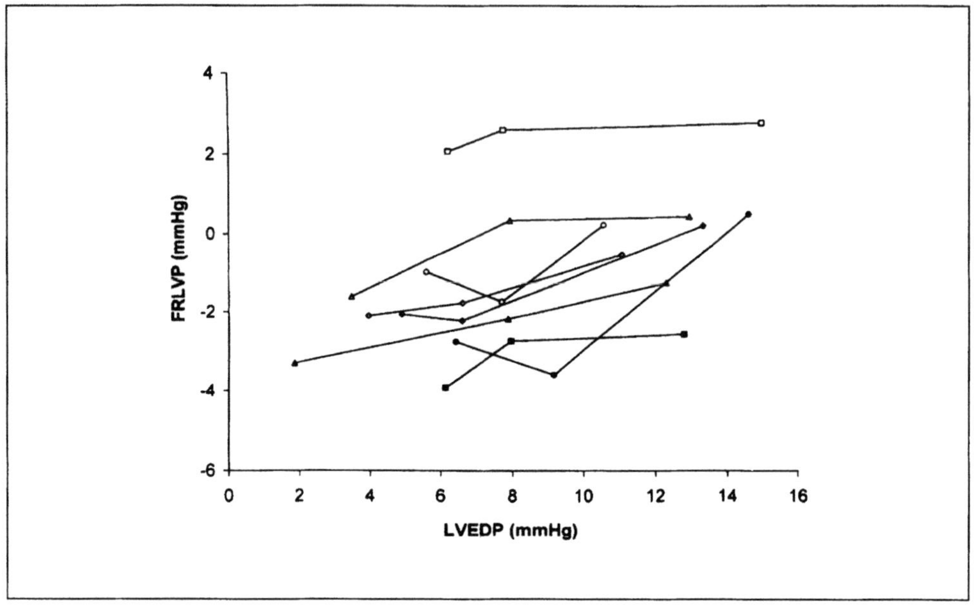

Fig. 2 Data points relating LVEDP to the fully relaxed LV pressure (FRLVP) in individual experiments as LV volume is altered by changing venous return. As LVEDP increases, the fully relaxed pressure also increases. (Reprinted by permission from Bell SP, Fabian J, Higashiyama A, Chen Z, Tischler MD, Watkins MW, LeWinter MM (1996) Restoring forces assessed with left atrial pressure clamps. Am J Physiol 270: H1015–1020.)

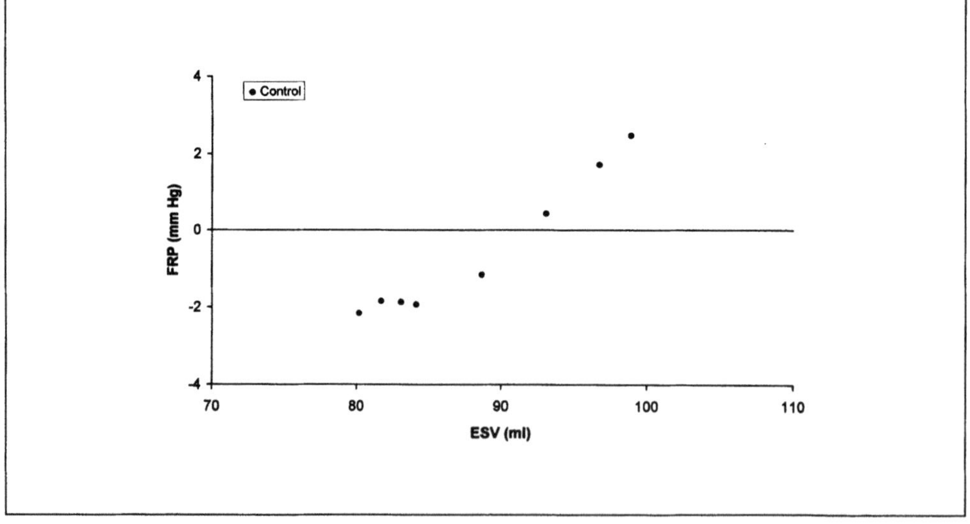

Fig. 3 An example of the relation between fully relaxed pressure (FRP) and end-systolic volume (ESV) as ESV is varied by caval and aortic constrictions in a normal (control) dog. ESV obtained from conductance catheter is uncalibrated in this example.

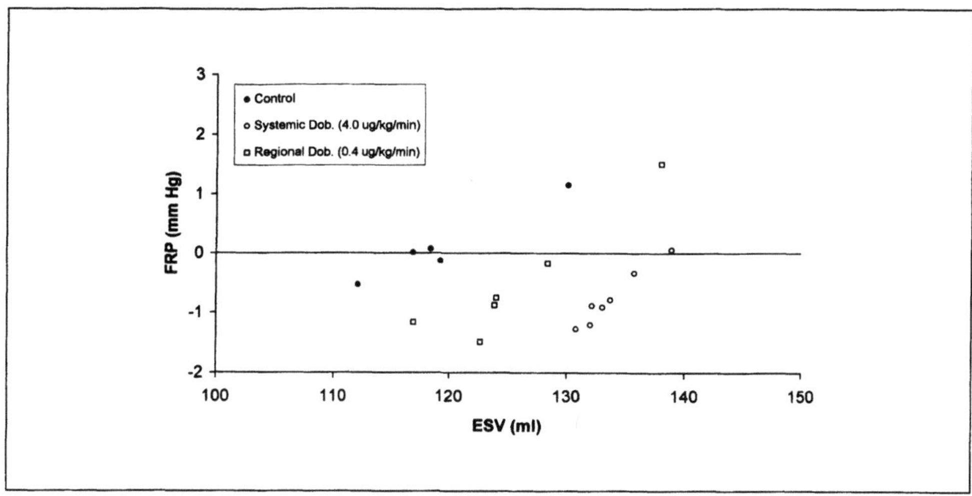

Fig. 4 An example of the effect of systemic (open circles) and regional (intracoronary, open squares) dobutamine administration on the relation between FRP and ESV (see text). Note downward displacement of the relation compared to control data (closed circles). ESV uncalibrated.

effects on the ability of the LV to generate RFs. An example is shown in Fig. 5, in which LVEDP is plotted against FRP during alterations in venous return. Note that the FRP fails to become negative even at very low LVEDP levels. The FRPV relation in a group of control dogs is plotted in Fig. 6, along with data from one of the tachycardia failure animals. Once again, the LV does not generate RFs even at very low ESVs. Interestingly, regional dobutamine displaced the FRPV relation downward toward a more normal position in one failure animal.

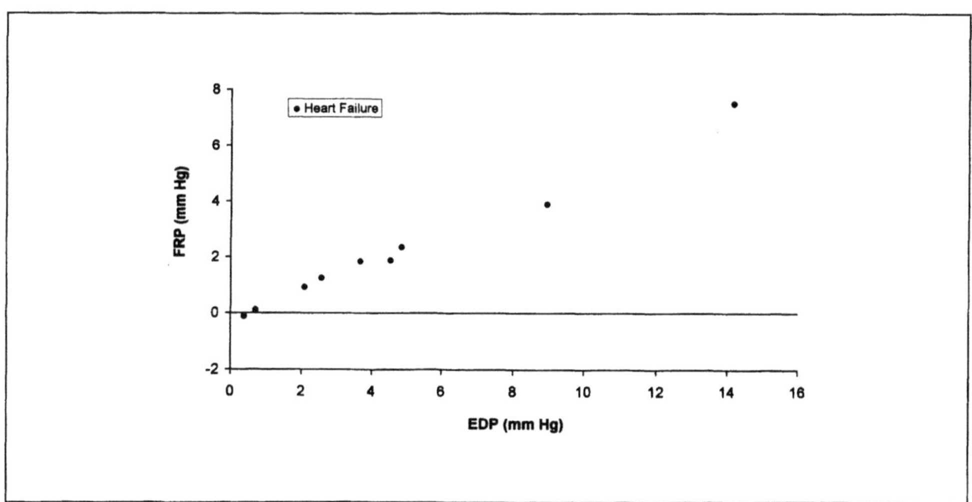

Fig. 5 An example of the relation between FRP and LVEDP in a tachycardia heart failure dog. Note that even at very low LVEDP, the FRP does not become significantly negative.

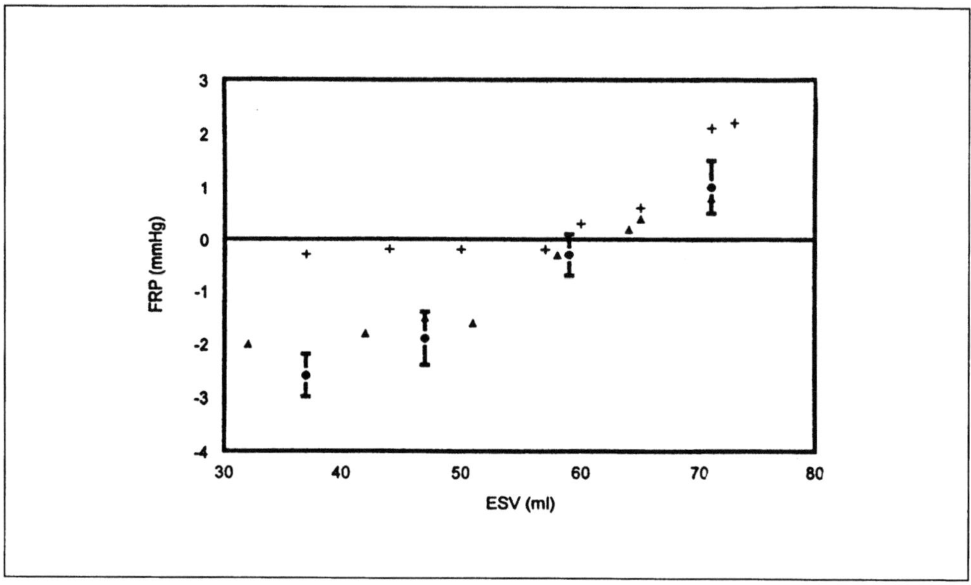

Fig. 6 Relation between ESV (calibrated) and FRP in a group of normal control dogs (circles, ± SE) and another tachycardia heart failure dog (crosses). Note that in the heart failure dog FRP fails to become significantly negative at ESV at which FRP is clearly negative in control dogs, indicating loss of ability to generate RFs. During regional dobutamine (triangles) the relation is shifted toward that present in the control dogs.

Discussion

RFs generated during contraction result in elastic recoil and ventricular filling by suction. Under some conditions in which ventricular volume is very small, suction can be the predominant mechanism of filling and appears to account for a significant fraction of the volume entering the ventricle during each diastole even at normal filling pressures (4, 11, 19, 21). RFs can be generated and stored within individual myocytes (14), possibly in the myocardial connective tissue matrix (18) and as a component of both transmural and three-dimensional systolic deformation of the LV, the latter including twist, or torsional rotation around the ventricular long axis (1, 5, 7, 8, 9). The relative contribution of these mechanisms and how they are integrated is unknown. Recent studies have delineated changes in the magnitude and timing of twist and untwisting as a function of loading conditions, contractility and ventricular volume (8, 17). Decreases in ESV increase twist (8); increases in contractility increase twist and prolong the onset of diastolic untwisting. Thus, interventions which increase twist and alter its timing are also those which would be expected to increase RFs. It has also been speculated that delaying the timing of untwisting has a specific role in generation of RFs by allowing further stretching of functional springs between the subepicardial and subendocardial layers of the myocardium (17).

Our LA servomotor system allows us to quantitatively study RFs in the intact LV without interfering with the normal mitral valve. In this regard, it is of interest that the magnitude of RFs we observe are significantly less than that observed previously in the prosthetic mitral valve preparation (15, 20). This does not necessarily imply that RFs are unimportant as a determinant of filling. Even a FRP of –2 mmHg is likely to be significant when it is kept in mind that this value is of the same magnitude as the normal early diastolic LA-LV pressure gradient that drives filling.

Two clinical studies in which LV pressure was measured during obstruction of the mitral valve by a balloon used for percutaneous valvuloplasty for mitral stenosis have been reported. Paulus et al. (16) did not record negative LV pressures during mitral obstruction. In contrast, Nakatani et al. (13) recorded a minimum LV pressure averaging –6 mmHg in their group of patients. In view of these widely discrepant results, it is very difficult to relate these findings to our results other than to note the obvious facts that our studies were performed in an open-chest, anesthetized preparation in which the heart was structurally normal, while the clinical studies were performed under much more physiologic conditions with a structurally abnormal heart. The reason for the discrepant results is unclear, but could conceivably be related to balloon inflation methodology or differences in patient characteristics.

Our results indicate that increases in heart rate produced by atrial pacing between about 100 and 150 beats minute do not influence the FRPV relation, i. e., this magnitude of increase does not alter the intrinsic ability of the LV to generate RFs. We suspect that the force-frequency relationship does not result in enough of an increase in contractility over this heart rate range in our preparation to result in a measurable change. Given the usual magnitude of RFs, it is possible that an unmeasurably small change using our techniques could have a significant effect on filling. Additionally, it is possible that acute increases in heart rate over a wider range might have been associated with a measurable effect on RFs. In contrast, increases in both global and regional anterior wall contractility shifted the FRPV relation downward, indicating an increase in the intrinsic ability of the LV to generate RFs.

One explanation for these findings is a change in twist or the timing of twist-untwisting that augments RFs. However, it is unlikely that such changes would be reflected as a component of the FRP, since they presumably would have dissipated during the course of relaxation. Alternatively, it is possible that systemic and regional dobutamine increase wall thickness (transmural deformation) in the fully relaxed state with resultant increased stretch of elastic elements in the wall which cause RFs. Since the increase in RFs occurred acutely, a potential mechanism for increased wall thickness is an increase in coronary blood volume. Clearly, additional studies will be required to precisely delineate how systemic and regional dobutamine increase RFs.

Although preliminary, our results in dogs with chronic tachycardia heart failure demonstrate a striking change in the FRPV relation, denoting a marked reduction in the intrinsic ability of the LV to generate RFs. Thus, loss of the ability to generate RFs may constitute a previously unappreciated mechanism of impaired filling during heart failure. One explanation for this observation is that it simply reflects depression of the force-frequency relationship accompanying heart failure. However, since we did not assess the influence of the force-frequency relationship on RF generation over a range appropriate to the heart failure dogs (i.e., between a typical physiologic basal rate of 60 beats/min and the rate at which our open-chest studies were performed, usually 90–100 beats/ min), we cannot comment on this point. Alternatively, the results in heart failure may simply reflect changes occurring in conjunction with chronically depressed contractility, i.e., the opposite of what was observed with dobutamine.

In summary, RFs represent a significant mechanism of filling in our preparation and their magnitude is related both to the ESV and to global and regional contractility. The force-frequency relationship does not appear to markedly influence RF generation, but studies encompassing a larger range of heart rate are required to fully elucidate this. Heart failure caused by chronic increases in heart rate appears to markedly depress RF generation, and therefore suction, as a mechanism of LV filling.

Acknowledgment   This research was supported by National Institutes of Health Grant RO1 HL-51201.

References

1. Arts T, Meerbaum S, Reneman RS, Corday (1984) Torsion of the left ventricle during the ejection phase in the intact dog. Cardiovasc Res 18: 183–193
2. Bell SP, Fabian J, Higashiyama A, Chen Z, Tischler MD, Watkins MW, LeWinter MM (1996) Restoring forces assessed with left atrial pressure clamps. Am J Physiol 270: H1015–1020
3. Brecher GA (1968) Critical review of recent work on ventricular diastolic suction. Circ Res 6: 554–566
4. Brutsaert DL, Sys SU (1989) Relaxation and diastole of the heart. Physiol Rev 69: 1228–1315
5. Buchalter MB, Weiss JL, Rogers WJ, Zerhouni EA, Weisfeldt ML, Beyar R, Shapiro EP (1990) Noninvasive quantification of left ventricular rotational deformation in normal humans using magnetic resonance imaging myocardial tagging. Circulation 81: 1236–1244
6. Cohn AE (1929) The development of the Harveian circulation. The Harvey Lectures 1927–1928. The Williams and Wilkins Co., Baltimore
7. DeAnda A Jr, Komeda M, Nikolic SD, Daughters GT II, Ingels NB, Miller C (1995) Left ventricular function, twist, and recoil after mitral valve replacement. Circulation 92 [suppl II]: II458–II466
8. Gibbons Kroeker CA, Tyberg JV, Beyar R (1995) Effect of load manipulations, heart rate, and contractility on left ventricular apical rotation. Circulation 92: 130–141
9. Ingels NB Jr, Hansen DE, Daughters GT II, Stinson EB, Alderman EL, Miller DC (1989) Relation between longitudinal, circumferential, and oblique shortening and torsional deformation in the left ventricle of the transplanted human heart. Circulation 64: 915–927
10. Ingels NB Jr, Daughters GT II, Nikolic SD, De Anda A, Moon MR, Bolger AF, Komeda M, Derby GC, Yellin EL, Miller DC (1994) Left atrial pressure-clamp servomechanism demonstrates LV suction in canine hearts with normal mitral valves. Am J Physiol 267: H354–H362
11. Ingels NB Jr, Daughters GT, Nikolic SD, DeAnda A, Moon MR, Bolger AF, Komeda M, Derby GC, Yellin EL, Miller DC (1996) Left ventricular diastolic suction with zero left atrial pressure in open chest dogs. Am J Physiol 270: H1217–1224
12. Katz LN (1930) The role played by the ventricular relaxation process in filling the ventricle. Am J Physiol 95: 542–550
13. Nakatani S, Beppu S, Nagata S, Ishikura F, Tamai J, Yamagishi M, Ohmori F, Kimura K, Takamiya M, Miyatake K (1994) Diastolic suction in the human ventricle: Observation during balloon mitral valvuloplasty with a single balloon. Am Heart J 127: 143–147
14. Niggli E, Lederer WJ (1991) Restoring forces in cardiac myocytes. Insight from relaxations induced by photolysis of caged ATP. Biophys J 59: 123–1135
15. Nikolic S, Yellin EL, Tamura K, Vetter H, Tamura T, Meisner JS, Frater RWM (1988) Passive properties of canine left ventricle: Diastolic stiffness and restoring forces. Circ Res 62: 1210–1222
16. Paulus WJ, Vantrimpont PJ, Rousseau MF (1992) Diastolic function of the nonfilling human ventricle. J Am Coll Cardiol 20: 1524–1532
17. Rademakers FE, Buchalter MB, Rogers WJ, Zerhouni EA, Weisfeldt ML, Weiss JL, Shapiro EP (1992) Dissociation between left ventricular untwisting and filling. Circulation 85: 1572–1581
18. Robinson RF, Cohen-Gould L, Remily RM (1985) Extracellular structures in heart muscle. In: Harris P, Poole-Wilson PA (eds) Advances in myocardiology. Plenum Publishing Corp., New York, vol 5, pp 243–255
19. Robinson TF, Factor SM, Sonnenblick EH (1986) The heart as a suction pump. Sci Amer 254 (June): 84–91
20. Yellin EL, Hori M, Yoran C, Sonnenblick EH, Gabbay S, Frater RWM (1986) Left ventricular relaxation in the filling and nonfilling intact canine heart. Am J Physiol 250: H620–H629
21. Yellin EL, Nikolic SD, Frater RWM (1990) Left ventricular filling dynamics and diastolic function. Prog Cardiovasc Dis 32: 247–271

Author's address:
Martin M. LeWinter, M.D.
Cardiology Unit
Fletcher Allen Health Care, MCHV Campus
111 Colchester Avenue
Burlington, VT 05401
USA

Beta-blocker treatment in heart failure.
Role of heart rate reduction

P. Lechat

Pharmacology Department, Pitié-Salpétrière Hospital, Paris, France

Abstract

The potential therapeutic effect of beta-blocker treatment in chronic heart failure is still actively being investigated through large scale clinical trials. The underlying cardioprotective mechanism relies upon protection against the deleterious consequences of cardiac sympathetic stimulation. Heart rate reduction induced by beta-blocker treatment may importantly contribute to such benefit especially by improving myocardial energetic balance and by inducing a less negative force-frequency relationship. Results from clinical trials such as CIBIS suggest that prognosis in chronic heart failure may partly depend on left ventricular function improvement, but additional data are needed to more precisely define the relationships between heart rate reduction, left ventricular function improvement, and survival.

Key words   Beta-blocker – heart failure – heart rate

Introduction

Heart failure is a consequence of initial damage on the myocardium which alters cardiac performance. Time course of the disease depends on extend of initial loss of contractile tissue and on the behavior of remaining myocytes which are submitted to an increased stress since loss of contractile tissue induces ventricle dilatation.

In order to maintain blood pressure, neuro-hormonal compensatory mechanisms such as sympathetic and renin-angiotensin aldosterone systems are stimulated which in turn further increase stress on myocardial cells and leads to progressive impairement of myocyte function and cell damage. However, the process leading to such an alteration is not fully understood.

Prevention of heart failure deterioration starts with suppression when possible of initial cause of injury, especially ischemia as a consequence of coronary artery disease.

Inhibition of the potential deleterious consequences of compensatory mechanisms actions has emerged as a new therapeutic concept. The dramatic benefit provided by angiotensin converting enzyme inhibitors at any stage of heart failure (14, 47, 48) has prompted such concept and stimulated intense experimental as well as clinical research in this direction. Inhibition of the other compensatory mechanisms is therefore currently being evaluated, especially blockade of adrenergic receptors. Beta-blockers that have then been evaluated in heart failure since the pioneer work of Waagstein in 1975 (53) are currently tested in large scale multicentric trials. The Mechanism of benefit remains, however, to be established and may partly be related to heart rate reduction.

Sympathetic tone in heart failure

Sympathetic activation consistently occurs in chronic heart failure both in early and advanced stages of the disease (10, 13, 23, 49, 50, 58). These results are mainly based on increased plasma levels of norepinephrine which represent a rough indirect indicator of sympathetic activity. Indeed, such an increase results from increased nerve traffic but also from an impairement of non-neural metabolism. Indeed plasma norepinephrine clearance is reduced (34) due to a decreased cardiac output and abnormal distribution of blood flow. However, determination of cardiac norepinephrine spill over, which is more accurately related to cardiac sympathetic drive (25, 38) and direct recording of sympathetic nerve traffic (20, 33), clearly documented the increased sympathetic activity in heart failure. The trigger for sympathetic activation comes from the baro-reflex control of blood pressure. The initial myocardial injury reduces blood pressure and then stimulates sympathetic tone through baro-receptor deactivation. In addition, in chronic heart failure, baroreflex function, which normally inhibits sympathetic outflow, loses its sensitivity to the normal physiological stimuli.

This increased sympathetic nerve activity depletes norepinephrine stores. Such a phenomenon is enhanced by a reduction of norepinephrine uptake in the failing human heart as demonstrated by Böhm et al. 1995 (8). Such norepinephrine store depletion in heart failure was recently well documented by Bristow et al. 1991 (5) in myocardium from heart transplant of end stage cardiac failure. The extent of this depletion (around 40 % of control levels) was similar in idiopathic dilated cardiomyopathy and in ischemic cardiomyopathy.

The increased sympathetic nerve traffic and the reduction of norepinephrine uptake both tend to increase the intra synaptic concentration of norepinephrine which induces the desensitization phenomenon of beta-adrenergic receptors caracterized by a reduction of the number of beta adrenergic receptors on the sarcolemmal membrane (6, 9). Bristow et al. 1982 (6), initially reported a 50 % decrease in beta-adrenergic density in freshly explanted human hearts with cardiomyopathy relative to normal donor organs, which was correlated with the degree of elevation of coronary sinus norepinephrine levels or tissue norepinephrine levels. Bristow et al. 1991 (5) showed that important differences exist in the regulatory behavior of components of the beta-adrenergic receptor-G protein-adenylate cyclase complex in idiopathic dilated cardiomyopathy compared to ischemic cardiomyopathy.

The down regulation phenomenon that is induced by the increase in intra synaptic concentration of norepinephrine, predominantly affects beta 1 adrenergic receptors which have a higher affinity for norepinephrine compared to beta 2 adrenergic receptors. At the ventricular level, in normal conditions, the modulation of contractile state by sympathetic activity is predominantly effected through beta 1 adrenergic receptors. In heart failure, with reduction of 50 % of beta 1 adrenergic receptors, the relative importance of the beta 2 adrenoceptors in the modulation of cardiac contractility could increase but the amount of such action remains to be clarified and might influence the choice of beta-adrenergic antagonist to be given in heart failure according to its seletivity on beta 1 versus beta 2 adrenergic receptors. In all cases, the process of down regulation of beta-adrenergic receptors as a consequence of increased norepinephrine release by sympathetic nerves is associated with a reduction of the inotropic response of Beta 1 stimulation by agonists such as isoprenaline or dobutamine. This loss of beta-adrenergic responsiveness appears specific since response to other inotropic stimuli (calcium, forskolin, digitalis) is preserved when these contractile responses are studied on isolated papillary muscles taken from explanted hearts from patients during cardiac transplantations (46).

Such loss of beta-adrenergic response upon sympathetic stimulation may be considered either as a component of the alteration of ventricular function in heart failure or as a protective mechanism against the cytotoxic effect of catecholamines. The first hypothesis is not likely to be the correct one since chronic administration of beta-adrenergic agonists or phosphodiesterase inhibitors in chronic heart failure have failed to improve patients prognosis and even have produced deleterious effects on survival (43). These results demonstrate that inotropic stimulation of the failing heart through an increase in intracellular cAMP leads to cardiac deterioration on a long-term basis. On the other hand, blockade of beta adrenergic receptors will primarily protect myocardial fibers against the deleterious consequences of catecholamine stimulation. This represents the fundamental basis for the rationale of beta-blocker administration in heart failure.

Mechanisms of beta-blockade induced benefit in heart failure

Inhibition of potential deleterious consequences of over stimulated beta-adrenergic receptors appears then to provide the basic hypothesis. Beta blockade should then reinforce the consequences of beta-receptor desensitization which must be considered as a beneficial adaptative mechanism. However, since beta-blocker therapy tends to restore the number of beta-receptors by the up-regulation mechanism (1, 36), even in myocardial tissue in heart failure, such treatment will have to achieve a sufficient high level in order to really block beta-receptors, even in case of restoration of their number.

Such an hypothesis can explain why the ability of up-regulation for a given beta-blocker is not related to its clinical efficacy in heart failure (24). Indeed the clinical response to therapy with beta-blockers is not related to the change in β-adrenergic receptor density. Some beta-receptor antagonists such as carvedilol that do not induce up-regulation of adrenergic beta-receptors can produce beneficial effects in heart failure both on functional state and prognosis (41, 42). In addition, changes in beta-adrenergic receptor density occur shortly after the initiation of β-blockade, but generally clinical and hemodynamic resonses are delayed (26, 52, 54).

Mechanism of benefit of beta-adrenergic blockade in heart failure appears then mainly related to a reduction of the effects of sympathetic stimulation of beta-adrenergic receptors. Indeed such chronic stimulation increases myocardial energetics and appears to exert a deleterious effect on myocardial fiber viability, favoring the progressive transformation of myocardial cell in noncontractile fibrous cells. Such a process, which might include apoptosis, leads to progressive decompensation of heart failure. This slow process of contractile fiber deterioration then represents the goal of preventive therapy of heart failure decompensation. In heart failure, myocardial cells are very likely chronically working near an ischemic state since sinus tachycardia and ventricle dilatation increase myocardial oxygen consumption and the increase of filling pressure reduces perfusion of sub-endo-cardial layers (27).

This chronic sub-ischemic state is very likely one of the most deleterious effect on myocardium, triggering the progressive fibrous degeneration of myocardial fibers through intra-cellular calcium overload. Administration of beta-blocker treatment will then prima-rily restore a more favorable energetic balance and afford protection against myocardial deterioration. Such effect will be initiated by a reduction of heart rate without too strong of a reduction of beta-adrenergic dependent inotropic support of ventricular contraction, i.e., without hemodynamic deterioration (cardiac output decrease and filling pressure increase).

Such loss of beta-adrenergic dependent inotropic support of cardiac contraction with beta-blocker treatment will be compensated by several mechanisms. One of them is the induction of a less negative force – frequency relationship. Indeed, such a relationship is inversed in chronic heart failure, both in humans and experimentally (40). This is related to alteration of the function of sarcoplasmic reticulum. Its calcium content is reduced in chronic heart failure due to a reduction of capacity of the ATPase Ca^{++} pump (37) which refills Ca during relaxation. A longer diastolic period induced by beta-blocker treatment should then allow sarcoplasmic reticulum to restore its calcium content.

Since the contractile force of myocardial cells mainly depends on the amount of Ca that is released by the sarcoplasmic reticulum during each cardiac cycle and since this amount is proportional to calcium content of sarcoplasmic reticulum (calcium induced-calcium release phenomenon), this can explain the potential increase in myocardial contractility with heart rate reduction in heart failure.

We can then hypothetize that the loss of adrenergic dependent contractile support of inotropism of myocardial fibers in heart failure will progressively be replaced by a better intrinsic myocardial contractile function under beta-blocker administration. Such changes will have to be induced by a progressive increment of doses of beta-blocker to avoid left ventricular function deterioration which is observed when such treatment is abruptly admin-istrated with a dose regimen similar to that used in hypertension or angina pectoris. When a progressive administration has been respected, an increase in left ventricular ejection fraction has been constantly reported in the clinical trials in heart failure with beta-blockers. However, such improvement takes more than one month to develop (26).

Other mechanisms can also participate to this hemodynamic improvement that is observed under beta-blocker therapy and caracterized by an increase in left ventricular ejec-tion fraction, an increase in cardiac output, and a decrease in ventricular filling pressures.

Heart rate reduction per se allows a better left ventricular filling, which can improve clinical tolerance to sub-maximal exercise that is impaired if tachycardia increases too much. Since sympathetic stimulation increases more intensively for a given exercise level in heart failure, antagonism of sympathetic drive during exercise will improve symptoms and quality of life.

Interaction with the immune process could also interfere with the beta-blocker induced benefit in heart failure. It has been recently shown that cytokine production could also participate to the auto-aggravating process that occurs in heart failure. Plasma concentrations of some cytokines, such as tumor necrosis factor, have been found elevated in patients with heart failure from idiopathic dilated cardiomyopathy (21). Moreover, immune reactivity to a subcutaneous test has been shown to improve after a six month duration of treatment with metroprolol (35). Mechanisms of such an interaction between beta-blockers and immune process are unclear and remain to be investigated. Beta-receptors that are present on surface membrane of lymphocytes could be involved in such actions. However, improvement of immune process under beta-blockade treatment may only be a consequence of hemodynamic improvement.

Another potentially important mechanism of induced benefit in heart failure is represented by a decrease in catecholamine release by sympathetic nerves which can potentially lead to myocyte damage since catecholamine metabolism induces oxydative stress (17). Beta-blockers can directly reduce norephinephrine release by sympathetic nerves by blocking pre-synaptic beta-receptors which are mostly of the beta 2 subtype. However their physiological and physiopathological importance remains not well known in man. Indirect reduction of nerve discharge will also occur if beta-blockade treatment improves cardiac performance and consequently reduces need for sympathetic compensation.

Oxydative metabolism of catecholamines by monoamine-oxidase results in catecholamine-O-quinone and radical species, such as the superoxide radical, which by dismutation, can form hydrogen peroxide, which is deleterious to membrane integrity. Catecholamine-O-quinone is expected to have various deleterious consequences.

It might not only effect the biological activity of a protein, but it might also provide an antigen, inducing an immunological response. The possibility should also be considered that oxygen radicals produced by polymorphonuclear leukocytes as a result of inflammation could also induce catecholamine oxidation resulting in a vicious cycle (17).

Several mechanisms of action may, therefore, participate to the benefit induced by beta-blockers in heart failure. Among them, heart rate reduction appears to play an important role. The relationships between heart rate reduction, left ventricular function improvement, and survival remain however to be intensively investigated during future trials in order to determine the best parameters of success of such a therapy.

The published studies provide, however, preliminary information on these potential relationships.

Heart rate reduction during beta-blocker therapy in heart failure

Heart rate is reduced under beta-blockade in heart failure and is rapidly obtained after onset of administration. Amplitude of such reduction at rest appears of the same order of that obtained in ischemic patients (without heart failure) or in hypertension. This means that beta-adrenergic receptors are not completely desensitized in heart failure and that beta-adrenergic stimulation is still effective. Amplitude of heart rate reduction, recorded at the end of the titration periods is rather variable (Table 1) among trials (2, 3, 7, 11, 16, 18, 19, 22, 29, 30, 39, 41, 44, 51, 55, 56) but without any significant difference between beta-blockers.

The only important difference is detected with beta-blockers with partial beta 1 agonist activity such as xamoterol. Such compound does not reduce heart rate during the nighttime. A large scale clinical trial testing xamoterol benefit in heart failure was prematurely stopped because of an excess of mortality in the xamoterol group (57). It then appears that such pharmacological profile of beta-blocker is not appropriate in heart failure and reinforces the potential deleterious effect of any sympathetic stimulation. The precise relationship between heart rate stimulation induced at night with xamoterol and survival impairement remains unknown.

Table 1   Beta-blocker induced heart rate change in randomized trials in heart failure

		Heart rate Baseline	On metoprolol	mean variation
Randomized trials with metoprolol				
Anderson	(2)		77 ± 15	–
Engelmeier	(19)	92 ± 15	–	–
Cucchini	1988 (16)	83 ± 15	64 ± 11	– 21
MDC	1993 (51)	90 ± 19	75 ± 14 (6 months)	– 15
Fisher	1994 (22)	82 ± 12	–	–
Eichhorn	1994 (18)	83 ± 17	68 ± 17	– 15
Randomized trials with nebivolol				
Lechat	1991 (30)	70 ± 12	64 ± 14	– 6
Wisenbaugh	1993 (55)	85 ± 12	71 ± 12	– 14
Randomized trials with bisoprolol				
CIBIS	1994 (11)	83 ± 14	67 ± 3	– 16
Randomized trials with bucindolol				
Pollock	1990 (44)	90 ± 21	82 ± 12	– 8
Woodley	1991 (56)	85 ± 14	72 ± 9	– 13
Bristow	1994 (7)			
(Holter data:	12.5 mg	86 ± 12	–	– 6 ± 7
mean 24 h	50 mg	87 ± 12	–	– 5 ± 8
heart rate)	200 mg	88 ± 12	–	– 7 ± 7
Study		Rest heart rate Baseline	On carvedilol	mean variation
Randomized trials with carvedilol				
Metra	1994 (39)	84 ± 14	70 ± 10	– 14
Olsen	1995 (41)	87 ± 17	67 ± 17	– 20
ANZ	1995 (3)	75 ± 13	66 ± 12	– 9
Krum	1995 (29)	89 ± 17	64 ± 11	– 25

Compounds that are devoided of intrinsic sympathomimetic activity decrease heart rate in heart failure patients during both day and night. This was clearly observed with bisoprolol in a subgroup of patients studied on Holter monitoring at baseline and two months after

Table 2   24 hour Holter recording in 79 patients from CIBIS

	Placebo (n = 39)			Bisoprolol (n = 40)		
	Median	Min	Max	Median	Min	Max
Baseline						
Diurnal heart rate	82	45	118	82	39	106
Nocturnal heart rate	67	45	129	68	28	95
After a 2 month period of treatment						
Diurnal heart rate	82	48	121	69	37	95
Nocturnal heart rate	69	47	124	59	41	102

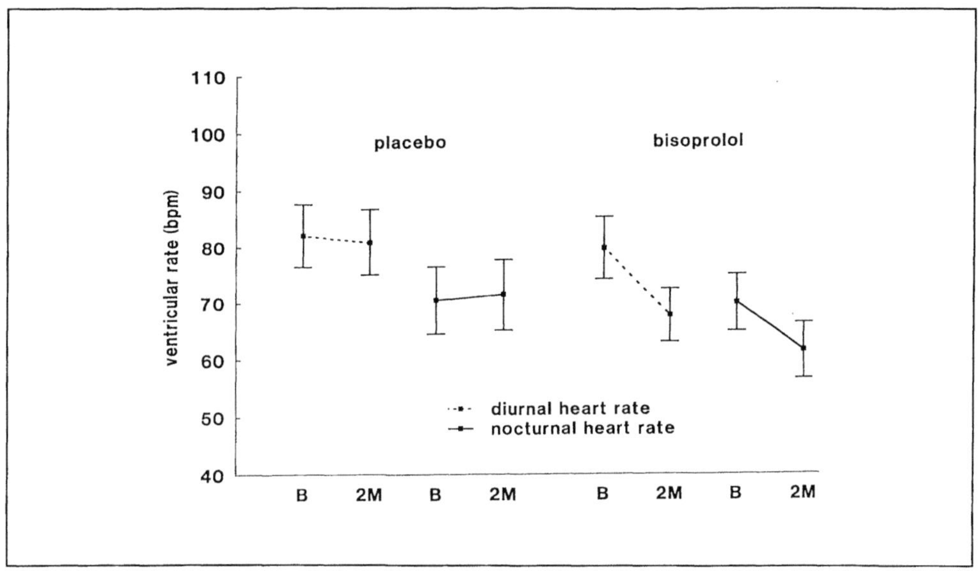

Fig. 1 Diurnal and nocturnal heart rate variations in a subgroup of patients included in the CIBIS study with 24 hour holter recording at baseline (B) and after a 2 month (2M) period of treatment: n = 40 in the placebo group, n = 39 in the bisoprolol group. Bars indicate 95 % confidence interval of the mean. Both diurnal and nocturnal heart rates were significantly reduced by bisoprolol treatment.

randomization in the CIBIS trial (Fig. 1 and Table 2). The dose-response (Heart rate) relationship is not however well – defined for most beta-blockers in heart failure.

Indeed, in most trials, dose increment is based on clinical tolerance and is not a forced titration. In the CIBIS study, at the end of the titration period, the mean administrated daily dose of bisoprolol was 3.8 ± 0.2 mg. Heart rate was reduced by – 16 ± 15 (SD) beats/min with bisoprolol, compared to – 1.5 ± 13 beats/min with placebo. Heart rate reduction was almost completely obtained by the second step of dose (2.5 mg/day). However a large inter-individual variability was observed. Such heart rate variation was not modified by concomittant digitalis or amiodarone treatment and was similar in ischemic and non-ischemic patients. A satisfactory evaluation of the heart rate response relationship with the dose is given by a parallel design such as in the study of Bristow et al. with bucindolol (7). In this study, heart rate reduction was similar in the different groups of dose (12.5 mg, 50 mg, 200 mg).

Beta-blocker induced reduction of heart rate appears to be partly related to baseline heart rate. This is due to the regression to the mean phenomenon but also to the fact that patients with highest baseline heart rates may have higher sympathetic activation and, thus, be more sensitive to beta-blockade. In the CIBIS study, the heart rate change over time recorded two months after randomization was significantly correlated with baseline in both study treatment groups: r = – 0.45 (p < 0.001) in the placebo group and r = – 0.59 (p < 0.001) in the bisoprolol group (Fig. 2, 32). However, when adjustment on regression to the mean was performed, the correlation remained significant only in the bisoprolol group. Such a result might provide a useful mean of clinical determination of patients that would most respond to beta-blocker and benefit from such a therapy on the long term. This will be particularly relevant if overall clinical benefit (quality of life and prognosis) is closely dependent on heart rate reduction.

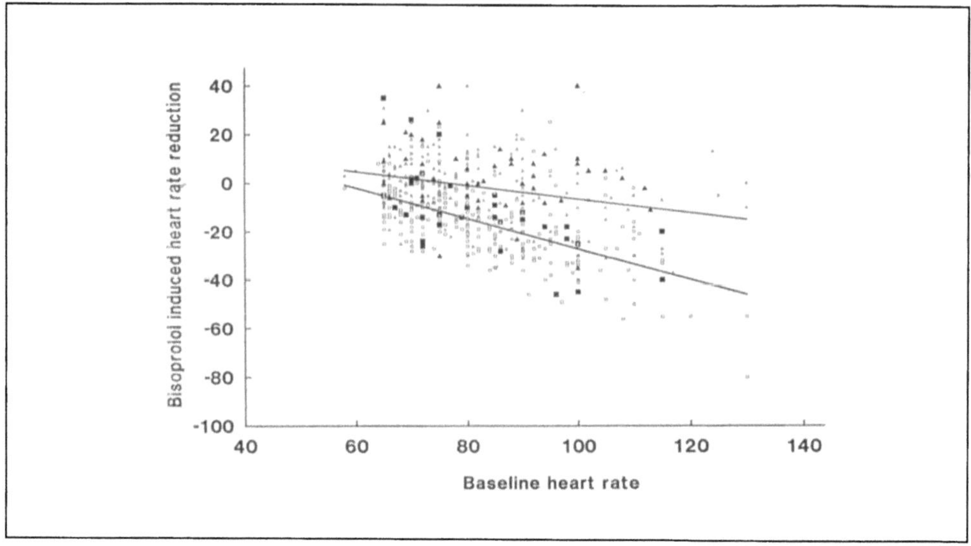

Fig. 2 Correlation between baseline heart rate and heart rate variation after a two month period of treatment in CIBIS study. The upper regression line is that obtained in the placebo group and expresses the regression to the mean related variation of heart rate. The lower regression line in that obtained in the bisoprolol group. Triangles represent patients in the placebo group. Squares represent patients in the bisoprolol group. Filled symbols represent patients who subsequently died during the CIBIS study after the initial first two months of treatment.

Heart rate change and left ventricular function improvement relationships

Beta-blocker treatment with progressive dose increment increases ejection fraction and stroke volume index and reduces left ventricle filling pressure. According to the results of 16 randomized trials, where information is available on ejection fraction after several months of treatment (31), the nonweighted mean of ejection fraction is 31 ± 4 % on beta-blocker and 23 ± 4 (mean $\pm$ sd) on placebo, representing an order of 20 % improvement. Such effect needs several weeks to develop and takes 2 to 3 months to reach its maximal. This is in opposition with heart rate reduction which is obtained after the first administration of beta-blocker. Relationships between both have provided inhomogenous results:
– with bucindolol, Bristow et al. did not find any relationship between heart rate and left ventricular ejection fraction variations after a three month period of treatment (7).
– with metoprolol, according to the data from MDC trial, Waagstein et al. observed that initial heart rate reduction was significantly correlated with left ventricular ejection fraction recorded 6 months after onset of treatment in both study treatment groups.

In the CIBIS study, left ventricular function could be studied by echocardiography in 160 patients still on treatment five months after randomization (32). Left ventricular fractional shortening significantly increased with bisoprolol compared to placebo. Among patients of the bisoprolol group, fractional shortening increase was not correlated to bisoprolol induced bradycardia recorded between baseline and at 5 months ($r = -0.11$, $p = 0.33$). With both groups considered together, (n = 160), the fractional shortening increase was not correlated to baseline heart rate but appeared significantly correlated to heart rate change over time ($r = -0.3$, $p = 0.02$). Such a correlation is obviously very weak and should be more precisely studied with Holter monitoring of heart rate. However, such a result suggests that heart rate reduction partly participates to left ventricular function improvement.

Beta-blocker induced heart rate reduction and prognosis

Very little information is available on such a relationship since among the different trials, only CIBIS was designed to demonstrate bisoprolol efficacy on mortality. In this trial, baseline heart rate was not significantly related to prognosis either in univariate or in multivariate Cox regression analysis. However, when heart rate change over time (baseline – two months after randomization) was added as a covariate in the multivariate Cox model, this covariate had the highest predictive value of survival (32).

This means that whatever the mechanism of beta-blocker induced benefit, heart rate reduction per se plays an important role. Such benefit may be obtained through improvement of left ventricular function (32), but more investigations are necessary to clarify the interrelationships between heart rate reduction, left ventricular function improvement, and survival during beta-blocker treatment in heart failure.

Mechanisms of benefit induced through heart rate reduction may also be related to heart rate variability increase. Such a parameter appears to be an independent marker of prognosis in post-myocardial infarction patients (28).

In heart failure, bisoprolol has been shown to increase heart rate variability, especially enhancing Vagally dependent heart rate variability (45). Such an effect was observed preferentially for lowest heart rates (15), which means that heart rate variability increase obtained with beta-blocker treatment is not entirely dependent on slowing of heart rate. Complementary investigations will be necessary to clarify the role of heart rate variability in heart failure during beta-blocker treatment.

All this information on mechanisms of beta-blocker induced benefit in heart failure will be especially provided by large scale trials with mortality as primary endpoint such as CIBIS II with bisoprolol (12) and BEST with bucindolol (4). The COMET trial comparing metroprolol and carvedilol will also provide further information on the potential difference of long term effects on survival according to the pharmacological profile of compounds and relationships between hemodynamic effects (including heart rate reduction) and survival improvement.

References

1. Aarons RD, Nies AS, Gal J, Hegestrand LR, Molinoff PB (1980) Elevation of beta-adrenergic receptor density in human lymphocytes after propranolol administration. J Clin Invest 65: 949–957
2. Anderson JL, Lutz JR, Gilbert EM, Sorensen SG, Yanowitz FG, Menlove RL, Bartholomew M (1985) A randomized trial of low-dose beta-blockade therapy for idiopathic dilated cardiomyopathy. Am J Cardiol 55: 471–75
3. Australia-New Zealand Heart Failure Research Collaborative Group (1995) Effects of carvedilol, a vasodilator-β-blocker, in patients with congestive heart failure due to ischemic heart disease. Circulation 92: 212–18

4. The Best Steering committee (1995) Design of the Beta-Blocker Evaluation Survival Trial. Am J Cardiol 75: 1220–1223

5. Bristow MR, Anderson FL, Port JD, Skesl L, Hershberger RE, Larrabee P, O'Connell JB, Renlund DG, Volkman K, Murray J, Feldman AM (1991) Differences in beta-adrenergic neuroeffector mechanisms in ischemic versus idiopathic dilated cardiomyopathy. Circulation 84: 1024–1039

6. Bristow MR, Ginsburg R, Minobe W et al. (1982) Decreased catecholamine sensitivity and β adrenergic receptor density in failing human hearts. N Engl J Med 307: 205–211

7. Bristow MR, O'Connell JB, Gilbert EM, French WJ, Leatherman G, Kantrowitz NE, Orie J, Smucker ML, Marshall G, Kelly P, Deitchman D, Anderson JL (1994) Dose-response of chronic β-blocker treatment in heart failure from either idiopathic dilated or ischemic cardiomyopathy. Circulation 89: 1632–42

8. Böhm M, LaRosie K, Schwinger R, Erdmann E (1995) Evidence for reduction of norepinephrine uptake sites in the failing human heart. JACC 25: 146–153

9. Brodde OE (1991) Beta 1 and 2 adrenoceptors in the human heart: Properties, function and alterations in chronic heart failure. Pharmacol Rev 43: 203–242

10. Chidsey CA, Braunwald E, Morrow AG (1965) Catecholamine excretion and cardiac stores of norepinephrine in congestive heart failure. Am J Med 39: 442–451

11. CIBIS Investigators and Committees (1994) A randomized trial of β-blockade in heart failure: The Cardiac Insufficiency Bisoprolol Study (CIBIS). Circulation 90: 1765–1773

12. The CIBIS II Scientific Committee (1997) Design of the Cardiac Insufficiency Bisoprolol Study (CIBIS II): Fundam Clin Pharmacol 11: 38–42

13. Cohn JN, Levin TB, Olivari MT et al. (1984) Plasma norepinephrine as a guide to prognosis in patients with chronic heart failure. N Engl J Med 311: 819–823

14. The Consensus Trial Study Group (1987) Effects of Enalapril on mortality in severe congestive heart failure: results of the Cooperative North Scandinavian Enalapril Survival Study (consensus). N Engl J Med 316: 1429–1435

15. Copie X, Pousset F, Lechat P, Jaillon P, Guize L, Le Heuzey JY and the Cardiac Insufficiency Bisoprolol Study Investigators (1996) Effects of beta-blockade with bisoprolol on heart rate variability in advanced heart failure: Analysis of scatterplots of RR intervals at selected heart rates. Am Heart J 132: 369–375

16. Cucchini F, Compostella L, Papalia D, De Domenico R, Iavernaro A, Zeppellini R (1988) Trattamento cronico della cardiomiopatia deilatativa con betabloccanti. G Ital Cardiol 18: 835–42

17. Dhalla KS, Rupp H, Beamish RE, Dhalla NS (1996) Mechanisms of alterations in cardiac membrane Ca^{2+} transport du to excess catecholamines. Cardiovascular Drugs and Therapy 10: 231–238

18. Eichhorn EJ, Heesch CM, Barnett JH, Alvarez LG, Fass SM, Grayburn PA, Hatfield BA, Marcoux LG, Malloy CR (1994) Effect of metroprolol on myocardial function and energetics in patients with nonischemic dilated cardiomyopathy: a randomized, double-blind, placebo-controlled study. J Am Coll Cardiol 24: 1310–20

19. Engelmeier RS, O'Connell JB, Walsh R, Rad N, Scanlon PJ, Gunnar RM (1985) Improvement in symptoms and exercise tolerance by metoprolol in patients with dilated cardiomyopathy: a double-blind, randomized, placebo-controlled trial. Circulation 72: 536–46

20. Ferguson DW, Berg WJ, Sanders JS (1990) Clinical and hemodynamic correlates of sympathetic neural activity in normal humans and patients with heart failure. J Am Coll Cardiol 16: 1125

21. Ferrari R, Bachetti T, Confortini R, Opasich C, Febo O, Corti A, Cassani G, Visioli O (1995) Tumor necrosis factor soluble receptors in patients with various degrees of congestive heart failure. Circulation 92: 1479–1486

22. Fisher ML, Gottlieb SS, Plonick GD, Greenberg NL, Patten RD, Bennett SK, Hamilton BP (1994) Beneficial effects of metoprolol in heart failure associated with coronary artery disease a randomized trial. J Am Coll Cardiol 23: 943–950

23. Francis GS, Benedict C, Johnstone DE, Kirlin PC, Nicklas J, Liang C, Kubo SH, Rudin-Toretsky E, Yusuf S, for the SOLVD investigators (1990) Comparison of neuroendocrine activation in patients with left ventricular dysfunction with and without congestive heart failure: a substudy of the studies of left ventricular dysfunction (SOLVD). Circulation 82: 1724–1729

24. Gilbert EM, Olsen SL, Mealey P, Volkman K, Larrabee P, Bristow MR (1991) Is beta receptor up-regulation necessary for improved LV function in dilated cardiomyopathy? Circulation 84 (suppl II): 469 Abstract

25. Hasking GJ, Esler MD, Jennings GI, Burton D, Johns JA, Korner PI (1986) Norepinephrine spill over to plasma in patients with congestive heart failure: evidence of increased overall and cardiorenal sympathetic nervous activity. Circulation 73: 615–621

26. Heilbrunn SM, Shah P, Bristow MR, Valantine HA, Ginsburg R, Fowler MB (1986) Increased beta-receptor density and improved hemodynamic response to catecholamine stimulation during long term metroprolol therapy in heart failure from dilated cardiomyopathy. Circulation 79: 483–490

27. Katz A (1988) Cellular mechanisms in congestive heart failure. Am J Cardiol 62: 3–8

28. Kleiger RE, Miller JP, Bigger JT, Moss AJ and the multicenter post infarction research group (1987) Dicreased heart rate variability and its association with increased mortality after myocardial infarction. Am J Cardiol 59: 256–262

29. Krum H, Sackner-Bernstein JD, Goldsmith RL, Kukin ML, Schwartz B, Penn J, Medina N, Yushak M, Horn E, Katz SD, Levin HR, Neuberg GW, DeLong G, Packer M (1995) Double-blind, placebo-controlled study of the long-term efficacy of carvedilol in patients with severe chronic heart failure. Circulation 92: 1499–1506

30. Lechat P, Boutelant S, Komajda M, Gagey S, Landault C, Maistre G, Grosgogeat Y (1991) Pilot study of cardiovascular effects of nebivolol in congestive heart failure. Drug Invest 3 (Suppl 1): 69–81

31. Lechat P, Packer M, Chalon S, Cucherat M, Arab T, Boissel JP (1998) Beta-blockade treatment in heart failure: Meta-analysis. Circulation (in press)

32. Lechat P, Escolano S, Golmard JL, Lardoux H, Witchitz S, Henneman JA, Maish B, Hetzel M, Jaillon P, Boissel JP, Mallet A on behalf of CIBIS investigators (1997) Prognostic value of bisoprolol induced hemodynamic effects in heart failure during the cardiac insufficiency Bisoprolol study. Circulation 96: 2197–2205

33. Leimbach WN, Wallin BG, Victor RG, Aylward PE, Sundlof G, Mark AL (1986) Direct evidence from intraneural recordings for increased central sympathetic outflow in patients with heart failure. Circulation 73: 913–919

34. Leuenberger U, Kenney G, Davis D, Clemson B, Zelis R (1992) Comparison of norepinephrine and isoproterenol clearance in congestive heart failure. Am J Physiol 263: H56–H60

35. Maisel A (1994) Beneficial effects of metoprolol treatment in congestive heart failure. Circulation 90: 1774–1780

36. Maki T, Naveri H, Leinonen H, Sovijäri A, Lewko B, Harkonen M, Kontula K (1990) Effect of propranolol and pindolol on the up-regulation of lymphocytic β adrenoceptors during acute submaximal physical exercise. A placebo controlled double blind study. J Cardiovasc Pharmacol 15: 544–551

37. Mercadier JJ, Lompre AM, Duc P et al. (1990) Altered sarcoplasmic reticulum Ca^{2+} ATPase gene expression in the human ventricle during end-stage heart failure. J Clin Invest 85: 305–309

38. Meredith IT, Eisenhofer G, Lambert GW, Dewar EM, Jennings GI, Esler MD (1993) Cardiac sympathetic nervous activity in congestive heart failure: Evidence for increased neuronal norepinephrine release and preserved neuronal reuptake. Circulation 88: 136–145

39. Metra M, Nardi M, Giubbini R, Deilas L (1994) Effects of short- and long-term carvedilol administration on rest and exercise hemodynamic variables, exercise capacity and clinical conditions in patients with idiopathic dilated cardiomyopathy. J Am Coll Cardiol 24: 1678–87

40. Mulieri LA, Hasenfuss G, Leavitt B, Allen PD, Alpert NR (1992) Altered myocardial force-frequency relation in human heart failure. Circulation 85: 1743–1750

41. Olsen SL, Gilbert EM, Renlund DG, Taylor DO, Yanowitz FD, Bristow MR (1995) Carvedilol improves left ventricular function and symptoms in chronic heart failure: a double-blind randomized study. J Am Coll Cardiol 25: 1225–31

42. Packer M, Bristow MR, Cohn J, Colucci W, Fowler MB, Gilbert EM, Shusterman NH, for the US carvedilol heart failure Study group (1996) The effect of carvedilol on morbidity and mortality in patients with chronic heart failure. N Engl J Med 334: 1349–1355

43. Packer M, Carver JR, Rodeheffer RJ, Ivanhoe RJ, Dibianco R, Zeldis SM, Hendrix GH, Bommer WJ, Elkayam U, Kukin ML, Mallis GI, Sollan JA, Shannon J, Tandon PK, DeMets DL, for the PROMISE Study Research Group (1991) Effect of oral milrinone on mortality in severe chronic heart failure. N Engl J Med 325: 1468–1475

44. Pollock SG, Lystash J, Tedesco C, Craddock G, Smucker ML (1990) Usefulness of bucindolol in congestive heart failure. Am J Cardiol 66: 603–7

45. Pousset F, Copie X, Lechat P, Jaillon P, Boissel JP, Hetzel M, Fillette F, Remme W, Guize L, Le Heuzey JY (1996) Effects of bisoprolol on heart rate variability in heart failure. Am J Cardiol 77: 612–617

46. Schwinger RHG, Böhm M, Pieske B, Erdmann E (1991) Different β-adrenoceptor-effector coupling in human ventricular and atrial myocardium. Eur J Clin Invest 21: 443–451

47. The SOLVD investigators (1991) Effect of enalapril on survival in patients with reduced left ventricular ejection fractions and congestive heart failure. N Engl J Med 325: 293–302

48. The SOLVD investigators (1992) Effect of enalapril on mortality and the development of heart failure in asymptomatic patients with reduced left ventricular ejection fractions. N Engl J Med 327: 685–691

49. Thomas JA, Marks BH (1978) Plasma norepinephrine in congestive heart failure. Am J Cardiol 41: 223–243

50. Vicquerat CE, Daly P, Swedberg K et al. (1985) Endogenous catecholamine levels in congestive heart failure: relation to severity of hemodynamic atnormality. Am J Med 78: 455–460

51. Waagstein F, Bristow MR, Swedberg K, Camerini F, Fowler MB, Silver MA, Gilbert EM, Johnson MR, Goss FG, Hjalmarson A (1993) Beneficial effects of metoprolol in idiopathic dilated cardiomyopathy. Lancet 342: 1441–46

52. Waagstein F, Caidahl K, Wallentin I, Bergh Ch, Hjalmarson A (1989) Long term beta-blockade in dilated cardiomyopathy: effects of short and long term metoprolol treatment followed by readministration of metoprolol. Circulation 80: 551–563

53. Waagstein F, Hjalmarson A, Varnauskas E, Wallentin I (1975) Effect of chronic beta-adrenergic receptor blockade in congestive cardiomyopathy. Br Heart J 37: 1022–1036

54. Whyte K, Jones CR, Howie CA, Deighton N, Summer DJ, Reid JL (1987) Hemodynamic, metabolic, and lymphocyte beta 2 adrenoceptor changes following chronic beta-adrenoceptor antagonism. Eur J Clin Pharmacol 32: 237–243
55. Wisenbaugh T, Katz I, Davis J, Essop R, Skoularigis J, Middlemost S, Röthlisberger C, Skudicky D, Sareli P (1993) Long-term (3-month) effects of a new beta-blocker (nebivolol) on cardiac performance in dilated cardiomyopathy. J Am Coll Cardiol 21: 1094–100
56. Woodley SL, Gilbert EM, Anderson JL, O'Connell JB, Deitchman D, Yanowitz FG, Mealey PC, Volkman K, Renlund DG, Menlove R, Bristow MR (1991) β-blockade with bucindolol in heart failure caused by ischemic versus idiopathic dilated cardiomyopathy. Circulation 84: 2426–41
57. Xamoterol in severe heart failure (1990) The Xamoterol in severe heart failure Study Group. Lancet 336: 1–6
58. Zelis R, Davis D (1986) The sympathetic nervous system in congestive heart failure. Heart Failure: 21–32

Author's address:
Philippe Lechat
Pharmacology Department
Pitié-Salpétrière Hospital
Paris
France

Digitalis therapy – Relevance of heart rate reduction

E. Erdmann

Klinik III für Innere Medizin der Universität zu Köln

Abstract

Although digitalis is of limited antiarrhythmic value in patients with atrial fibrillation, it does control ventricular heart rate in the majority of patients at rest. It may be necessary, to add a β-blocking agent or a calcium antagonist to control ventricular heart rate during exercise. This therapeutic approach should be controlled by exercise testing.

In heart failure patients with sinus rhythm digitalis decreases heart rate, has anti-adrenergic effects, and restores baroreceptor and parasympathetic activity. These actions are seen only in patients with severe heart failure due to left ventricular enlargement and low ejection fraction. In mild heart failure as well as in diastolic heart failure or cor pumonale, digitalis does not seem to be of clinical value. Thus, the use of digitalis in patients with sinus rhythm should be restricted to those with severe heart failure.

Key words Heart rate – heart failure – digitalis – antiadrenergic effects

Introduction

More then 200 years ago Dr. William Withering introduced the use of foxglove in dropsical cases (22) – what we would call heart failure today. Since then, the efficacy of digitalis as an antiarrhythmic drug and as the drug of choice for the treatment of chronic heart failure has remained controversial (2, 7, 8, 17). Numerous studies, reviews, and points of view have been published on this subject (4, 5, 9, 10, 12, 15, 19). This account concentrates on three problems only: 1. The use of digitalis in atrial fibrillation. 2. Does digitalis reduce heart rate acutely and chronically? 3. Which patients may need digitalis?

The use of digitalis in atrial fibrillation

Every physician treating patients with tachyarrhythmia due to atrial fibrillation knows that in the majority of cases ventricular heart rate decreases after the use of digitalis. The older

Table 1 Heart rate in atrial fibrillation at rest and during exercise (n = 12) (18)

	Rest	submax. Exercise
Digoxin	88 ± 19	170 ± 20
Diltiazem	86 ± 12	154 ± 23

Table 2 Heart rate in atrial fibrillation at rest and during exercise (n = 10) (14)

	exercise rest	anaerobic threshold (min^{-1})	peak
no medication	85	127	175
digoxin (0.25 mg)	75	120	174
propranolol (3 x 20 mg)	63	99	138
verapamil (3 x 80 mg)	70	107	138

physicians used the pulse deficit as a marker for the beneficial action of the cardiac glycoside. In some patients, digitalis alone will not be sufficient to decrease ventricular rate down to about 70/min at rest. In these cases small doses of β-blocking agents (2 x 50 mg of metoprolol p.o. daily or 5 mg of bisoprolol once daily) usually are adequate to control the heart rate (3, 18). Instead, one could also add diltiazem or verapamil, 2–3 times 80 mg p.o. daily. The latter medication is also often used in patients with intermittent atrial fibrillation to maintain sinus rhythm. One should note, however, that in patients with moderate or severe heart failure, even these low doses of calcium-antagonists may aggravate heart failure. Therefore, one should use the lowest possible doses at the beginning of this therapy. Acutally, a distinction has to be made between high heart rate in atrial fibrillation without heart failure and a similar when the heart is failing. Calcium antagonists are contraindicated in heart failure due to reduced pump function – that is low EF.

Lately, it has been reported, the digitalis may be adequate to control ventricular rate at rest. During exercise, however, digitalis does not suffice. Several studies to this effect indeed have shown that calcium antagonists as diltiazem or verapamil may be superior to digitalis to control ventricular rate at submaximal exercise (14, 18) (Table 1). The same seems to be true for β-blocking agents (Table 2). Thus, the usual way to treat patients with tachyarrhythmic atrial fibrillation is to give digitalis at a dose sufficient to set ventricular heart rate at around 70/min at rest and to add a β-blocking agent or a calcium-antagonist (verapamil or diltiazem) until heart rate during submaximal exercise is also controlled adequately. Whenever the ejection fraction is low (< 35 %) one should not use calcium-antagonists in order to not aggravate heart failure.

The above mentioned procedure intends to decrease high heart rates, as it is well known, that patients feel agitated with tachyarrhythmia, the cardiac output is low under these circumstances due to the too short filling time of the left ventricle, and oxygen supply to the myocardium may be low during tachyarrhythmia. In atrial fibrillation, these pathophysiological changes may lead to heart failure even, if the cardiac muscle itself is not affected. Thus, most physicians today will agree that high heart rates in atrial fibrillation have to be lower; this, indeed, is the aim of treatment. In sinus rhythm, however, the situation is not that clear.

Does digitalis reduce heart rate?

Acute heart rate is not decreased very much after digitalis in sinus rhythm, if a carotid sinus syndrome and a sick sinus syndrome are excluded. If however, patients with apparent heart failure, who do have an increased heart rate (Table 3), are investigated very accurately before and after normal doses of digitalis, one usually notices a reduction of sinus rate by about 10 % (Table 4) (5). This has been shown in heart failure patients in many investigations. The more serious the condition of left ventricular failure, the greater the effect of digitalis on sinus rate seems to be. A second apparently important effect of digitalis is the increase in heart rate variability and the reduction of noradrenalin concentrations as a marker of neuroendocrine activity in heart failure (Tables 3–5). Ferguson and coworkers (5, 6) indeed could measure muscle sympathetic nerve activity in normal subjects and in heart failure patients (Table 4). They convincingly showed that the blunted effect of baroreceptor deactivation after nitroprusside application can be restored after digitalis (Table 5). Cardiac glycosides also decrease muscle sympathetic nerve activity (MSNA). Similar investigations demonstrating the acute antiadrenergic effects of digitalis have been published by several authors. Recently, Krum and coworkers (11) could demonstrate the antiadrenergic effects of long-term digitalis therapy. Norepinephrine levels are significantly decreased by digitalis, so is heart rate. Along with this, a restored baroreflex activity as well as a restored parasympathetic activity has been measured in 26 patients after digitalis treatment for 4–6 weeks.

Table 3 Heart rate data in controls and in congestive heart failure (1)

	24 h HR (beats/min)	24 h HR SD (ms)
Control (n = 20)	73.1 ± 9	233.2 ± 26
CHF (n = 20)	84.2 ± 11	97.5 ± 41

Table 4 Effects of digitalis on heart rate in chronic heart failure (5)

	before	after digitalis
HR (min–1)	91.1	83.7*
CI (I min–1m2)	2.05	2.49*
MSNA (U/100 beats)	831.0	474.4*

Table 5 Responses to baroreceptor deactivation (nitroprusside) (6)

	Normal subjects (n = 10)		Heart failure (n = 10)	
	Control	Nitroprusside	Control	Nitroprusside
Heart rate (beats/min)	68 ± 3	81 ± 4	91 ± 6	97 ± 4
MAP (mm Hg)	90 ± 2	80 ± 3	89 ± 2	77 ± 3
MSNA(U/min)	326 ± 74	746 ± 147	936 ± 155	1179 ± 221

Thus, is has been proven that digitalis in heart failure decreases sinus rate acutely and chronically. This action is probably due to its anti adrenergic activity leading to a restored parasympathetic activity and baroreflex activity. At present, it is rather uncertain, whether the beneficial effects of digitalis are due to its inotropic actions (20).

Which patients may need digitalis?

Recently, some of the data of the DIG trial have been released (Table 6) (23). 6800 patients with an ejection fraction below 45 % (28 % on average) have been treated in 301 centers. The overall effect on mortality, however, was not different from the placebo. Thus, one has to look critically for the reasons of this apparently inefficacious drug.

Table 6   DIG trial (n = 6800, 301 centers, EF < 45 % mean: 32 %)

age:	64 years
ischemic cardiomyopathy:	60 %
dilated cardiomyopathy:	40 %
digoxin doses:	0.125–0.5 mg/day
digoxin levels:	0.5–1 ng/ml (63 %)
duration of the trial:	37 (28–58) months
diuretics:	82 %
ACE-I:	94 %
NYHA I:	14 %
NYHA II:	54 %
NYHA III:	30 %
NYHA IV:	2 %
overall mortality:	no effect
mortality due to heart failure:	– 20 % (p < 0.03)
hospitalization due to heart failure:	– 28 % (p < 0.03)
arrhythmias and MI:	increased (n.s.)

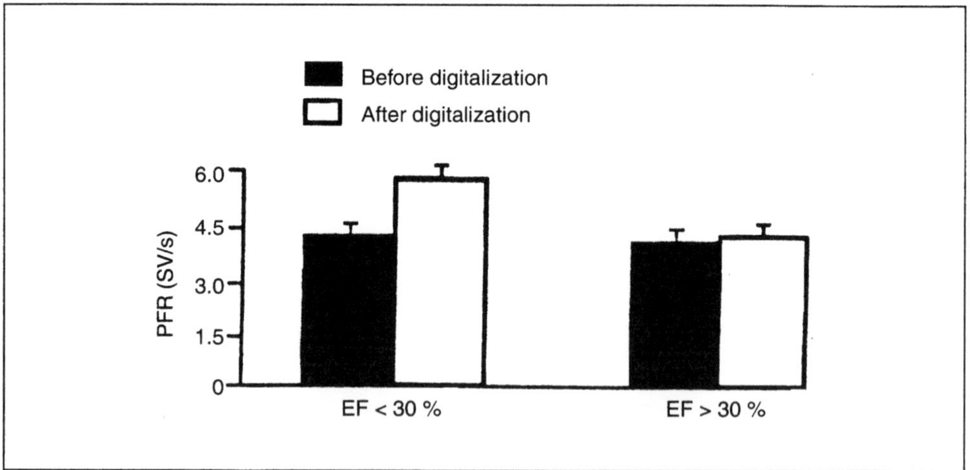

Fig. 1 Digitalis and ventricular function (PFR = peak filling rate normalized to mitral stroke volume) (21)

Table 7 Peak hemodynamic response to digoxin in 11 patients (8)

	Responders (n = 6)			Nonresponders (n = 5)		
	Control	Digoxin	p Value	Control	Digoxin	p Value
HR (beats/min)	107 ± 24	98 ± 29	< 0.05	85 ± 12	85 ± 13	NS
AP (mm Hg)	97 ± 21	96 ± 14	NS	94 ± 10	106 ± 24	NS
PCWP (mm Hg)	28 ± 5	18 ± 2	< 0.004	17 ± 5	17 ± 6	NS
RAP (mm Hg)	9 ± 3	5 ± 2	< 0.003	6.0 ± 2	5.0 ± 5	NS
CI (liters/min per m2)	2.1 ± 0.3	3.1 ± 0.02	< 0.02	3.1 ± 0.6	3.4 ± 0.6	NS
TSVR (dynes.s.cm–5)	1775 ± 317	1229 ± 236	< 0.04	1285 ± 282	1332 ± 218	NS
LVSWI (g.m/m2)	19 ± 8	37 ± 20	< 0.03	36 ± 15	50 ± 27	NS
EF (%) (n = 8)	20 ± 6	28 ± 6	< 0.03	28 ± 17	30 ± 20	NS

It seems to be important that 65 % of all patients in the DIG trial had heart failure NYHA I and II. Only 32 % had heart failure NYHA III-IV. Digitalis, however, decreased mortality in patients with severe heart failure significantly (p < 0.03) and decreased hospitalisation due to heart failure by 28 % (p < 0.03). Thus, digitalis may be efficacious only in patients with severe heart failure. This opinion is being supported by several investigations (Fig. 1). Gheorghiade et al. (8, 9) most convincingly demonstrated this when looking at the hemodynamic parameters of patients responding to digoxin and those not responding to digoxin (Table 7). Their measurements clearly indicated that heart rate decreased in these patients (if it was high to begin with), left ventricular filling pressure decreased, if it was high to begin with, and cardiac index increased, if it was low. In those patients, whom they called non-responders, who had lower heart rates at the beginning as well as high cardiac output, there were no beneficial effects of digitalis.

Several well-controlled prospective studies indicate the severe symptomatic chronic heart failure is best treated by diuretics, digitalis, and ACE inhibitors. Even in the era of ACE inhibitors, digitalis is needed in these patients. In the DIG trial, too many patients with asymptotic or mild heart failure (69 %) were treated. These patients, we know now for certain, do not need digitalis, if they are in sinus rhythm. They usually do not have a high heart rate as they do not suffer from an increased neurohormoral activity. In mild heart failure, in diastolic heart failure, and in chronic cor pulmonale with right heart failure, digitalis does not seem to be of clinical value (13, 19).

References

1. Casolo G, Balli E, Taddei T, Amuhasi J, Gori C (1989) Decreased spontaneous heart rate variability in congestive heart failure. Am J Cardiol 64: 1162–1167
2. Erdmann E (1995) Digitalis – friend of foe? Europ Heart J 16: 16–19
3. Falk RH, Knowlton AA, Bernard SA, Gotlieb NE, Battinelli NJ (1987) Digoxin for converting recent-onset atrial fibrillation to sinus rhythm 106: 503–506
4. Falk RH, Leavitt JI (1991) Digoxin for atrial fibrillation: a drug whose time has gone? Ann Intern Med 114: 573–575
5. Ferguson DW, Berg WJ, Sanders JS, Roach PJ, Kempf JS, Kienzle MG (1989) Sympathoinhibitory responses to digitalis glycosides in heart failure patients. Circulation 80: 65–77
6. Ferguson DW, Berg WJ, Roach PJ, Oren RM, Mark AL (1992) Effects of heart failure on baroreflex control of sympathetic neural activity. Am J Cardiol 69: 523–531
7. Fleg JL, Lakatta EG (1984) How useful is digitalis in patients with congestive heart failure and sinus rhythm? Int J Cardiol 6: 295–305
8. Gheorghiade M, St. Clair J, St. Clair C, Beller GA (1987) Hemodynamic effects of intravenous digoxin in patients with severe heart failure initially treated with diuretics and vasodilators. J Am Coll Cardiol 9: 849–857

9. Gheorghiade M, Hall V, Lakier JB, Goldstein S (1989) Comparative hemodynamic and neurohormoral effects of intravenous captopril and digoxin and their combinations in patients with severe heart failure. J Am Coll Cardiol 13: 134–142
10. Kimmelstiel C, Benotti JR (1988) How effective is digitalis in the treatment of congestive heart failure? Am Heart J 4: 1063–1070
11. Krum H, Bigger T, Rochelle L, Goldsmith EDD, Packer M (1995) Effect of long-term digoxin therapy on automatic function in patients with chronic heart failure. J Am Coll Cardiol 25: 289–294
12. Lauer MS, Eagle KA, Buckley MJ, DeSanctis RW (1989) Atrial fibrillation following coronary artery bypass surgery. Progr Cardiovasc Dis 31: 367–378
13. Mathur PN, Powles ACP, Pugsley S, McEwan P, Campbell EJM (1981) Effect of digoxin on right ventricular function in severe chronic airflow obstruction. Ann Intern Med 95: 283–288
14. Matsuda M, Matsuda Y, Yamagishi T et al. (1991) Effects of digoxin propranolol, and verapamil on exercise in patients with chronic isolated atrial fibrillation. Cardiovasc Res 25: 453–457
15. Packer M, Leier CV (1987) Survival in congestive heart failure during treatment with drugs with positive inotropic actions. Circulation 75: IV-55
16. Packer M, Gheorghiade M, Young JB et al. for the RADIANCE study (1993) Withdrawal of digoxin from patients with chronic heart failure treated with angiotensin-converting-enzyme inhibitors. N Engl J Med 329: 1–7
17. Poole-Wilson PA, Robinson K (1989) Digoxin – a redundant drug in congestive cardiac failure. Cardiovasc Drugs Ther 2: 733–741
18. Roth A, Harrison E, Mitani G, Cohen J, Rahimtoola SH, Elkayam U (1986) Efficacy and safety of medium- and high-dose diltiazem alone and in combination with digoxin for control of heart rate at rest an during exercise in patients with chronic atrial fibrillation. Circulation 73: 316–324
19. Schüren KP, Hüttemann U (1974) Chronisch obstruktive Lungenerkrankungen: Die hämodynamische Wirkung von Digitalis beim chronischen Cor pulmonale in Ruhe und unter Belastung. Klin Wschr 52: 736–746
20. Schwinger RHG, Böhm M, Erdmann E (1990) Effectiveness of cardiac glycosides in human myocardium with and without "downregulated" beta-adrenoceptors. J Cardiovasc Pharmacol 15: 692–697
21. Vitarelli A, Fedele F, Dagianti A, Penco M, Pastore LR, Dagianti A (1995) A reexamination of the hemodynamic effects of digitalis relative to ventricular dysfunction. Cardiology 86: 94–101
22. Withering W (1785) An account of the foxglove and some of its medical uses. M. Swinney, Birmingham
23. The Digitalis Investigation Group (DIG) (1997) The effect of digoxin on mortality and morbidity in patients with heart failure. N Engl J Med 336: 525–533

Author's address:
E. Erdmann
Klinik III für Innere Medizin
der Universität zu Köln
Joseph-Stelzmann-Str. 9
50924 Köln
Germany

β-Blocker treatment of chronic heart failure with special regard to carvedilol

C. Maack, M. Böhm

Medizinische Universitätsklinik und Poliklinik, Homburg/Saar

Introduction

Congestive heart failure is a major public health problem in most Western countries. In the United States, approximately three million people suffer from heart failure, 10 % of whom are admitted to a hospital each year (57). Although in recent decades considerable changes in medical therapy have been achieved, especially by angiotensin converting enzyme (ACE) inhibitors (19, 58), mortality of heart failure still remains very high. In patients of New York Heart Association (NYHA) functional class II there is a mortality of about 10 % (2). In order to improve this poor prognosis, additional pharmacological interventions to counteract the pathophysiological changes occurring in heart failure are still important.

Waagstein et al. (1975) were the first to treat patients with idiopathic dilated cardiomyopathy (IDC) with β-blockers in a small open trial (68). They observed improvements in exercise tolerance and ventricular function and a reduction of heart size in these patients. Due to their negative inotropic actions, β-blockers had not been considered to be an appropriate treatment of heart failure. But in 1979, in a retrospective analysis using matched historical controls, Swedberg et al. (60) suggested that β-blockers have a favorable effect on mortality in patients with heart failure. In 1980, these authors reported deleterious effects of β-blocker withdrawal and subsequent improvement after readministration in a group of 15 patients with IDC (6). In another noncontrolled study of patients with IDC, this group reported that long-term (6–62 months) β-blockade resulted in an improvement of systolic and diastolic myocardial function and functional class (62). These favorable initial studies have spawned a number of randomized, double-blinded, placebo-controlled trials of heart failure, investigating the effects of β-blockers on various hemodynamic factors, symptoms, functional class, exercise capacity, and survival.

Pathophysiology of the beta-adrenergic system and mechanisms of beta-receptor blockade

In the early stages of heart failure several neuroendocrine mechanisms beneficial in acute hemodynamic shock are activated via maintaining arterial blood pressure and blood flow to vital organs, thereby supplying these organs with sufficient amounts of oxygen. When chronically activated, these compensatory mechanisms, i.e., an activation of the renin-angiotensin-aldosterone system and of the sympathetic nervous system, have a negative

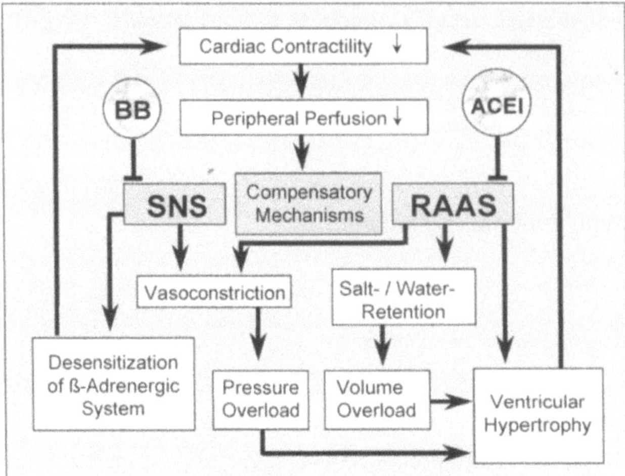

Fig. 1   Pathophysiological processes in heart failure leading to cardiac contractile dysfunction.

impact on cardiac function. Thus, the aim of β-blocker- and angiotensin converting enzyme (ACE)-inhibitor therapy is an interruption of the vicious circle that leads to a continuous impairment of myocardial function (Fig. 1).

Plasma norepinephrine levels are chronically elevated in patients with heart failure and the amount of elevation correlates with their poor prognosis (17). The resulting increase in stimulation of the β-adrenergic system leads to a desensitization of the adenylyl cyclase of the heart (36), which is due to a decrease in β-adrenoceptor density on the surface of the cardiac myocytes (9), an increased expression of the α-subunit of the inhibitory G-protein (Giα, 7), and a phosphorylation of the adrenoceptors by increased activity and expression of the β-adrenergic receptor kinase (βARK, 65). The functional relevance of these cellular changes is reflected by a decreased response of the heart to catecholamines *in vitro* (7) and *in vivo* (28). Furthermore, the chronic β-adrenergic activation causes an increase in heart rate, which leads to reduced myocardial blood flow due to a shortened diastolic coronary vascular perfusion time. This has a negative impact on the balance of myocardial energy expenditure. The catecholamine-induced increase in calcium influx contributes to the high energy expenditure and leads to an intracellular acidosis with impairment of oxydation phosphorylation (54) and an activation of calcium dependent proteases, which might contribute to the development of myocardial necrosis. The detrimental effect of persistent tachycardia on myocardial function is documented by the fact that in several animal models, heart failure can be induced by rapid left ventricular pacing. In normal human hearts, a rise in stimulation frequency is followed by an increase in cardiac contractility. This positive force frequency relationship is blunted in the failing human heart, which can be observed in *in vivo* (24) and *in vitro* (44) experiments. Thus, tachycardia results in a decreased myocardial contractility in the failing human heart.

These mechanisms clearly indicate the detrimental effects of chronic sympathetic activation on cardiac function and are a rationale for a β-blocker therapy in patients with heart failure, as these compounds intervene with the pathophysiological changes that occur in heart failure. An overview of the most common agents used in patients with heart failure and their pharmacological properties is given in Table 1. Metoprolol and bisoprolol have a higher affinity to the β_1- than to the β_2-adrenoceptor. As in the human heart the majority of the β-adrenoceptors consists of the β_1-adrenoceptor population, these agents exert their pharmacological actions primarily in the heart. Adverse effects, such as bronchoconstric-

Table 1 Pharmacological profile of ß-blockers commonly used in heart failure

	β_1-Selectivity	Vasodilatation	α-Receptor-Antagonism	Antioxidant Properties
Metoprolol	++	–	–	–
Bisoprolol	++	–	–	–
Carvedilol	–	+	+	+

tion or worsening of peripheral arterial disease, are mainly due to the blockade of β_2-adreno-ceptors and, thus, occur to a smaller degree with these selective compounds. Carvedilol is a non-selective β-blocker, but in addition to β-blockade this agent causes peripheral vasodilatation due to vascular α-adrenoceptor blockade. None of the listed agents exerts intrinsic sympathomimetic activity (ISA). Partial agonists that exert ISA, like xamoterol, can increase heart rate and contractility to a small degree through a weak stimulation of adenylyl cyclase.

The application of a β-blocker leads to a reduced heart rate, resulting in a lower myocardial energy expenditure (23), prolonged diastolic filling (1), and increased effective myocardial blood flow due to the prolonged coronary vascular diastolic perfusion time (25). The importance of reducing heart rate is documented by the fact that therapy with xamoterol led to an increase in mortality in patients with severe heart failure. In these patients, especially at night, a higher heart rate could be observed due to the intrinsic sympathomimetic activity of this agent (46).

Fig. 2 Effects of metoprolol, carvedilol or placebo on left ventricular ejection fraction and β-adrenoceptor density in patients with heart failure (from 32).

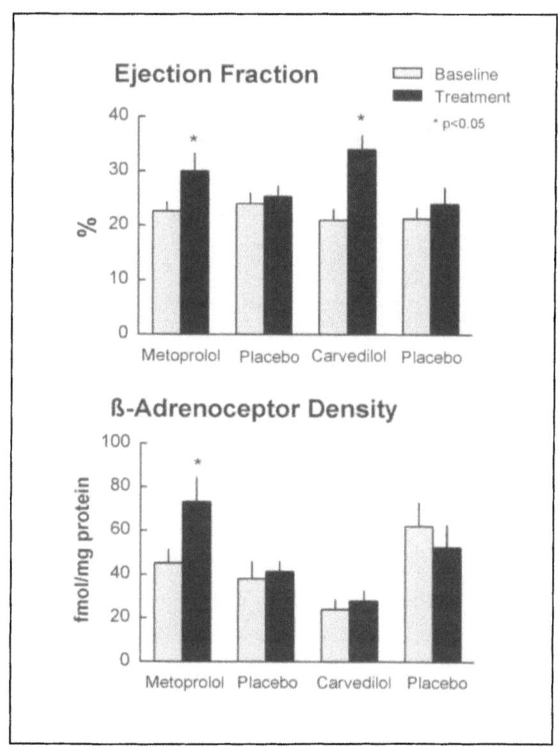

Furthermore, plasma norepinephrine levels are reduced by β-blockers (31), but only carvedilol was shown to reduce cardiac norepinephrine release (30). However, in both cases the myocardium is protected from the cardiotoxic effects of norepinephrine (20, 38). In contrast to carvedilol therapy, metoprolol therapy caused an increase in left ventricular β-adrenoceptor density (32) and downregulated the increased expression of the inhibitory G-protein (56). This indicates that these two agents differ in β-adrenoceptor interaction (72). However, it is unlikely that β-adrenoceptor upregulation plays a crucial role in amelioration of left ventricular function, as left ventricular ejection fraction can be improved by carvedilol therapy (Fig. 2). In addition, a decreased β-adrenoceptor density can be upregulated within hours to days (71), whereas a functional improvement usually occurs not earlier than three months after the onset of β-blocker therapy (33).

Thus, one should consider other mechanisms contributing to the improvement of ventricular function. Kukin et al. (39) compared the effects of metoprolol and the combination of metoprolol and doxazosin (α-blocker) on ventricular function and hemodynamics in patients with heart failure, in order to estimate the relevance of α-receptor blockade. After six weeks of therapy a marked decline in vascular resistance and an increase in cardiac index was observed (Fig. 3). These beneficial effects on hemodynamics were not different in the two groups. Thus, α-receptor blockade (i.e., by carvedilol) appears to have no crucial impact on hemodynamics in long-term therapy.

Of the listed compounds (Table 1) only carvedilol exerts antioxidant activity. This ability of carvedilol to prevent oxygen free radical damage or to scavenge free radicals directly

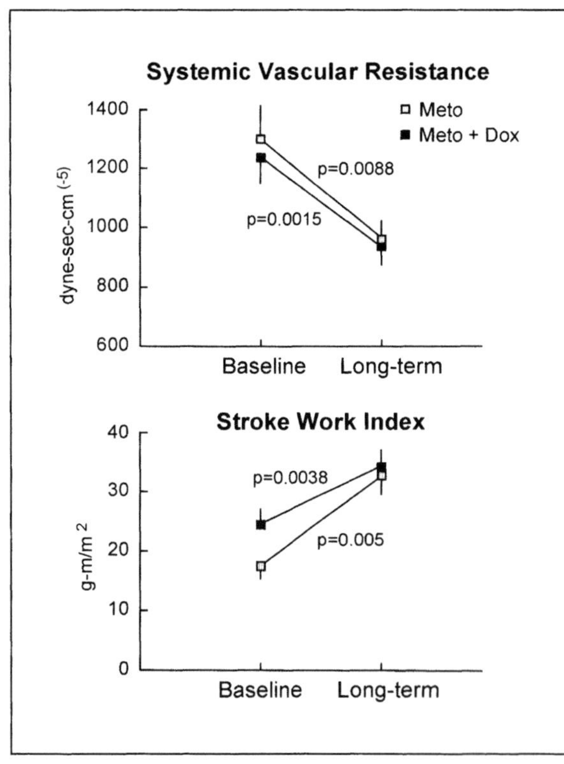

Fig. 3 Effects of β- or β- plus α-blockade in patients with heart failure (from 39).

was demonstrated by several *in vitro* experiments (73, 74). Oxygen free radicals occur not only in the reperfusion of ischemic myocardium (phenomenon of "myocardial stunning"; 8), but also in the plasma of patients with heart failure, where an increased amount of malondialdehydes as a sign for lipid peroxidation due to free radicals was observed. The degree of free radical damage inversely correlates to left ventricular function in these patients (Fig. 4; 5). Oxygen free radicals are involved in the pathogenesis of apoptosis. In the myocardium of patients with heart failure, higher rates of apoptosis compared to normal controls have been observed (45, 48). It is not entirely clear if and to what extent apoptosis contributes to cardiac dysfunction in heart failure. However, carvedilol was shown to reduce free radical-induced apoptotis in reperfused ischemic myocardium (75). But besides the induction of apoptosis, which is an active progress that requires denovo protein synthesis, oxygen free radicals can also lead to a direct impairment of myocardial function (27). Carvedilol, but not metoprolol, led to an improvement of cardiac contractility in human myocardium exposed to free radicals (27). Oxygen free radicals have also been implicated in the pathogenesis of vascular smooth muscle cell proliferation. Both *in vitro* (63) and *in vivo* (47) experiments demonstrated a concentration-dependent inhibition of vascular smooth muscle cell proliferation by carvedilol. Thus, carvedilol treatment could delay the progression of coronary atheromas and alter vascular remodeling processes that occur in chronic heart failure due to ischemic heart disease.

Taken together, the multiple experimental data suggest an explanation for the beneficial effects of β-blockers observed in clinical trials, which ultimately are the crucial criteria for successful treatment of heart failure.

Fig. 4 **A)** Amount of oxygen free radical damage (lipid peroxidation) in patients with heart failure compared to normal controls; **B)** Extent of lipid peroxidation in relation to left ventricular ejection fraction in patients with heart failure (from 5).

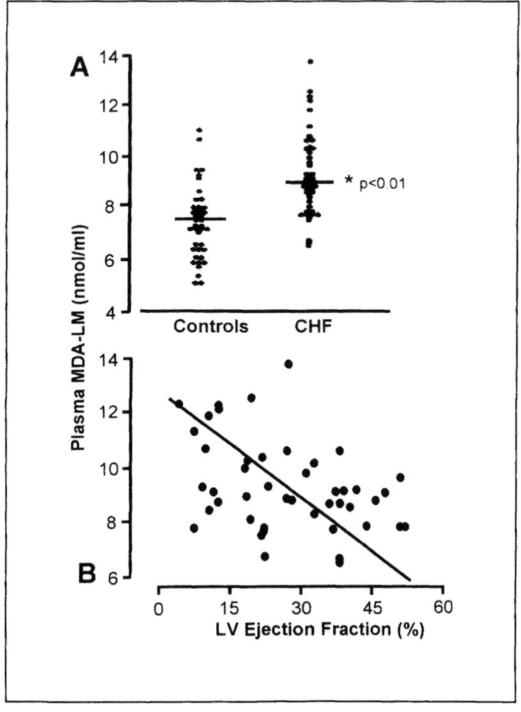

Aims of treatment of heart failure and its evaluation

The objectives of the treatment of heart failure can be defined as to prolong active life and improve quality of life (14). To achieve these goals, major adverse events, such as hospitalization or recurrent myocardial infarction, should be prevented. Preventing the progression of cardiac dysfunction is an integral part of achieving these aims. To estimate the success of heart failure treatment, several subjective and objective parameters can be used. Among the subjective parameters there are clinical estimations of functional classes (NYHA scores) and the general assessment by the physician or patient. The objective parameters consist of the estimation of certain hemodynamic parameters, such as arterial blood pressure, heart rate, ventricular ejection fraction and volumina, but also of the determination of major adverse events such as hospitalization, recurrent myocardial infarction, need for cardiac transplantation or death.

Subjective parameters

Most clinical trials with β_1-selective blockers demonstrated an improvement of symptoms. Metoprolol treatment significantly improved NYHA functional class in patients with idiopathic dilated cardiomyopathy (IDC) (MDC study, 66) as well as with ischemic cardiomyopathy (ICM) (26). This holds true also for bisoprolol in a trial of 641 patients with both IDC and ICM (CIBIS I, 13). In the US trials (50) and in most of the smaller trials with carvedilol, a significant improvement of NYHA functional class was noted. In contrast, the ANZ (3) revealed no significant improvement of NYHA functional class after 18 months of treatment with carvedilol.

Objective parameters

Hemodynamics

By inhibiting the effects of catecholamines on cardiac β-adrenergic receptors, β-blockers are potential negative inotropic compounds and for these reasons had been suggested to be contraindicated in patients with heart failure. Waagstein et al. (67) compared acute and long-term (6 months) effects of metoprolol treatment in patients with heart failure. Figure 5 gives an overview of the results. After acute administration of 5 mg of metoprolol intravenously, a significant decrease in heart rate and a slight reduction of systolic blood pressure could be observed, resulting in a significant decrease of cardiac index. Left ventricular enddiastolic pressure (LVEDP), a sign for cardiac preload, rises consecutively. These changes in hemodynamics are typical effects of a negative inotropic compound. In contrast, after 6 months of long-term therapy with initial doses of 5 mg of metoprolol and a slow uptitration to doses of 2x50 or even 2x100 mg, the hemodynamic situation changed completely. Despite a further decrease in heart rate, systolic blood pressure and cardiac index increased significantly, resulting in a pronounced decrease of LVEDP. These results indicate two things: first, in long-term treatment the negative inotropic effect of the β-blocker converts

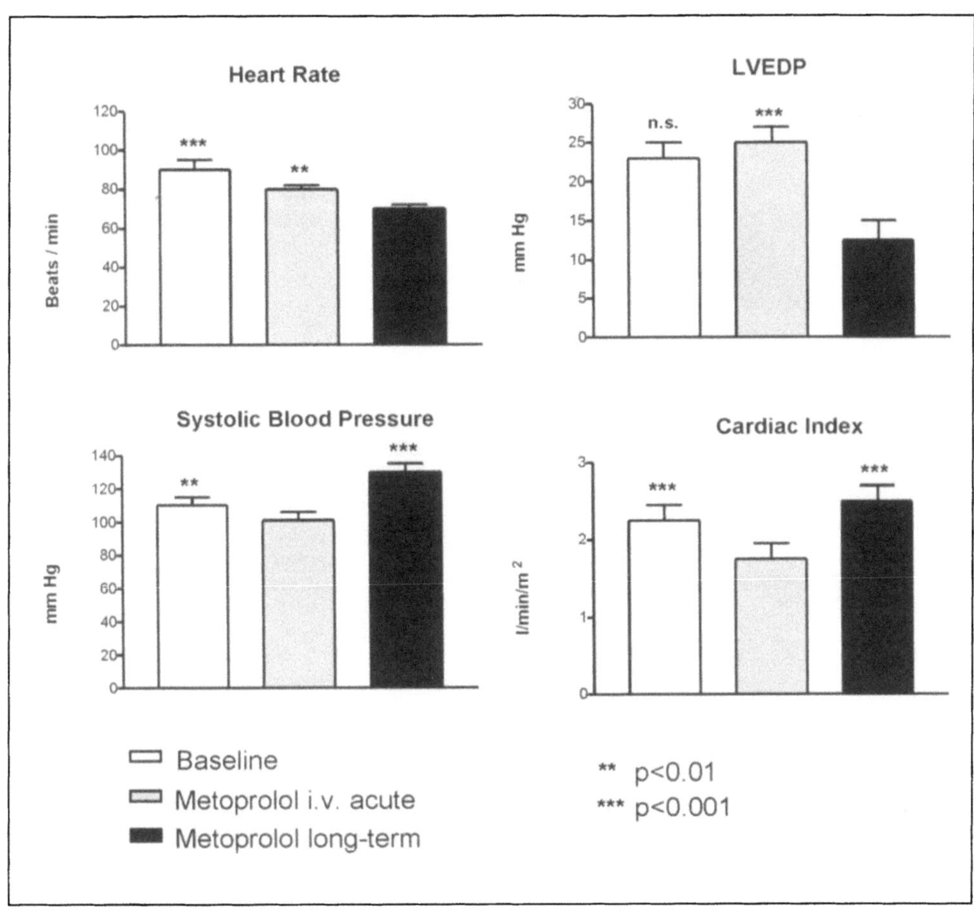

Fig. 5   Effect of short- and long-term metoprolol treatment on various hemodynamic parameters (from 67).

into maintenance of contractility. Second, the results clearly demonstrate that high initial doses or uncautious uptitration of doses might lead to forward failure with decreased cardiac output or to backward failure with pulmonary edema and elevated left ventricular filling pressures. Thus, β-blocker therapy in patients with heart failure must be initiated very carefully.

Already in 1987 comparable results occurred in patients with coronary artery disease after myocardial infarction who were treated with carvedilol. Lahiri et al. (40) observed a concentration-dependent decrease in endsystolic as well as in enddiastolic volumes (Fig. 6). Withdrawal of carvedilol resulted in a subsequent increase of these parameters. As these data were achieved already two weeks after the onset of therapy, the α-adrenoceptor blocking properties with vasodilatation as a consequence could be responsible for this relatively acute reduction of pre- and afterload. These pharmacological properties of carvedilol might be of particular importance during the initiation and titration period of treatment, as this agent might be better tolerated due to its acute hemodynamic effects.

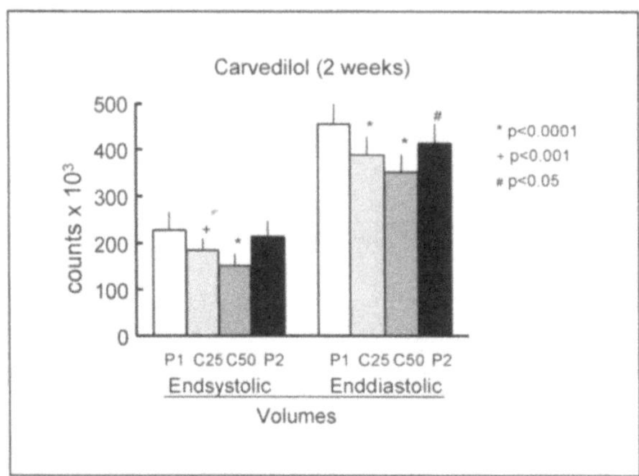

Fig. 6 Effects of various concentrations of carvedilol on left ventricular volumes in patients with stable angina pectoris. Patients entered a 2-week phase taking placebo (P1). They then received carvedilol, 25 (C25) and then 50 mg (C50) twice daily for two weeks on each dose, followed by another 2-week phase of placebo (P2) (from 40).

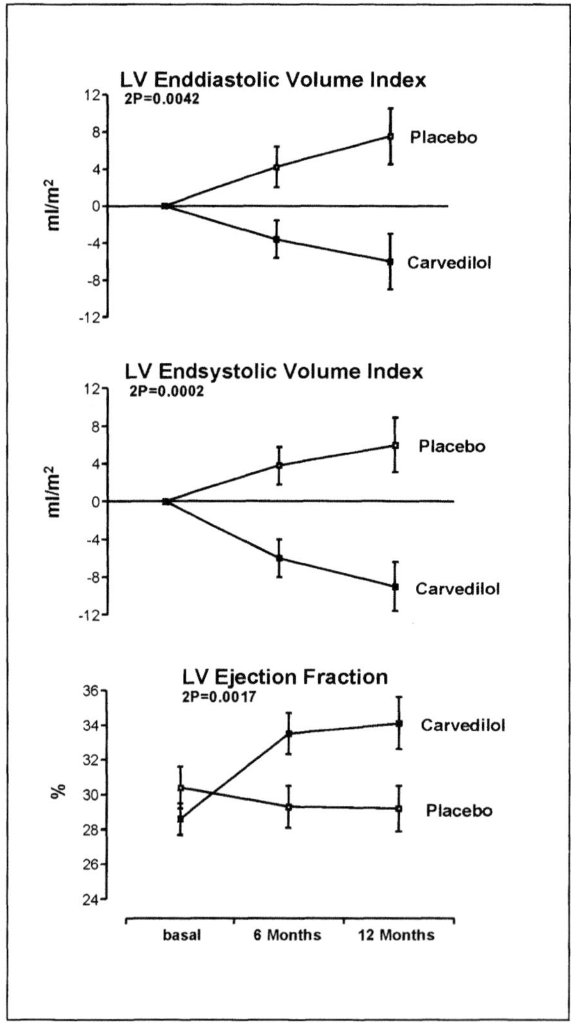

Fig. 7 Effect of carvedilol treatment on left ventricular volume indexes and ejection fraction in patients with heart failure (from 22).

Ventricular function and remodeling

Although there is evidence for the development of tolerance to the vasodilating effects of α-adrenoceptor blocking agents (4, 43), 12 months of carvedilol treatment in patients with heart failure demonstrated a progredient positive impact on left ventricular volumes (22). In a substudy of the ANZ trial of carvedilol in patients with heart failure due to ischemic heart disease, the effects of this treatment on left ventricular (LV) endsystolic and enddiastolic volumes and on LV ejection fraction were determined. Despite a basal treatment including ACE inhibitors, there was a continuous increase in LV endsystolic and enddiastolic volume index. In contrast, in patients receiving carvedilol these parameters decreased significantly compared to controls (Fig. 7). Left ventricular ejection fraction increased by 4.9 % in the carvedilol group compared with the placebo group, in which this parameter remained unaffected. These data suggest that in patients with heart failure a progressive left ventricular dilatation can occur despite a lack of deterioration of LV ejection fraction. These observations are in accordance with earlier results from patients after myocardial infarction (29). In those patients left ventricular volumes could be identified as important prognostic markers with regard to mortality (34, 69). In studies on patients after myocardial infarction the ACE inhibitor captopril was shown to attenuate left ventricular dilatation (55) and to reduce mortality (64). The causal relationship between ventricular dilatation and mortality could be due to the observation that ventricular remodeling may result in both pump failure and sudden death (15). These results clearly suggest the important role of ventricular remodeling in the context of the development of heart failure after ischemic events. Hence, when considering the effect of an intervention on left ventricular ejection fraction as a marker of left ventricular function, it is important to consider the associated changes in left ventricular volumes (22). The main ANZ carvedilol trial (3) demonstrated a 26 % reduction in a combined end point of death or hospital admission after 20 months of treatment. Thus, the beneficial effect of carvedilol on left ventricular remodeling reported in the ANZ substudy (22) would be consistent with favorable effects of this agent on mortality.

These benefits of β-blocker treatment are limited neither to heart failure resulting from ischemic heart disease nor to treatment with carvedilol. Hall et al. (33) could demonstrate that in patients with heart failure due to both ischemic heart disease and idiopathic dilated cardiomyopathy, long-term (18 months) metoprolol treatment resulted in a significant reduction of left ventricular volumes and mass. Left ventricular shape became less spherical and assumed a more normal elliptical shape. These morphological changes were paralleled by an improvement of left ventricular ejection fraction. Both the studies on metoprolol (33) and on carvedilol (22) indicate that the addition of long-term β-blockade to background therapy with ACE inhibitors confers additional benefit by reducing ventricular remodeling. Thus, these observations suggest that β-blocking agents may not simply slow remodeling, but may actually reverse it (33). Further studies elucidating the pathophysiological mechanisms can be expected.

In more than 20 trials that investigated β-blocker treatment in patients with heart failure, a mean increase in left ventricular ejection fraction of 7.7 % could be observed (35). This improvement of hemodynamics was independent of the underlying genesis of heart failure (IDC or ICM), the amount of left ventricular ejection fraction at baseline, and the kind of β-blocker that was used (metoprolol, bisoprolol or carvedilol). As previously mentioned, the time course of change in ventricular function is of particular importance. Hall et al. (33) could demonstrate that at day 1 of metoprolol treatment left ventricular ejection fraction was depressed but returned to baseline by month 1 and improved between month 1 and 3 (Fig. 8). By the third month of therapy there was a significant increase in left ventricular ejection fraction in the metoprolol group patients compared with those in the stan-

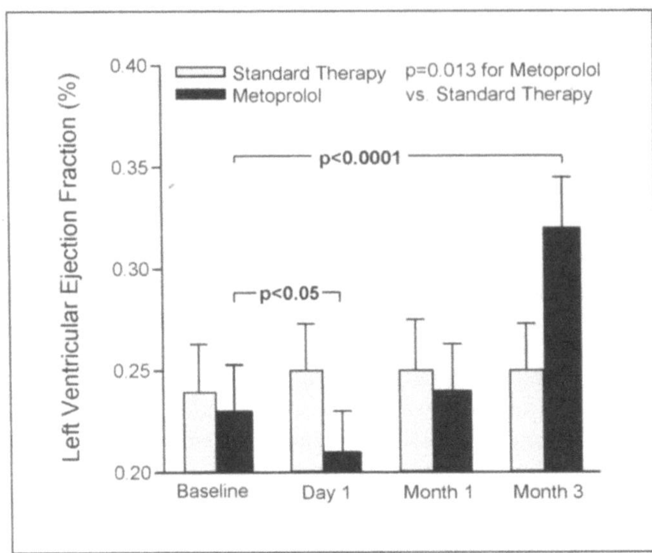

Fig. 8 Changes in left ventricular ejection fraction from baseline to day 1, month 1, and month 3 in the metoprolol and standard therapy group (from 33).

dard therapy group. These results are consistent with the observations of Waagstein et al. (67, see above) regarding ventricular filling pressures and cardiac index and may be an explanation for the common problem that many patients with heart failure report temporal deterioration of symptoms at the onset of β-blocker therapy. Thus, it is very important to initiate a β-blocker therapy in these patients at very low doses in order to avoid a decompensation of heart failure due to the pharmacologically acute effects of β-blockers. Nevertheless, to achieve optimal effects of treatment, low initial doses should be titrated up to the maximum tolerated dose within several weeks.

Exercise tolerance

The role of exercise tolerance as a criterion for successful treatment of heart failure is controversial. Clinical trials have not sufficiently demonstrated a correlation between exercise tolerance and mortality (59). Furthermore, it is questionable whether the tolerance of maximal exercise is important for improving quality of life, or whether the estimation of submaximal exercise tolerance (i.e., by the 6 minute walk distance) is a more adequate way to determine one's ability to cope with situations in every day life. In this context Hash and Prisant (35) compared the results of most studies on β-blockers in heart failure regarding maximal and submaximal exercise tolerance. They found that β-blockers have a greater effect on submaximal exercise than on maximal exercise capacity. An improvement of maximal exercise capacity could only be observed by the treatment with metoprolol, whereas carvedilol only improved submaximal exercise tolerance. The absence of improvement in maximal exercise capacity has been attributed to the attenuation of peak exercise heart rate by β-blockers. Bristow et al. (11) found a significant direct correlation between the reduction in maximum exercise time and reduction in peak exercise heart rate. The fact that in some studies improvement in maximal exercise can be achieved under β-blockade despite attenuation of maximal exercise heart rate suggests that in these patients the treatment with β-blockers led to an improved cardiac contractility.

The different effects of metoprolol and carvedilol on exercise capacity might be due to the differences in the β-adrenoceptor interaction between these two compounds. As previously described, there is a 60 to 70 % reduction of cardiac β_1-adrenoceptor density in patients with severe heart failure. In addition, the responsiveness of β_2-adrenoceptors is reduced by 30 % due to uncoupling from the adenylyl cyclase system (32), and the α-subunit of the inhibitory G-protein is overexpressed (7). Metoprolol therapy leads to a reversal of these pathological changes and to an improved response of the heart to catecholamines (37) and milrinone (6), an inhibitor of the 3'5'-adenosinmono-phosphate (cAMP)-phosphodiesterase (PDE III). This indicates that a blockade of cardiac β-adrenoceptors by metoprolol can be overcome by high levels of catecholamines, and the increased positive inotropic effect of catecholamines appears to be due to the improvements of the β-adrenergic system (increased β-adrenoceptor density and decreased levels of G_i α). White et al. (70) examined the relation between cardiac β-adrenoceptor density and maximal exercise capacity in 72 patients with idiopathic dilated cardiomyopathy. They observed that of all variables, maximal exercise oxygen consumption had the highest correlation with β-adrenoceptor density. In the same study, metoprolol treatment, but not carvedilol treatment, led to an increase in left ventricular β-adrenoceptor density. When taking into account that maximal exercise capacity is only improved by metoprolol treatment, whereas carvedilol improves submaximal exercise capacity, it can be concluded that "peripheral adaptations (i.e., by the intrinsic vasodilating effects of carvedilol) play a more important role in the ability to sustain submaximal exercise, with β-adrenergic signal transduction being more important in the cardiac response to peak exercise" (70).

Mortality

As described, β-blocker treatment in patients with heart failure improves symptoms and cardiac function. It seems likely that these beneficial effects could also cause a prolongation of survival. However, this cannot be taken as proven. Milrinone, an inhibitor of the phosphodiesterase (PDE III) improved symptoms and exercise capacity in patients with heart failure, but caused an increase in mortality of these patients (PROMISE trial, 49). Recent data of the DIG study (21) demonstrated that treatment with digoxin improved symptoms and reduced hospitalization in patients with heart failure, but had no effects on survival. Thus, Lipicky and Packer (41) state that, in the area of heart failure, no surrogate end point currently exists that can be used to assess the effect of a drug on survival.

The MDC trial (66) enrolled 383 patients with heart failure due to idiopathic dilated cardiomyopathy, of whom 94 % were in NYHA functional class II or III. Patients were treated with either metoprolol or placebo for 18 months. Although there was no reduction of overall mortality (even a slight increase), the combined endpoint of death or need for transplantation was reduced by metoprolol treatment by 34 % (relative %).

The CIBIS I trial (13) included mainly patients in NYHA functional class III, and half of the study population had heart failure due to ischemic heart disease. After 23 months of treatment there was no reduction in overall mortality. However, when looking at subgroup analysis, bisoprolol treatment significantly reduced mortality in patients without a history of myocardial infarction by 50 %, whereas in patients with heart failure and a history of myocardial infarction bisoprolol had no effect on mortality. As no stratification based on etiology of heart failure was performed at randomization and thus patients did not entirely undergo coronary angiography, one has to be careful in interpreting these results.

The ANZ study on carvedilol (3) consisted exclusively of patients with mild heart failure due to ischemic heart disease. The treatment with carvedilol caused a 26 % reduction of the combined end point death or hospitalization after 19 months, but again no decrease of overall mortality. This result may be due to the fairly good overall prognosis of patients in the study population. The ANZ trial was part of a prospective study in the context of the US carvedilol heart failure program. Besides the ANZ study, patients were assigned to one of four treatment protocols on the basis of their exercise capacity. Thus, the US trials consisted of patients with mild (18), moderate (10, 51), and severe (16) heart failure. After 6.5 months of treatment, the overall mortality in all four protocols was reduced by 67 % by the treatment with carvedilol, independent of the underlying etiology of heart failure (IDC or ICM) and of the severity of heart failure (50, Fig. 9). This finding led the Data and Monitoring Board to recommend termination of the study before its scheduled completion. Pfeffer and Stevenson (53) criticized that this was not the result of a single, definitve trial with adequate power to detect changes in mortality, and that there was a censoring of seven deaths during the run-in period. This two-week period was designed to test the patient's ability to tolerate the drug that was being tested. However, this 0.6 % mortality during the run-in period of the US carvedilol trial is comparable to the mortality of the run-in period of the SOLVD treatment trial (58).

Cleland et al. (14) summarized the data of the four large trials on three different β-blockers (metoprolol, bisoprolol, and carvedilol) with more than 2500 patients suffering from heart failure altogether. The mortality on placebo was 12.8 % falling to 8.3 % on a β-blocker over a follow-up of about 13 months, resulting in a relative risk reduction of about 37 % and an absolute benefit of 45 lives saved per 1000 treated. This absolute benefit is similar to that of ACE inhibition in the SOLVD treatment trial (58), in which about 35 lives had been saved per 1000 treated with enalapril at 15 months. In the SOLVD treatment trial, one-year mortality of 16 % on placebo fell to 12 % on enalapril. When extrapolating the 7.8 % mortality on placebo in the US carvedilol trial to a duration of one year, the result is comparable to the mortality of the active treatment group of the SOLVD treatment trial. In all four trials most patients in the placebo groups received standard therapy including ACE inhibitors. Therefore the effect of a β-blocker can be viewed as an additional benefit.

In the meantime, large trials with bisoprolol (CIBIS II, 12) and metoprolol (MERIT-HF, 42) have been undertaken. Bisoprolol led to a 34 % decrease of overall-mortality in mainly NYHA III patients suffering from heart failure of ischemic and non-ischemic cause. For metoprolol, a 34 % reduction of mortality in patients in NYHA class II-III (IDC and ICM)

Mortality	Placebo	ß-Blocker	Risk reduction
US Carvedilol Studies:			
n=1052 (53% NYHA II; 44% NYHA III; 3%NYHA IV)			
Total	7.8%	3.2%	65% (p<0.0001)
NYHA II	6.0%	2.0%	60% (p<0.05)
NYHA III-IV	11.0%	4.0%	67% (p<0.05)
IDC	6.7%	2.5%	65% (p<0.05)
ICM	9.0%	3.9%	65% (p<0.01)
CIBIS II: n=2647 (83% NYHA III; 17% NYHA IV)			
Total	17.3%	11.8%	34% (p<0.0001)
MERIT-HF: n=3991 (41% NYHA II, 56% NYHA III, 3.6% NYHA IV)			
Total	11.0%	7.2%	34% (p=0.00009)

Fig. 9 Mortality results from heart failure trials with carvedilol (50), bisoprolol (CIBIS II, 12) and metoprolol (MERIT-HF, 42).

has been observed (Fig. 9). In both studies, sufficient data concerning the effects of these agents on mortality in NYHA IV patients are not available. Very recently, the COPERNIKUS study has been terminated. In this study, carvedilol has led to an improved survival in patients with severe heart failure (NYHA IV) (unpublished data).

Carvedilol was the first β-blocking agent that had been permitted for the treatment of stable chronic heart failure in the USA and most western countries in 1997. In 1999, metoprolol and bisoprolol have also been permitted for this indication.

Future studies

To estimate whether the different pharmacological properties of metoprolol and carvedilol have different effects on survival, a comparing trial (COMET) has been initiated. Patient recruitment was complete in 1998. The CAPRICORN trial will test whether carvedilol influences ventricular remodeling and the progress of left ventricular dysfunction to manifest heart failure in patients after myocardial infarction.

Doses

As already mentioned in the section "Hemodynamics", a β-blocker has a potential negative inotropic effect. Thus, in patients with heart failure, it is of great importance to initiate

Fig. 10 Mortality in the US carvedilol trials of the US Carvedilol Heart Failure Program.

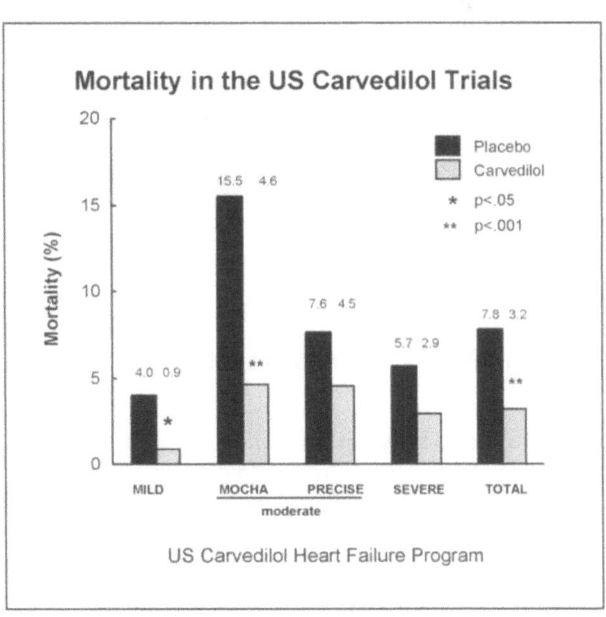

Table 2 Doses of β-blocker treatment of heart failure

	Test Dose**	Starting Dose	Titration***	Target Dose
Metoprolol*	10 mg	1 x 10 mg	→	200 mg***
Bisoprolol	1.25 mg	1 x 1.25 mg	→	10 mg***
Carvedilol	3.125 mg	2 x 3.125 mg	→	2 x 25 mg****
*slow release	**under observation of a physician		***Doubling of dose approx. every 14 days, depending on the clinical condition	****or highest tolerated dose, respectively

treatment with a β-blocker at very low doses in order to avoid decompensation. The treated patient should be in a stable condition for at least two weeks and should receive standard therapy consisting of diuretics, digitalis, and ACE inhibitors. As patients with heart failure have a poor prognosis and tend to decompensate already at slight worsening of cardiac function, a β-blocker should be regarded as additional treatment and should not replace any of the standard drugs. In the US trials even a β-blocker with beneficial hemodynamic properties such as carvedilol led to increased hospitalization in patients with severe heart failure (NYHA III–IV), although in less severe heart failure hospitalization was reduced. As long-term treatment with carvedilol exerted beneficial effects regarding survival in patients with mild, moderate, and severe heart failure (Fig.10), the temporary aggravation of symptoms does not necessarily indicate a lack of efficacy, but is rather a sign for the biphasic character of pharmacological activity of β-blockers, which was also mentioned in the section "Hemodynamics". Regarding the study of Hall et al. (30, Fig. 8), a beneficial effect of a β-blocker on ventricular function cannot be expected before the third month of treatment. As the hemodynamic parameters are consistent with clinical observations, during this critical period of the first three months a rather careful observation of the patient is indicated.

Table 2 summarizes the dose pattern of β-blocker treatment of heart failure. Of great importance is the initiation of therapy with very low doses. According to clinical response, the dose should be doubled at 2-week intervals towards the target dose. In patients who experience worsening symptoms of chronic heart failure, the doses of ACE inhibitor or diuretic, or both, should be increased, whereas the doses of these agents should be reduced in the event of symptomatic hypotension. Figure 11 illustrates that the effects of β-blocking therapy on ejection fraction and mortality were dose-dependent. Thus, achieving the target dose is of importance for the therapeutical success of β-blocker treatment.

Which patients should be treated?

Patients with chronic heart failure should be in a stable condition before they are put on β-blockers. Patients with bronchial asthma should not receive a β-blocker. Tachycardia can be a sign for an increased sympathetic activation. In patients with an increased heart rate at rest a β-blocker might be of special benefit as these patients profit especially from the negative chronotropic effect of this compound. In the mortality studies of β-blockade, the mean age of patients has ranged from 49 years to 67 years, whereas the mean age of chronic

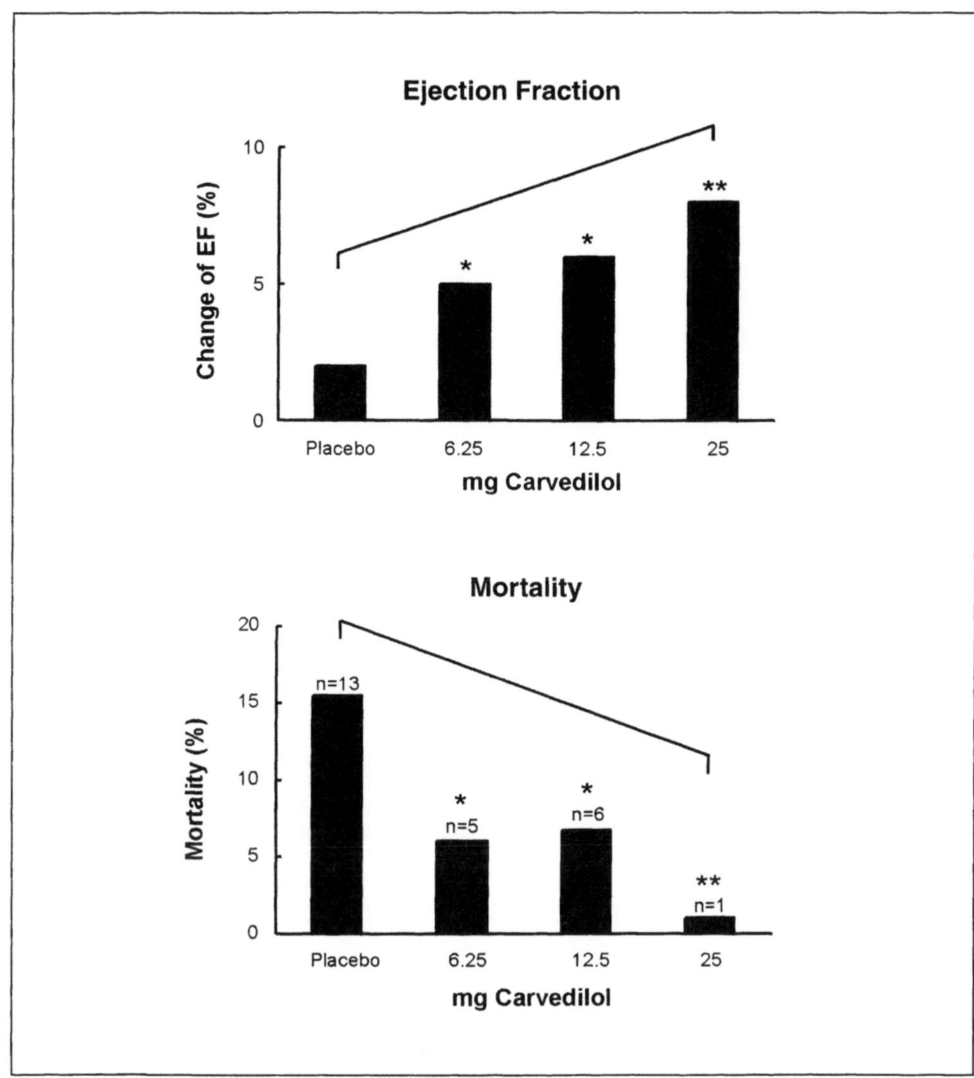

Fig. 11   Effect of various concentrations of carvedilol on left ventricular ejection fraction and mortality (from 10).

heart failure patients in the community is 74 years (52). However, the US carvedilol trials suggest that the mortality benefits were similar in patients above and below the median age. Thus, a patient's age appears to have no impact on the efficacy of β-blocking treatment of heart failure. The underlying etiology of heart failure could also be relevant. In the carvedilol US trials as well as in CIBIS II and MERIT-HF, the benefit of β-blockers concerning survival was independent of the underlying etiology of heart failure. Taken together, no final conclusion regarding the choice of a β-blocker at a certain etiology of heart failure can be drawn from the results of the mentioned trials. Thus, further results from future trials (i.e., COMET) must be analyzed.

Summary

The treatment of heart failure with β-blockers is rational, as it is a pharmacological prevention of the deleterious effects of elevated plasma norepinephrine levels on cardiac function that occur in patients with heart failure. Clinical trials demonstrated a beneficial effect of β-blocker treatment on symptoms, ventricular function, hospitalization, and survival. Thus, β-blockers can be used in addition to standard therapy consisting of diuretics, digitalis, and ACE inhibitors. Careful initiation and uptitration of the applicated doses is of great importance.

References

1. Andersson B, Hamm C, Persson S et al. (1994) Improved exercise hemodynamic status in dilated cardiomyopathy after beta-blockade treatment. J Am Coll Cardiol 23: 1397–1404
2. Australia-New Zealand Heart Failure Research Collaborative Group (1995) Effects of carvedilol, a vasodilator-beta-blocker, in patients with congestive heart failure due to ischemic heart disease. Circulation 92: 212–218
3. Australia-New Zealand Heart Failure Research Collaborative Group (1997) Randomized, placebo-controlled trial of carvedilol in patients with congestive heart failure due to ischemic heart disease. Lancet 349: 375–380
4. Awan NA, Needham KE, Evenson MK et al. (1981) Therapeutic application of prazosin in chronic refractory congestive heart failure: tolerance and "tachyphylaxis" in perspective. Am J Med 71: 153–160
5. Belch JJF, Bridges AB, Scott N, Chopra M (1991) Oxygen free radicals in congestive heart failure. Br Heart J 65: 245–248
6. Böhm M, Deutsch HJ, Hartmann D, La Rosée K, Stäblein A (1997) Improvement of postreceptor events by metoprolol treatment in patients with chronic heart failure. J Am Coll Cardiol 30: 992–996
7. Böhm M, Gierschik P, Jakobs KH, Pieske B, Schnabel P, Ungerer M, Erdmann E (1990) Increase of Gia in human hearts with dilated but not ischemic cardiomyopathy. Circulation 82: 1249–1265
8. Bolli R (1990) Mechanisms of myocardial stunning. Circulation 82: 723–738
9. Bristow MR, Ginsburg R, Minobe W, Cubiciotti RS, Sageman WS, Lurie K, Billingham ME, Harrison DE, Stinson EB (1982) Decreased catecholamine sensitivity and ß-adrenergic receptor density in failing human hearts. N Engl J Med 307: 205–211
10. Bristow MR, Gilbert EM, Abraham WT, Adams KF, Fowler MB, Hershberger RE, Kubo SH, Narahara KA, Ingersoll H, Krueger S, Young S, Shusterman N (1996) Carvedilol produces dose-related improvements in left ventricular function and survival in subjects with chronic heart failure. MOCHA Investigators (Comment). Circulation 94: 2807–2816
11. Bristow MR, O'Connel JB, Gilbert EM et al. (1994) Dose-response of chronic β-blocker treatment in heart failure from either idiopathic dilated or ischemic cardiomyopathy. Circulation 89: 1632–1642
12. CIBIS II-Investigators and Committees (1999) The Cardiac Insufficiency Bisoprolol Study II (CIBIS II): a randomised trial. Lancet 353: 9–13
13. CIBIS Investigators and Committees (1994) A randomized trial of β-blockade in heart failure. The Cardiac Insufficienty Bisoprolol Study (CIBIS). Circulation 90: 1765–1773
14. Cleland JGF, Bristow MR, Erdmann E, Remme WJ, Swedberg K, Waagstein F (1996) Beta-blocking agents in heart failure-should they be used and how? Eur Heart J 17: 1629–1639
15. Cohn JN (1994) Vasodilators in heart failure: conclusions from V-HeFT II and rationale for V-HeFT III. Drugs 47 (suppl 4): 47–58
16. Cohn J, Fowler MB, Bristow MR, Colucci WS, Gilbert EM, Kinal V et al. (1997) Safety and efficacy of carvedilol in severe chronic heart failure. J Card Failure 3: 173–179
17. Cohn JN, Levine TB, Olivari MT, Gerberg V, Lura D, Francis GS, Simon AB, Rector T (1984) Plasma norepinephrine as a guide to prognosis in patients with chronic congestive heart failure. N Engl J Med 311: 819–823
18. Colucci WS, Packer M, Bristow MR, Cohn J, Fowler MB, Gilbert EM et al. (1996) Carvedilol inhibits clinical progression in patients with mild heart failure. Circulation 94: 2800–2806
19. The CONSENSUS Trial Study Group (1987) Effects of enalapril on mortality in severe congestive heart failure. Results of the Cooperative North Scandinavian Enalapril Survival Study (CONSENSUS). N Engl J Med 316: 1429–1435

20. Cruickshank JM, Neil-Dwyer G, Degaute JP et al. (1987) Reduction of stress/catecholamine-induced cardiac necrosis by beta1-selective blockade. Lancet 1: 585–589

21. The Digitalis Investigation Group (DIG) (1997) The effect of digoxin on mortality and morbidity in patients with heart failure. N Engl J Med 336 (8): 525–533

22. Doughty RN, Whalley GA, Gamble G et al. on behalf of the Australia-New Zealand Heart Failure Research Collaborative Group (1997) Left ventricular remodeling with carvedilol in patients with congestive heart failure due to ischemic heart disease. J Am Coll Cardiol 29: 1060–1066

23. Eichhorn EJ, Bedotto JB, Malloy CR et al. (1990) Effects of β-adrenergic receptor blockade on myocardial function and energetics in congestive heart failure. Circulation 82: 473–483

24. Feldman MD, Alderman JD, Aroesty JM, Royal HD, Ferguson JJ, Owen RM, Grossman W, McKay RG (1988) Depression of systolic and diastolic myocardial reserve during atrial pacing tachycardia in patients with dilated cardiomyopathy. J Clin Invest 82: 1661–1669

25. Ferro G, Duilio C, Spinelli L et al. (1991) Effects of beta-blockade on the relation between heart rate and ventricular diastolic perfusion time during exercise in systemic hypertension. Am J Cardiol 68: 1101–1103

26. Fisher ML, Gottlieb SS, Plotnick G et al. (1994) Beneficial effects of metoprolol in heart failure associated with coronary artery disease: a randomized trial. J Am Coll Cardiol 23: 943–950

27. Flesch M, Maack C, Cremers B, Bäumer AT, Südkamp M, Böhm M (1999) Effect of β-blockers on free radical-induced cardiac contractile dysfunction. Circulation 100: 346–353

28. Gage J, Rutman H, Lucido D, Le Jemtel TH (1986) Additive effects of Dobutamine and amrinone on myocardial contractility and ventricular performance in patients with severe heart failure. Circulation 74: 367–373

29. Gaudron P, Eilles C, Kugler I, Ertl G (1993) Progressive left ventricular dysfunction and remodeling after myocardial infarction. Potential mechanisms and early predictors. Circulation 87: 755–763

30. Gilbert EM, Abraham WT, Olsen S, Hattler B, White M et al. (1996) Comparative hemodynamic, left ventricular functional and antiadrenergic effects of chronic treatment with metoprolol versus carvedilol in the failing heart. Circulation 94: 2817–2825

31. Gilbert EM, Anderson JL, Deitchman D et al. (1990) Long-term beta-blocker vasodilator therapy improves cardiac function in idiopathic dilated cardiomyopathy: a double-blind, randomized study of bucindolol versus placebo. Am. J. Med. 88: 223–229

32. Gilbert EM, Olsen SL, Renlund DG, Bristow MR (1993) Beta-adrenergic receptor regulation and left ventricular function in idiopathic dilated cardiomyopathy. Am J Cardiol 71: 23C–29C

33. Hall SA, Cigarroa CG, Marcoux L, Risser RC et al. (1995) Time course of improvement in left ventricular function, mass and geometry in patients with congestive heart failure trearted with beta-adrenergic blockade. J Am Coll Cardiol 25: 1154–6131

34. Hammermeister KE, De Rouen TA, Dodge HT (1979) Variables predictive of survival in patients with coronary disease: selection by univariate and multivariate analyses from the clinical, electrocardiographic, exercise, arteriographic and quantitative angiographic evaluations. Circulation 59: 421–430

35. Hash TW, Prisant LM (1997) β-blocker use in systolic heart failure and dilated cardiomyopathy. J Am Coll Cardiol 37: 7–19

36. Hausdorff WP, Caron MG, Lefkowitz RJ (1990) Turning off the signal: desensitization of β-adrenergic receptor function. FASEB J 4: 2881–2889

37. Heilbrunn SM, Shah P, Bristow MR, Valantine HA et al. (1989) Increased β-receptor density and improved hemodynamic response to catecholamine stimulation during long-term metoprolol therapy in heart failure from dilated cardiomyopathy. Circulation 79: 483–490

38. Imperato-McGinley J, Gautier T, Ehlers K et al. (1987) Reversibility of catecholamine-induced dilated cardiomyopathy in a child with pheochromocytoma. N Engl J Med 316: 793–797

39. Kukin ML, Kalman J, Mannino M, Freudenberger R et al. (1996) Combined alpha-beta-blockade (doxazosin and metoprolol) compared with beta-blockade alone in chronic congestive heart failure. Am J Cardiol 77: 486–491

40. Lahiri A, Rodrigues EA, Al-Khawaja I et al. (1987) Effect of a new vasodilating beta-blocking drug, carvedilol, on left ventricular function in stable angina-pectoris. Am J Cardiol 59: 769–774

41. Lipicky RJ, Packer M (1993) Role of surrogate end points in the evaluation of drugs for heart failure. J Am Coll Cardiol 22 (suppl A): 179A–184A

42. MERIT-HF Study Group (1999) Effect of metoprolol CR/XL in chronic heart failure: Metoprolol CR/XL Randomised Intervention Trial in Congestive Heart Failure (MERIT-HF). Lancet 353: 2001–2007

43. Metra M, Nardi M, Giubbini R (1994) Effects of short- and long-term carvedilol administration on rest and exercise hemodynamic variables, exercise capacity and clinical conditions in patients with idiopathic dilated cardiomyopathy. J Am Coll Cardiol 24: 1678–1687

44. Mulieri LA, Hasenfuss G, Leavitt B, Allen PD, Alpert NR (1992) Altered myocardial force-frequency relation in human heart failure. Circulation 85: 1743–1750

45. Narula J, Haider N, Virmani R, DiSalvo TG, Kolodgie FE, Hajjar RJ, Schmidt U, Semigran MJ, Dee GW, Khaw BA (1996) Apoptosis in myocytes in end-stage heart failure. N Engl J Med 335: 1182–1189

46. Nicholas G, Oakley C, Pouleur H et al. (1990) Xamoterol in severe heart failure. Lancet 336: 1–6

47. Ohlstein EH, Douglas SA, Sung C-P et al. (1993) Carvedilol, a cardiovascular drug, prevents vascular smooth muscle cell proliferation, migration and neointimal formation following vascular injury. Proc Natl Acad Sci USA 90: 6189–6193

48. Olivetti G, Abbi R, Quaini F Kajstura J, Cheng W, Nitahara JA, Quaini E, Di Loreto C, Beltrami CA, Krajewski W, Reed JC, Anversa P (1997) Apoptosis in the failing human heart. N Engl J Med 336: 1131–1141

49. Packer M, Arver JR, Rodeheffer RJ, Ivanhoe RJ et al. for the PROMISE Study Research Group (1991) Effect of oral milrinone on mortality in severe chronic heart failure. N Engl J Med 325: 1468–1475

50. Packer M, Bristow MR, Cohn JN et al. for the US carvedilol study group (1996) The effect of carvedilol on morbidity and mortality in patients with chronic heart failure. N Engl J Med 334: 1349–1355

51. Packer M, Colucci WS, Sackner-Bernstein JD, Liang CS et al. for the PRECISE Study Group (1996) Double-blind, placebo controlled study of the effects of carvedilol in patients with moderate to severe heart failure: the PRECISE trial. Circulation 94: 2793–2799

52. Parmershwar J, Shackel MM, Richardson A, Poole-Wilson PA, Sutton GC (1992) Prevalence of heart failure in three general practices in north west London. Br J General Pract 42: 287–289

53. Pfeffer MA, Stevenson LW (1996) β-adrenergic blockers and survival in heart failure. N Engl J Med 334: 1396–1397

54. Schwartz A, Lindenmayer GE, Harigaya S (1968) Respiratory control and calcium transport in heart mitochondria from the cardiomyopathic hamster. Trans N Y Acad Sci 30 (Suppl 2): 951

55. Sharpe N, Murphy J, Smith H, Hannan S (1988) Treatment of patients with symptomless left ventricular dysfunction after myocardial infarction. Lancet 255–259

56. Sigmund M, Jakob H, Becker H (1996) Effects of metoprolol on myocardial β-adrenoceptors and Gia-proteins in patients with congestive heart failure. Eur J Clin Pharmacol 51: 127–132

57. Smith WM (1985) Epidemiology of congestive heart failure. Am J Cardiol 55: 3–8A

58. The SOLVD Investigators (1991) Effects of enalapril on survival in patients with reduced left ventricular ejection fractions and congestive heart failure. N Engl J Med 325: 293–302

59. Swedberg K (1994) Exercise testing in heart failure: a critical review. Drugs 47 (suppl 4): 14–24

60. Swedberg K, Hjalmarson A, Waagstein F, Wallentin I (1979) Prolongation of survival in congestive cardiomyopathy by beat-receptor blockade. Lancet 1: 1374–1376

61. Swedberg K, Hjalmarson A, Waagstein F, Wallentin I (1980) Adverse effects of beta-blocker withdrawal in patients with congestive cardiomyopathy. Br Heart J 44: 134–142

62. Swedberg K, Hjalmarson A, Waagstein F, Wallentin I (1980) Beneficial effects of long-term beta-blockade in congestive cardiomyopathy. Br Heart J 44: 117–133

63. Sung C-P, Arleth AJ, Ohlstein EH (1993) Carvedilol inhibits vascular smooth muscle cell proliferation. J Cardiovasc Pharmacol 21: 221–227

64. Sutton MSJ, Pfeffer MA, Plappert T et al. (1994) Quantitative two-dimensional echocardiographic measurements are major predictors of adverse cardiovascular events after acute myocardial infarction. Circulation 89: 68–75

65. Ungerer M, Böhm M, Elce JS, Erdmann E, Lohse MJ (1993) Altered expression of ß-adrenergic receptor kinase and β1-adrenergic receptors in the failing human heart. Circulation 87: 454–463

66. Waagstein F, Bristow MR, Swedberg K et al. (1993) Beneficial effects of metoprolol in idiopathic dilated cardiomyopathy. Lancet 342: 1441–1446

67. Waagstein F, Caidahl K, Wallentin I et al. (1989) Long-term beta-blockade in dilated cardiomyopathy: effects of short- and long-term metoprolol treatment followed by withdrawal and readministration of metoprolol. Circulation 80: 551–563

68. Waagstein F, Hjalmarson A, Varnauskas E, Wallentin I (1975) Effect of chronic beta-adrenergic receptor blockade in congestive cardiomyopathy. Br Heart J 37: 1022–1036

69. White HD, Norris RM, Brown MA, Brandt PWT, Whitlock RML, Wild CJ (1987) Left ventricular end-systolic volume as the major determinant of survival after recovery from myocardial infarction. Circulation 76: 44–51

70. White M, Yanowitz F, Gilbert EM et al. (1995) Role of β-adrenergic receptor downregulation in the peak exercise response in patients with heart failure due to idiopathic dilative cardiomyopathy. Am J Cardiol 76: 1271–1276

71. Whyte K, Jones CR, Howie CA et al. (1987) Haemodynamic metabolic and lymphocyte beta2-adrenoceptor changes following chronic beta-adrenoceptor antagonism. Eur J Clin Pharmacol 32: 237–243

72. Yoshikawa T, Port JD, Asaro K, Bristow MR et al. (1996) Cardiac adrenergic receptor effects of carvedilol. Eur Heart J 17 (Suppl B): 8–16

73. Yue TL, Cheng H-J, Lysko PG et al. (1992) Carvedilol, a new vasodilator and beta-adrenoceptor antagonist, is an antioxidant and free radical scavenger. J Pharmacol Exp Ther 263: 92–98
74. Yue T-L, Liu T, Feuerstein G (1992) Carvedilol, a new vasodilator and beta-adrenoceptor antagonist, inhibits oxygen radical mediated lipid peroxidation in swine ventricular membranes. Pharmacol Communications 1: 27–35
75. Yue TL, Ma XL, Wang X, Romanic AM, Liu G-L, Louden C, Gu J-L, Kumar S, Poste G, Ruffolo RR, Feuerstein GZ (1998) Possible involvement of stress-activated protein kinase signaling pathway and Fas receptor expression in prevention of ischemia/reperfusion-induced cardiomyocyte apoptosis by carvedilol. Circ Res 82: 166–174

Authors' address:
Prof. Dr. Michael Böhm
Dr. Christoph Maack
Medizinische Universitätsklinik und Poliklinik
(Innere Medizin III)
66421 Homburg/Saar
Germany

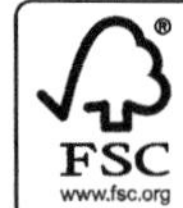